MW01382514

NORMAN BETHUNE IN SPAIN

The Cañada Blanch / Sussex Academic Studies on Contemporary Spain

General Editor: Professor Paul Preston, London School of Economics

Margaret Joan Anstee, *JB – An Unlikely Spanish Don: The Life and Times of Professor John Brande Trend.*

Richard Barker, *Skeletons in the Closet, Skeletons in the Ground: Repression, Victimization and Humiliation in a Small Andalusian Town – The Human Consequences of the Spanish Civil War.*

Germà Bel, *Infrastructure and the Political Economy of Nation Building in Spain, 1720–2010.*

Gerald Blaney Jr., *"The Three-Cornered Hat and the Tri-Colored Flag": The Civil Guard and the Second Spanish Republic, 1931–1936.*

Michael Eaude, *Triumph at Midnight in the Century: A Critical Biography of Arturo Barea.*

Francisco Espinosa-Maestre, *Shoot the Messenger?: Spanish Democracy and the Crimes of Francoism – From the Pact of Silence to the Trial of Baltasar Garzón*

Soledad Fox, *Constancia de la Mora in War and Exile: International Voice for the Spanish Republic.*

Helen Graham, *The War and its Shadow: Spain's Civil War in Europe's Long Twentieth Century.*

Angela Jackson, *'For us it was Heaven': The Passion, Grief and Fortitude of Patience Darton – From the Spanish Civil War to Mao's China.*

Gabriel Jackson, *Juan Negrín: Physiologist, Socialist, and Spanish Republican War Leader.*

Sid Lowe, *Catholicism, War and the Foundation of Francoism: The Juventud de Acción Popular in Spain, 1931–1939.*

David Lethbridge, *Norman Bethune in Spain: Commitment, Crisis, and Conspiracy.*

Olivia Muñoz-Rojas, *Ashes and Granite: Destruction and Reconstruction in the Spanish Civil War and Its Aftermath.*

Linda Palfreeman, *¡SALUD!: British Volunteers in the Republican Medical Service during the Spanish Civil War, 1936–1939.*

Cristina Palomares, *The Quest for Survival after Franco: Moderate Francoism and the Slow Journey to the Polls, 1964–1977.*

David Wingeate Pike, *France Divided: The French and the Civil War in Spain.*

Hugh Purcell with Phyll Smith, *The Last English Revolutionary: Tom Wintringham, 1898–1949.*

Isabelle Rohr, *The Spanish Right and the Jews, 1898–1945: Antisemitism and Opportunism.*

Gareth Stockey, *Gibraltar: "A Dagger in the Spine of Spain?"*

Ramon Tremosa-i-Balcells, *Catalonia – An Emerging Economy: The Most Cost-Effective Ports in the Mediterranean Sea.*

Maria Thomas, *The Faith and the Fury: Popular Anticlerical Violence and Iconoclasm in Spain, 1931–1936.*

Dacia Viejo-Rose, *Reconstructing Spain: Cultural Heritage and Memory after Civil War.*

Richard Wigg, *Churchill and Spain: The Survival of the Franco Regime, 1940–1945.*

NORMAN BETHUNE IN SPAIN

Commitment, Crisis, and Conspiracy

DAVID LETHBRIDGE

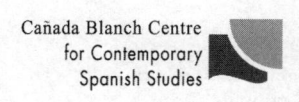

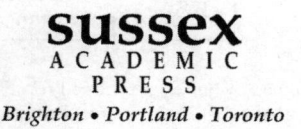

Copyright © David Lethbridge, 2013.

The right of David Lethbridge to be identified as Author of this work has been asserted in accordance with the Copyright, Designs and Patents Act 1988.

2 4 6 8 10 9 7 5 3 1

First published in 2013 in Great Britain by
SUSSEX ACADEMIC PRESS
PO Box 139
Eastbourne BN24 9BP

and in the United States of America by
SUSSEX ACADEMIC PRESS
920 NE 58th Ave   Suite 300
Portland, Oregon 97213-3786

and in Canada by
SUSSEX ACADEMIC PRESS (CANADA)
8000 Bathurst Street, Unit 1, PO Box 30010, Vaughan, Ontario L4J 0C6

Published in collaboration with the
Cañada Blanch Centre for Contemporary Spanish Studies.

Excerpt from *War is Beautiful*, copyright © 2008, by James Neugass, reprinted by permission of The New Press, www.thenewpress.com.

All rights reserved. Except for the quotation of short passages for the purposes of criticism and review, no part of this publication may be reproduced, stored in a retrieval system, or transmitted, in any form or by any means, electronic, mechanical, photocopying, recording or otherwise, without the prior permission of the publisher.

British Library Cataloguing in Publication Data
A CIP catalogue record for this book is available from the British Library.

Library of Congress Cataloging-in-Publication Data
Lethbridge, David, 1950–
Norman Bethune in Spain : commitment, crisis, and conspiracy / David Lethbridge.
page   cm. — (Cañada Blanch/Sussex Academic studies on contemporary Spain)
Includes bibliographical references and index.
ISBN 978-1-84519-547-2 (h/b : alk. paper) —
ISBN 978-1-84519-548-9 (p/b : alk. paper)
   1. Bethune, Norman. 2. Physicians—Canada—Biography. 3. Physicians—Spain—Biography. 4. Spain—History—Civil War, 1936–1939—Medical care. I. Title.
R464.B4L48 2013
946.081'7—dc23
[B]   2012039183

MIX
Paper from
responsible sources
FSC   FSC® C013056
www.fsc.org

Typeset & designed by Sussex Academic Press, Brighton & Eastbourne.
Printed by TJ International, Padstow, Cornwall.

Contents

The Cañada Blanch Centre for Contemporary Spanish Studies	ix
Foreword by Linda Palfreeman	xiii
Author's Preface	xvi
Acknowledgements	xviii
List of Illustrations	xix

PART ONE Wounded

1 A Rotten Childhood	3
2 Nothing He Would Not Do	20
3 Last Night Rose Low and Wild and Red	38

PART TWO Capitalism Breeds Fascism the Way a Fly Breeds Maggots

4 The Double Pyramid	51
5 Men of Iron, Men of Gold	58
6 The Frankenstein Project	61
7 Imperialism Prefers Fascism	65
8 The Butchers' Revolt	72
9 Imperialist Betrayal	79
10 They Killed My Soul	86

PART THREE Life's Blood

11 The Plan	91
12 Based on Blood: A New Type of Human Relationship	102
13 I Would Not Be Anywhere Else	118
14 Slaughter of the Innocents	129
15 Every Minute is Beautiful	138
16 The Blood of the Dead	147
17 I Killed My Own Son	157

| 18 | The Conspiracy | 168 |
| 19 | They Are In Me, They Have Changed Me | 179 |

PART FOUR   In Defense of the Republic

20	A Tumultuous Welcome	195
21	Sharply Raising the Question of Class Struggle	206
22	You See Now Why I Must Go	212
23	People Let Me Tell You, Now Is the Time to Wake Up	217
24	Will You Come?	224

PART FIVE   Aubade

| 25 | A Dream of Himself | 231 |

Notes	233
Index	258
About the Author	266

The Cañada Blanch Centre for Contemporary Spanish Studies

In the 1960s, the most important initiative in the cultural and academic relations between Spain and the United Kingdom was launched by a Valencian fruit importer in London. The creation by Vicente Cañada Blanch of the Anglo-Spanish Cultural Foundation has subsequently benefited large numbers of Spanish and British scholars at various levels. Thanks to the generosity of Vicente Cañada Blanch, thousands of Spanish schoolchildren have been educated at the secondary school in West London that bears his name. At the same time, many British and Spanish university students have benefited from the exchange scholarships which fostered cultural and scientific exchanges between the two countries. Some of the most important historical, artistic and literary work on Spanish topics to be produced in Great Britain was initially made possible by Cañada Blanch scholarships.

Vicente Cañada Blanch was, by inclination, a conservative. When his Foundation was created, the Franco regime was still in the plenitude of its power. Nevertheless, the keynote of the Foundation's activities was always a complete open-mindedness on political issues. This was reflected in the diversity of research projects supported by the Foundation, many of which, in Francoist Spain, would have been regarded as subversive. When the Dictator died, Don Vicente was in his seventy-fifth year. In the two decades following the death of the Dictator, although apparently indestructible, Don Vicente was obliged to husband his energies. Increasingly, the work of the Foundation was carried forward by Miguel Dols whose tireless and imaginative work in London was matched in Spain by that of José María Coll Comín. They were united in the Foundation's spirit of open-minded commitment to fostering research of high quality in pursuit of better Anglo-Spanish cultural relations. Throughout the 1990s, thanks to them, the role of the Foundation grew considerably.

In 1994, in collaboration with the London School of Economics, the Foundation established the Príncipe de Asturias Chair of Contemporary Spanish History and the Cañada Blanch Centre for Contemporary Spanish Studies. It is the particular task of the Cañada Blanch Centre for Contemporary Spanish Studies to promote the understanding of twentieth-century Spain through research and teaching of contemporary Spanish history, politics, economy, sociology and culture. The Centre possesses a valuable library and archival centre for specialists in contemporary Spain. This work is carried on through the publications of the doctoral and post-doctoral researchers at the Centre itself and through the many seminars and lectures held at the London School of Economics. While the seminars are the province of the researchers, the lecture cycles have been the forum in which Spanish politicians have been able to address audiences in the United Kingdom.

Since 1998, the Cañada Blanch Centre has published a substantial number of books in collaboration with several different publishers on the subject of contemporary Spanish history and politics. A fruitful partnership with Sussex Academic Press began in 2004 with the publication of Christina Palomares's fascinating work on the origins of the Partido Popular in Spain, *The Quest for Survival after Franco: Moderate Francoism and the Slow Journey to the Polls, 1964–1977*. This was followed in 2007 by Soledad Fox's deeply moving biography of one of the most intriguing women of 1930s Spain, *Constancia de la Mora in War and Exile: International Voice for the Spanish Republic* and Isabel Rohr's path-breaking study of antisemitism in Spain, *The Spanish Right and the Jews, 1898–1945: Antisemitism and Opportunism*. 2008 saw the publication of a revised edition of Richard Wigg's penetrating study of Anglo-Spanish relations during the Second World War, *Churchill and Spain: The Survival of the Franco Regime, 1940–1945* together with *Triumph at Midnight of the Century: A Critical Biography of Arturo Barea*, Michael Eaude's fascinating revaluation of the great Spanish author of *The Forging of a Rebel*.

Our collaboration in 2009 was inaugurated by Gareth Stockey's incisive account of another crucial element in Anglo-Spanish relations, *Gibraltar. A Dagger in the Spine of Spain*. We were especially proud that it was continued by the most distinguished American historian of the Spanish Civil War, Gabriel Jackson. His pioneering work *The Spanish Republic and the Civil War*, first published 1965 and still in print, quickly became a classic. The Sussex Academic Press/Cañada Blanch series was greatly privileged to be associated with Professor Jackson's biography of the great Republican war leader, Juan Negrín.

2011 took the series to new heights. Two remarkable and complementary works, Olivia Muñoz Rojas, *Ashes and Granite: Destruction and Reconstruction in the Spanish Civil War and its Aftermath* and Dacia Viejo-Rose, *Reconstructing Spain: Cultural Heritage and Memory after Civil War*, opened up an entirely new dimension of the study of the early Franco regime and its internal conflicts. They were followed by Richard Purkiss's analysis of the Valencian anarchist movement during the revolutionary period from 1918 to 1923, the military dictatorship of General Primo de Rivera and the Second Republic. It is a fascinating work which sheds entirely new light both on the breakdown of political coexistence during the Republic and on the origins of the violence that was to explode after the military coup of July 1936. The year ended with the publication of *France Divided: The French and the Civil War in Spain* by David Wingeate Pike. It made available in a thoroughly updated edition, and in English for the first time, one of the classics of the historiography of the Spanish Civil War.

An extremely rich programme for 2012 opened with Germà Bel's remarkable *Infrastructure and the Political Economy of Nation Building in Spain*. This startlingly original work exposed the damage done to the Spanish economy by the country's asymmetrical and dysfunctional transport and communications model. It was followed by a trio of books concerned with the International Brigades and the Republican medical services in the Spanish Civil War: Angela Jackson's rich and moving account of an extraordinary life – that of the left-wing nurse Patience Darton; the comprehensive account of the Republican medical services by Linda Palfreeman and the fascinating life of Tom Wintringham by Hugh Purcell and Phyl Smith.

They were followed by Helen Graham's *The War and its Shadow*, an extraordinarily original analysis of the afterlife of the Spanish Civil War, not just during the long dictatorship which was the institutionalization of Franco's victory but in Spain's present-day democracy. Especially striking is the way in which she relates the horrors of the Spanish Civil War to the mass violence taking place across Europe in the inter-war period. That work was matched in importance by Maria Thomas's ground-breaking work on the anti-clericalism that remains at the heart of many of the bitter on-going polemics about the Spanish war. *The Faith and the Fury: Popular Anticlerical Violence and Iconoclasm in Spain, 1931–1936* is an illuminating and even-handed account which fills a major gap in the literature.

An equally nutritious programme is envisaged for the series in 2013. It opens with two important works. David Lethbridge's perceptive study of the time spent in Spain by the remarkable Canadian surgeon Norman Bethune is a crucial addition to the literature on the Republican medical services during the Spanish Civil War. Alongside previous volumes in the series by Angela Jackson and Linda Palfreeman, David Lethbridge has made an outstanding biographical contribution. The series also welcomes Francisco Espinosa-Maestre, one of the most important historians of the Francoist repression during the Spanish conflict and its aftermath. He is best known for his many books on the terror in southern Spain but his contribution to the series is a unique addition to the literature. *Shoot the Messenger* lays out twelve cases in which investigation into atrocities committed in Spain has been blocked by various legal subterfuges and threats. It goes a very long way to explaining the maintenance of silence about the crimes of Franco.

PAUL PRESTON
Series Editor
London School of Economics

Foreword by Linda Palfreeman

Norman Bethune was a gifted and pioneering surgeon, inventor, artist and orator and, above all, a dedicated humanist whose complex, contradictory and often controversial character was ultimately guided by an enormous and overriding compassion towards those in need. While much has been written about this remarkable Canadian, in the following pages David Lethbridge reveals aspects of Bethune's life and work that make this book a valuable contribution to the existing literature.

With his authoritative analysis of the psychological trauma of Bethune's formative years, Lethbridge affords us valuable insight to the psyche of this great man – the man behind the legendary hero that he was later to become. And in uncovering the tormented, loveless childhood that was both to haunt and to shape Bethune's adult life and relationships, the author helps us to understand the sometimes volatile, erratic and self-destructive behavior that curtailed the surgeon's otherwise boundless energy and self-less devotion to his patients – especially to children, to whose care and protection he was particularly committed.

An equally salient aspect of this book is its unique focus on the surgeon's time in Spain during the Spanish civil war – a tremendously significant period in Bethune's life and one during which he made transcendent contributions to medicine and to humanity. Previous works have centred on Bethune's early medical successes at home in his native Canada and his heroic achievements later as military medical officer in China, during the Second Sino-Japanese invasion. Little close examination has been made of his accomplishments in Spain – a deficit that the present work seeks admirably to fill.

In what Lethbridge explains as a conscious rejection of the oppressive religious fanaticism of his parents, Henry Norman Bethune took up both the name and the profession of his surgeon grandfather. After recovering from a near-fatal pulmonary tuberculosis, Norman Bethune devoted himself to the treatment of other victims of the disease, specializing in thoracic surgery, first at the Royal Victoria Hospital, and later at the Hôpital du Sacré-Coeur, in Montreal.

After rising to eminence in his field, Norman Bethune continued to advance and perfect surgical technique, though he became disillusioned with an economic and political system that returned patients to the very conditions that had originated their illness. He challenged the Canadian medical establishment and provoked the antagonism of his peers by proposing radical reforms of the health services and advocating free access to medical care for those who could not afford it. Leading by example, Bethune founded a clinic that operated under these premises and a school offering art classes to underprivileged children. Lack of resources meant that these initiatives were sadly short-lived. Bethune's experiences led him, during this time, to align himself with the Communist Party, which he eventually joined in 1935.

Select biographical detail of Bethune's early life is included in this work with a single aim in mind – to enable the reader to understand who Norman Bethune was (and what had made him that way) by the time that civil war erupted in Spain in the summer of 1936.

When the conflict began, all kinds of services had to be created or reorganized and one of those that required greater effort was, undoubtedly, the medical service. Thanks to the insurgents' unprecedented large-scale bombardment of the civilian population, it soon became clear that the Republic would be unable to cope with the vast number of wounded – of both a military and non-military nature – and on 26 July, the Spanish government made a worldwide plea for help. Norman Bethune was one of those who responded to that call. He was convinced of the imperious need to confront fascism in Spain and acutely aware that the outcome would have lasting repercussions for the future of Europe and America.

At the invitation of the Committee to Aid Spanish Democracy (CASD), Bethune went out to Spain at the end of October 1936 – initially with the responsibility of coordinating medical aid sent from Canada to the Republic. However, the visionary surgeon already had other plans in mind. Lethbridge reveals that, contrary to popular belief, it was whilst he was still in Canada that Bethune, realizing the imminent need, had already planned to create a blood transfusion service in Spain and had obtained approval from the Communist Party to do so before he set sail.

With funds from the CASD, Bethune set about securing equipment and recruiting personnel with the necessary skills to expand the rudimentary Blood Transfusion Service in Madrid into what became known as the *Servicio Hispano-Canadiense de Transfusión de Sangre*. Later, Bethune acquired a Ford station-wagon which he fitted with a refrigerator, sterilizing equipment, transfusion sets, bottles and flasks for the storage of extracted blood, etc., bringing to fruition his ultimate objective of giving the blood transfusion service the mobility essential to be able to carry out emergency transfusions at the front.

Foreword by Linda Palfreeman **xv**

This pioneering mobile blood transfusion service is recognized as Bethune's single greatest achievement in Spain. What has, until now, remained largely unexplored, however, is the extent to which Bethune and his team contributed to the scientific advancement of blood transfusion and to the development of techniques for the extraction, storage and preservation of blood, including experimental work on the use of use of blood from human cadavers. Meticulous research enables Lethbridge to present previously un-edited documentary evidence of this pioneering work.

The author also reproduces Bethune's detailed and heart-rending account of an event that caused a profound and lasting effect upon him – the scenes of tragic human misery that ensued from the taking of Malaga by the fascist forces. Faced with thousands of terrified refugees fleeing from the town, Bethune and his assistants T. C. Worsley and Hazen Sise were forced to abandon their mission to get supplies of refrigerated blood to the front. Instead, they spent three days ferrying the sick and wounded – mainly children – to hospital in Almeria.

In exploring the nature of Bethune's relationships with his colleagues at the Blood Transfusion Institute, and in particular with secret Party member, Henning Sorensen, Lethbridge unravels the details of the conspiracy that led to Bethune's eventual removal from Spain – a conspiracy based largely on groundless suspicions and personal jealousies, motivated to some extent by Bethune's romantic involvement with Swedish journalist Kasja Rothman.

Despite his eventual expulsion from Spain, and still thoroughly committed to the cause, Bethune embarked upon an exhaustive propaganda tour of North America to raise funds and public awareness on behalf of the Spanish Republic before travelling to China in January 1938, to join the Chinese Communists in their struggle against the invading Japanese. In the summer of 1939 Bethune was appointed Medical Advisor Mao's Eighth Route Army. Later that year, whilst operating on a soldier in typically primitive conditions, he cut his finger and subsequently contracted septicaemia, from which he died on November 12, 1939.

The singular events described in this particular episode of Norman Bethune's life are brought sharply into focus by the author, within the coherent framework of their wider historical and political context, providing not only a piece of groundbreaking historical research but also a compelling read.

Author's Preface

"Anyone turning biographer commits himself to lies, to concealment, to hypocrisy, to flattery, and even to hiding his own lack of understanding, for biographical truth is not to be had, and even if it were it couldn't be used." So Sigmund Freud once wrote to his friend Arnold Zweig, the novelist.[1] Was he right? Perhaps. He was right in so many things that we prefer to deny.

Much has been written about Norman Bethune. Quite possibly lies and concealment, hypocrisy and flattery have played their part; accidentally or otherwise. And yet the basic story of the revolutionary doctor whose fierce star blazed across three continents, and who was ultimately eulogized by Chairman Mao as the most selfless of men, is well known.

But there is also the Bethune whom we do not know.

Born to fanatical religious zealots, deeply wounded by the cold and unloving mother he came to call "the Dragon," and the weak, vacillating, and contemptible father whom he hated, Bethune struggled throughout his life to overcome his deep emotional scars. Sexually inhibited, given to outbursts of near psychopathic rage, this wounded doctor healed himself through healing others.

By the mid-1930s, Bethune had emerged as a renowned surgeon fighting the twin plagues of disease and fascism. When Franco launched an offensive against the legitimate government of Spain, Bethune traveled quickly to Madrid. He organized a mobile transfusion service and, often under fire, brought blood to the wounded at the front; an accomplishment for which he became justifiably famous.

But in all the many books written about Bethune, his work in Spain tends to fall uncomfortably between his medical success in Montreal and his legendary commitment to Mao's Eighth Route Army. That is to say, it becomes the victim of a sort of historical parenthesis; Spain is seen simply as a step towards China, a lesser achievement, outshone by later glory.

Here we shall correct this impression. Bethune's outstanding achievement in Spain will be brought into sharp focus and treated as it deserves to be: as a fully autonomous project.

And we shall attempt to break new ground.

The usual claim that Bethune met Graham Spry – a high-ranking func-

Author's Preface   **xvii**

tionary in the Canadian social democratic party, the CCF – quite serendip-
itously when he answered Spry's advertisement in a newspaper, and that this
accident led to Bethune's leaving for Spain, will be challenged. Testimony
exists that Bethune had known Spry for several months and that his departure for Spain had little to do with him. Moreover, written documents
indicate that Bethune had already planned to institute a blood transfusion
service in Spain while still in Canada, and that he had sought and received
approval from the Communist Party for this purpose

The role that Bethune played in the discovery of a practical method for
performing cadaver blood transfusion as close to the battle line as possible
will be fully documented.

Intriguing evidence that Henning Sorensen – Bethune's right-hand man
in Spain – was a secret member of the Communist Party of Canada, and was
in the same secret Party cell as Bethune, will be explored. If indeed Sorensen
knew Bethune well before Spain, new light would be shone on Sorensen's
role in the conspiracy that ended Bethune's tenure in Spain.

The profound effect that the Malaga atrocity had on Bethune, and the
role it played in Bethune's effort to build "children's cities" outside the war
zones where the young could live free from danger, will be detailed. This
was a project of much importance to Bethune, and which expressed his deep
unconscious and conflicted obsession with the health and happiness of children.

Importantly, the nature and complexity of the conspiracy that led to
Bethune's ejection from Spain will be unraveled, the conspirators named,
and their later testimony challenged on the grounds of internal inconsis-
tency or outright perjury.

Furthermore, we will attempt to reveal the complexity of Bethune's
internal development. We will examine Bethune's childhood and early
years, in an effort to know Bethune as he really was and not the hero he
became in hindsight; *to get inside him*, so to speak and to understand a little
better this tortured doctor who both found himself and lost himself in the
furnace of Spain. We will present the whole man – torn and hurt, lost, lacerated and misused – cutting to the core of his interiority. In short, we will
seek to uncover the complex truth of Bethune's unique activity and personality as it intersects with history.

Finally, we shall provide the necessary historical context – so often
lacking – that explains why Britain and the other imperialist powers took
the side of Franco politically, ideologically and materially, and instituted
the notorious "non-intervention pact."

Acknowledgements

Grateful acknowledgement is due to:

The Canadian Plains Research Center for permission to quote from *Passion and Conviction: The letters of Graham Spry*, by Rose Potvin, Regina, 1992.

Lawrence and Wishart for permission to quote from *Eurocommunism and the State*, by Santiago Carrillo, London, 1977.

The *Canadian Bulletin of Medical History* for permission to reproduce, in slightly different form, my article "'The Blood Fights on in Other Veins': Norman Bethune and the Transfusion of Cadaver Blood in the Spanish Civil War," Vol. 29, 1 (2012).

The New Press for permission to quote from *War is Beautiful: An American Ambulance Driver in the Spanish Civil War,* by James Neugass, New York, 2008.

The following individuals and institutions provided me with access to their archives or their files, their personal reminiscences or their advice. I would like to take this opportunity to thank all of them, and above all, Larry Hannant.

Patricia Albers, Richard Baxell, Betty-Jean Bjornson, Jim Carmody, Michael Crook, Pierre Delva, José Diz, Helena Jordo-Zieske, Irene Kon, Dovid Kunigis, Bill Livant, Bernard Lutz, Linda Palfreeman, Michael Petrou, Peter Pinkerton, Paul Preston, Paul Schmidt, Marian Shaw, Larry Stephenson, Roderick Stewart, Glen Thompson, and Amanda Vaill. The librarians at the Library and Archives Canada, the librarians at the Lilly Library at Indiana University, the archivists at the National Film Board of Canada, the librarians at Okanagan College, the librarians at the Osler Library of the History of Medicine, the librarians at the University of California, Los Angeles, the Marx Memorial Library, and the Communist Party of Canada.

I would like to offer my gratitude to Anthony Grahame, Editorial Director at Sussex Academic.

On a more personal level, I would like to dedicate this work to my loving companion of all these many years, Sharon Lethbridge.

List of Illustrations

The author and publisher gratefully acknowledge the following for permission to reproduce copyright material. The publishers apologize for any errors or omissions in the above list and would be grateful to be notified of any corrections that should be incorporated in the next edition or reprint of this book.

All images courtesy of Library and Archives Canada unless otherwise indicated.

The plate section is after page 140.

1   Mural Scene III. "Journey in Thick Woods – Childhood." Detail. Does this dragon represent Bethune's mother? *Courtesy of Larry Hannant.*
2   Professional photograph of Bethune taken in Paris (late February 1937).
3   Bethune transfusing blood into a wounded soldier.
4   Bethune transfusing blood into the foot of a patient.
5   Bethune with ambulance and unknown woman, possibly a Spanish nurse.
6   Bethune examining the remains of a downed Nazi aircraft. The British government consistently denied any evidence of German or Italian military presence in Spain.
7   Bethune observing a game of checkers. Haldane is on the right.
8   Bethune resting on the way to a front-line hospital.
9   The Canadian Blood Transfusion team. From right to left: Sorensen, Bethune, Sise, and unknown Spaniard.
10 Bethune standing beside the new Renault truck purchased in Marseilles (January 1937).
11 Group of Malaga refugees resting.
12 Refugee mother feeding baby.
13 Sise and Worsley in the Renault on the Malaga–Almeria road.
14 Malaga refugees walking the *Caravana de la Muerte*.
15 Front cover of Bethune's passionate indictment *The Crime on the Road: Malaga–Almeria*. The book was published simultaneously in English, Spanish, and French. *Courtesy of Paul Preston.*

LIST OF ILLUSTRATIONS

16 Bethune during filming of *Heart of Spain* (April or May 1937).

17 Bethune at the front with Sorensen and May (April or May 1937).

18 Hitler warmly greeting Franco (1938). *Photograph by Ned Bayne. Courtesy of Paul Preston.*

PART ONE

Wounded

A Rotten Childhood

A rotten childhood: that is what Bethune told Richard Brown he'd had when they were traveling together in China.[1] He said much the same thing to Harriett Hammond, a young woman he met in Boston.[2] Dr. Edward Archibald, chief surgeon at the Royal Victoria Hospital in Montreal revealed: "I knew that Norm had some problems resulting from his home environment."[3] How do they know? It was not a question of interpretation: Bethune told them. It gnawed at him; and he spoke of it to many.

Bethune was born on 4 March 1890.[4] Apart from a few highly selective reminiscences, his childhood died with him. He left no early diary, nor any letters to guide us. His first home was the Presbyterian manse in Gravenhurst, Ontario.[5] The family had been living there since June 1889 but did not stay long – moving on only three years after Bethune's arrival – but it was here that Bethune briefly lived with his aging grandfather whom he loved, soon to die in a Toronto nursing home. And it was in this house that he discovered that his mother was a denizen of Hell, a fierce and unforgiving Dragon.

When, much later, in 1934, Bethune and Elizabeth Wallace were lovers, he said to her that his mother was a Dragon: a designation whose meaning bears no connotation of fondness.[6] A dragon is a beast whose breath is corrosive fire, a monster with leather-like wings who swoops suddenly down upon its prey, of claws and fangs that rip and tear. In any event, it is a word that is redolent with symbolism and an image that first emerged concretely when he was struck down with disease. In September 1926, at the age of thirty-six, Bethune was diagnosed with tuberculosis. He was admitted to the Trudeau Sanatorium in northern New York State.[7] It can be questioned whether his tuberculosis would ultimately have been fatal; there have been opinions that his condition was not that grave.[8] On the other hand, the disease in itself was incurable with the methods at hand. It scarcely matters: what is important is that Bethune *lived* his tuberculosis as a death. Deep in despair, a chance reading of a recent book by Dr. John Alexander gave him some desperate hope.[9] Bethune demanded a meeting with the sanatorium's medical staff. They pointed out the risks involved in Alexander's procedure: a hollow needle would be inserted between the ribs over the diseased lung;

air would be pumped into the chest cavity collapsing the lung and allowing it to heal. But there was always the possibility that the needle would penetrate too far and puncture the lung. Bethune rose instantly, tore open his shirt and bared his chest, announcing, "Gentlemen, I welcome the risk!"[10]

A chest x-ray was scheduled. The operation was performed. An hour after the procedure, Bethune complained of shortness of breath: he was unsure whether he would survive or die. Lying down on his cot, in one of the many outlying cottages where patients at the Trudeau lived, Bethune had a moment of impelling vision: he saw his life entire unfolding as a disturbing dream. He left the cottage, staggered down to the sanatorium's laundry room and obtained a roll of wrapping paper. He tacked the paper as a single sheet around each of the cottage's four walls, cutting out holes for the doors and windows.[11] Using colored chalks, he began to draw an allegory of the episodes of his life; a series of murals which ended with his death.

The mural series – which Bethune entitled *Nine Painful Scenes* – resembles a waking dream, an externalized fantasy with elements of nightmare, drawn in despair and foreshadowing imminent death. As with any dream, it requires interpretation. We shall be concerned with only the first and third of these scenes which are, perhaps, of the most value and provide the greatest yield: these are the scenes of his earliest childhood: in both he is repeatedly attacked by dragons and beasts from Hell.[12]

The first panel of the sequence, entitled *Womb and Foetus*, depicts Bethune's prenatal existence. The uterus is drawn as a dark circular cave. The infant Bethune appears as fully formed; his mouth is wide open in a horrified silent cry and his expression one of agonizing distress. His arms are raised toward a gigantic red pterodactyl, a prehistoric dragon beast, its long ferocious beak lined with sharp teeth, which is quite clearly attacking him. There is no sign of comfort here, no representation of refuge. If the dragon had not been present, the empty blackness of the cave would itself be a lonely, hollow place with no indication of any maternal warmth or presence. There is not even an umbilical cord uniting this terrified child-fetus to the protection of its mother's body. The symbolism is clear enough: the dragon is the mother; the mother, the dragon.

The third panel, *Journey in Thick Wood: Childhood*, reveals not one dragon, but a dozen nightmare beasts. Significantly, each of the major creatures in this scene carries a naked boy in its claws: a large blue dragon carries the child upside down and from behind, as does another blue creature swooping down from an enormous dark and menacing tree. A red dragon to the right of the tree, with maternal breasts and a savage beak, holds a small boy by the head; the child's arms are crossed in front of him, possibly even bound; the naked genitals are visible between the boy's legs. In the largest image, the child Bethune is bleeding while bat-like creatures tear his neck and he is held in the talons of a huge blue dragon. Since all of these creatures hold the various boys with their backs toward them – and this is entirely obvious in the depiction of the child carried upside down, with his small face toward the ground and his legs bent – there is a suggestion of almost sexual violation. The picture as a whole seems to indicate a childhood filled with nightmare and horror, cruel beasts and dragons lurking in every corner of this landscape. A dark womb gives way to a dark wood.

Now it is true that Bethune has added the words of various diseases such as "measles" or "diphtheria" beside the images of these dragons, as if these beasts represented the variety of children's illnesses prevalent at the time. But this is an illusion, an unconscious defensive maneuver; these medical labels are designed to draw attention *away* from the fact that Bethune represents his childhood as an unending series of monstrous attacks. In any event, what Bethune has drawn is a depiction of a terrible, frightening childhood devoid of any indication of happiness, innocence, or joy. The infantile journey is a torment. He even wrote, beneath this panel, in reference to these various violations by the dragon-mother: "The wounds and scars of their attack, he'll carry to the grave."[13] Symbolic though this may be, it is nonetheless an accurate rendering.

Who was this wounding mother? Elizabeth Ann Goodwin was born in 1852, the daughter of an English cabinet-maker whose name was Henry.[14] She distributed religious tracts in the streets of London at the age of ten; a strange, even dangerous occupation for a little girl. Who put her up to this we cannot say. At twenty-one she took ship for Hawaii, intent on converting the natives to Presbyterianism.[15] Was she indeed a missionary? There is apparently "no record of Elizabeth Goodwin as a missionary in relevant archives."[16] No matter. Perhaps she landed on the Islands with an individual calling, unsponsored by the church. Perhaps she was merely some unknown pastor's assistant, her activities thought unworthy of record. In any event, she was filled with "a vast determination to save the heathen and spread the word of Christ."[17] As the daughter of a cabinet-maker, in nineteenth-century England, she was undoubtedly uneducated. Superstition and dogma took the place of knowledge. More than that, she "looked on learning and books as a temptation of the devil."[18] Goodwin was a proponent of Dwight Lyman Moody's brand of missionary evangelism.[19] A three hundred pound former shoe salesman of limited intelligence, he preached a form of religion that relied upon a literal acceptance of the biblical text. Vigorously opposed to the work of Darwin and the teaching of evolution,[20] he considered the reading of any but the most simple-minded religious texts as spiritually dangerous: "people read infidel books and they wonder why they are unbelievers."[21] Moody toured Great Britain to increasingly massive crowds. Was Elizabeth Goodwin present when Moody arrived, full-blown on the sails of victory, into London's impoverished East End? This woman, trawling the streets from childhood, seeking out the down-trodden and the gullible, arms full of absurd evangelical tracts, would she not be attracted to these overflowing mass meetings? We are surely justified in imagining she would. Nor should we be surprised that she set out for Hawaii – fired with a renewed missionary zeal – at the end of the very same year, 1873, as Moody's most successful evangelical campaign.

It was in Hawaii that she met Malcolm Bethune.[22] Born in 1857, he was twenty-three.[23] He had left Toronto less than a year before, had sailed to Australia where he had failed in a brief stint as a sheep farmer, and had written home a pathetic letter begging for money.[24] His wallet refilled and his spirits renewed, he had stopped in Hawaii and decided to invest in orange groves; a project which came to nothing. How he met Elizabeth Goodwin is nowhere recorded. All we are told is that, although he had never shown "the least desire to be an evangelist,"[25] Goodwin quickly converted him, that he "abandoned all thoughts of orange groves and fortunes,"[26] and that he renounced "his former way of life."[27] Smitten by Goodwin and God, he proposed.

Back in Toronto, Malcolm was admitted to Knox Theological College in 1888, the same year he and Elizabeth's first child Janet was born.[28] Goodwin, now Bethune, was thirty-eight when she brought her second child, Norman, into the world. She was not young. She was toughened by many years as a missionary. The man she had evangelized and converted to the faith had finally found himself a vocation; at thirty-three, five years her junior, he had been the Reverend Malcolm Bethune for only three years. No doubt she was pleased to have provided her husband with a son.

Elizabeth Bethune had a formidable strength, but given the times it could not express itself directly. Even though she had evangelized her husband, and in this sense was responsible for what he had become, she must be forever a power behind the throne. She was condemned by the prevailing social ideology, and self-condemned through her own religious conviction, to be always the shadow of her husband, the mere wife and helpmate of the most Reverend Bethune. This was not a role that she relished. True, there were compensations: whenever her husband was laid low by some minor illness, or made dumb by influenza, she would nurse him with practiced care all the while preparing the blistering sermon she herself would deliver from the pulpit and in his place.[29] This was the time of her glory. Dressed from head to heel in deepest black, she mounted the few steps to the platform, the Bible clutched in her dry hand, and stared

A Rotten Childhood

down at the congregation below. For an hour they were hers! But an hour was hardly sufficient; it passed all too quickly, and soon enough her husband rose again and she was eclipsed once more. Her strength had always been a hard strength, stiff with the rectitude of the pious and now, since her marriage, there was added to it a secret and unspoken bitterness. It was *she* who was the evangelist, *she* who was the mouth and tongue of God; now she had been reduced to mere echo of the very man she herself converted. Certainly it was true that she had been relegated – even *reduced* – to the role of a minister's wife, but she would not play the role lightly. Others would suffer.

Given the period, and their specific milieu, it may be that it was the father's necessary position to legitimize the new-born child through the public process of naming him. If there were arguments over the name, we do not know; but this hard mother would have her way regardless of the father's wishes. Her first son would be named *Henry* Norman Bethune, after *her* father; a small victory, but one with some significance: it had long been the Bethune tradition to name grandsons for grandfathers. If the Reverend Malcolm suffered this reversal as an indignity, that was too bad.

We are told that she "made life miserable" for her husband; he was not her only victim.[30] Every day, at every meal, and again before bedtime, she would read the Bible to the three children – Janet, Henry Norman, and Malcolm Jr. But Norman was the true target: he was, perhaps unfortunately, her "favorite son," and "always her reading was directed solely at him; she tried to do with Bethune what she had done to the father."[31] On Sundays, true to Moody's bleak doctrine, the children were forbidden to play, and had to sit, mute and still, dressed in their uncomfortable church clothes while the mother read endlessly to them from the Bible, her eyes focused on Bethune, forcing him into immobility. Since she regarded books as the temptation of the devil, we can imagine how few volumes graced the family shelves in Bethune's earliest years. Certainly we know that as a boy Bethune began to accumulate books, which his mother would stuff with endless evangelical tracts, a practice she continued even when he was married.[32] In her malign fervor, she never stopped trying to convert him. Much later, when Bethune was suffering from tuberculosis and believed he was near death, the mother, descending upon his weakened body like a dragon sensing its prey, told him that his illness was God's punishment and that God had "caught up to him."[33] On yet another occasion – it is unclear when, but quite likely not until the father had died and Bethune had joined the Communist Party – she told him that he was no longer her son and that she had disowned him.[34]

It would be absurd to imagine that such a woman, such a "hard relentless woman,"[35] a woman capable of telling her deathly sick son that God had finally ensnared him and that, in effect, a place was waiting for him soon in Hell, a dragon-woman who gave her husband and children a miserable life, would have been anything other than an unempathic and disturbing mother to her infant son. She had children because it was expected of her. It was her duty as a Christian wife to produce children both for her husband, and for the glory of God. And so the children were produced, regularly and mechanically, at predetermined intervals: Janet in 1888, Norman in 1890, Malcolm in 1892. They are not children born of passion; they are children of duty: they will be dutifully and mechanically cared for. Nor would her hardness be softened by the arrival of her infants: she never ceased to take a dragon's role. She did not so much fall in love with her husband as effect a conversion within him. First and foremost she was an evangelist, with all the zealotry and bigotry of the ignorant. Her primary duty is not to love her children but to *save* them, to make them suitable for God; to prepare them, even in their swaddling clothes, for the shroud – for an encounter with a jealous deity in the world of the dead. Wife of a man she has herself, through force of will alone, turned into an ordained Reverend, the task of producing and raising children for this converted husband is nothing but a necessary maternal detour to her true work as an advance agent for the conquering army of the Lord.

Bethune, like any infant, had needs well beyond the basic requirements to be fed, to be cleaned, to be relieved of distress. Efficiency, and the forms of care that derive from a purely mechanical duty are inadequate in themselves. For an infant to become a value in its own eyes, it must first have been valorized through the kindness of the mother. The more that kindness is manifest, the greater is the infant's self-valorization; it feels its value through the tenderness of the mother's attentions. In this way the infant receives her pride, and pride is born inside him as the mirror of her valorization. But *this* mother is not a mirror. When the infant Bethune looks up to her he does not find himself reflected. He sees only her demands, her implacable, hard, and dutiful intensity. It is not his own image, reflected back to him, that he internalizes, but the mother's refusal of him. He reaches out to her in love, as all infants do, but it is not love that he finds. *This is the first great disappointment*.

Love rejected brings both disappointment and rage. For fear of driving the mother away, the rage must be both hidden and denied, but it never disappears. For fear of losing the mother, of losing the loving tenderness he passionately desires but which is never forthcoming, he must dissemble his own feelings; but it is a losing game and the denied rage inside only increases. The infant assured of love is integrated in itself through the

A Rotten Childhood

valorization it sees mirrored in its mother's gaze. But the infant denied this essential love is forever dependant on an *imaginary* mother; dependant on a desire for a nonexistent mother whose love would make it whole but whose absence throws up a mirage which is as forever tantalizing as it is permanently out of reach. The mother that the infant Bethune confronts in reality is never the mother he encounters in desire. This is truly Hell: haunted by the mother that does not exist and tormented by the one that does. In short, it *hurts* to be with this mother.

Throughout his infancy, and throughout all the early years of his childhood, he cannot gain her approval, only her unloving attention. This hard mother is a dragon to Bethune: suddenly swooping down upon him from above, snatching him up in her talons, shrieking. What else is a dragon to a child? At three years old, or four, a small boy falls in love with his mother: the physical destination of his own passionate phallic upsurge. But *this* mother will not be the object of her son's attentions. Lacking in empathy, incapable of tenderness, she returns, so to speak, his valentines unopened. *This is the second great disappointment.* The rage inside deepens and, without losing any of its primal intensity, gives birth to resentment. Many years later, Bethune will say to his wife Frances: "Women are beasts. Women are flowers; get their fragrance and leave them alone."[36] He does not fully mean what he says – indeed, it is entirely insincere – and we are denied its context, but nevertheless this desperate statement reflects Bethune's underlying rage and fear; his ambivalence and dependence. He cannot love her and he cannot leave her.

Important as the mother is to the infant, he does not experience life entirely through her alone. An important question arises: can the Reverend Malcolm act as an ally to protect the little Bethune against the mother? Can he be for his son a haven, a calm port in which to seek refuge? What the young Bethune will need, particularly given the nature of the mother's fierce unlove, is an idealizing image, a father on whom he can rely as a source of perceived perfection, calmness, and strength; someone with whom he can temporarily merge and who can function as an alter ego. If the Reverend Malcolm can be that ally, he can provide his son not only with a power to resist this formidable mother, but an image of what he could be in the future.

Bethune was not so lucky. This father was not the father he needed. Calmness, perfection, and strength were hardly the Reverend Malcolm's strong suits. He was as much a fanatic as the mother, perhaps more so as he came to his fanaticism late, and by second hand; he was recruited into fanaticism from failure. And yet, at the same time, underlying the fanaticism, and at its secret core, there is a disturbing *weakness*. If the mother, in her cherished role as matriarch, made life miserable for the Reverend Malcolm, he allowed this misery to continue, he acquiesced to it, and was complicit with it.[37] Dr. Brown recalled that Bethune "seemed to think that he had a very bad childhood":[38] he can hardly be accused of exaggeration. Remembered after half a life, Bethune looked back upon his earliest years with the same intensity of anguish that enveloped him in the nursery at Gravenhurst.

No doubt the father believed that he loved his son, as did the mother; we must grant them this much. But to be loved by these mad preachers brings more pain than joy. The little Bethune wants to love them, just as he needs their love. He wants to be encircled by a sweet valorization, by the mutuality of idealizing pride, to be caressed, at the very least, by a tenderness that will bind him to them. But all the wanting in the world will not change their fierce and stubborn unlove; their gaze lies elsewhere − on the corruption and sin they discover lurking over every horizon. Soon enough they will discern the same degraded impulses pulsating in the rebellious heart of their son.

The mother is terrifying; the father both fanatical and weak. Any child, torn between two impossibilities, will try to live by discovering a new road forward. Shuttling back and forth between this unempathic mother and this volatile, weak and ultimately contemptible father, Bethune is almost lost. He is saved by his grandfather.

In a family largely of clerics, the first Norman Bethune, the Reverend Malcolm's father, practiced medicine.[39] In the same year that he entered divinity school, Malcolm invited his aged father to come and live with his new family. They were together for four years, in Toronto and then finally in Gravenhurst.[40] The grandfather was Bethune's calm companion throughout his infancy. The old man's infirmities kept him in the house; he sat on the sofa, dozing from time to time, napping like his infant grandson. He was always there. He existed, for Bethune, as his sole source of comfort. Sometimes he would take him for walks in the garden, limping heavily, but supporting himself with the wooden cane that always fascinated the little boy. Hopelessly vacillating between the coldness of the mother and the weakness of the father, it was in the grandfather that Bethune found the possibility of hope and pride. And then the catastrophe happened. Bethune was too young to recognize the increasing decline of the grandfather; there was a series of paralyzing strokes. The grandfather was taken away from the manse in circumstances that his grandson could not comprehend, and died alone in a Toronto nursing home.[41] No doubt there was a funeral: the Reverend Malcolm Bethune would have attended, gathered together with the remnants of his family. At the gravesite, the small and hopelessly

A Rotten Childhood   **11**

bereaved grandson, stood alone between the silent darkness of his parents, forsaken of love.

And then Bethune was truly lost. It was not enough that the mother's relentless unlove was the very cradle of his lostness; in the years to come, and especially in his adolescence, she would tell him openly that he *was* lost, that she was praying for his soul both night and day, praying for him to find the road back to salvation.[42] She made the choice quite plain: believe as she believed, accept ignorance over truth, superstition over reason, dogma over freedom, or be damned. You will be lost, lost forever, not just lost to me, but lost for all eternity unless you come back, willingly, into my arms. Clearly the choice was not a choice or, more to the point, it was a choice between two impossibilities: be free and therefore damned forever, or return to the fetal darkness of the dragon's cave.

Faced with this impossibility, Bethune was unable to accept his mother's unceasing attempts to evangelize him, but also and at the same time unable to completely throw it off. It was not so much a matter of religion but of the chains of love and hate that bound him to her. He comprehended this lostness in himself, he felt it and could almost touch it, although he could not know it; its origins lay too far back in the past, in a dreamtime whose temporality was unconscious even to itself.

The nature of Bethune's lostness haunted him throughout his life. In 1935, following the collapse of his two marriages to Frances Penney, he had become infatuated with Marian Scott, whom he called "Pony."[43] While she was briefly staying in London, he sent her a pretended "handbill." At the top of the page was the single word: "Lost." The text read, in part:

> In the neighborhood of Ecclestone Square, on July 17th, A Canadian bred Pony . . . Stands about five and a half hands high. White face, gentle disposition. Was the companion of a small boy who is inconsolable over his loss. Any information received leading to her recovery will be handsomely rewarded.[44]

The "small boy who is inconsolable over his loss" was, of course, Bethune himself; an odd phrase to use for a would-be lover courting a woman, but unconsciously revelatory of the small boy that he once had been, and still in some sense was: lost, and inconsolable over his loss. This lostness emerged most fully whenever love, or even its possibility, became manifest. Some part of himself, deeply wounded in his infancy, inevitably connected the experience of love with the experience of lostness and with the internal image of the small boy. In a line from a subsequent letter to Scott, Bethune wrote: "Put away this small child of our love you are holding so quietly and tenderly in your cupped hands."[45] Here, love itself was identified with a "small child" and it is almost possible to feel directly, in this sad line, Bethune's childhood need to be held quietly and tenderly by some loving parental hand; a need that was consistently denied him.

Lost in childhood, denied the necessary love of his mother, he was equally bereft of a father on whose strength he could rely: his only strength was fanaticism. Before Bethune can even understand what is being said he is intimately familiar with his father's zealotry. On Sunday mornings, dressed in his absurd little suit with a white lace collar, he observed his father raging on from the pulpit.[46] Bethune understands not a word of this, but he sees the fanaticism in his father's eyes and in his voice: he will come to understand it very well, and to loathe it. This father was nothing if not a "stern and determined preacher,"[47] and a consummate fanatic. Bethune always felt this. It stayed with him as he recognized, years later, when he said: "I feel the same fanaticism in me that was in my father."[48]

Where was this fanatic father during all those endless and unforgiving Bible readings? Not a morsel of food was allowed to touch the boy's lips until he had endured yet another of the mother's endless cycle of gospel recitations. There were no bed-time stories, not even in infancy, that were not discourses from the testament; the little eyes were not allowed to flutter closed until every verse was concluded. For the first eight years – and we shall see that everything then changes – the mother demanded that the young Bethune memorize the Apostle's Creed and no less than thirty-two Psalms.[49] She may already have suspected that he believed not a word of any of this, but nothing and no one will brook her fierce determination: her son must be destined for pre-eminence in the ministry. It did not matter whether the father agreed with any of the mother's claims upon his son, we know how weak he was; it was *her* will that would be done, not *his*.

So strong upon the pulpit, so weak within the home, the Reverend Malcolm could not protect Bethune from his mother, or even from himself. Certainly it was true that when young Bethune required punishment his father would fly into a towering rage, put him over his knee, and mete out a stern walloping.[50] In itself it was nothing: such discipline was entirely to be expected among the boys of Bethune's milieu. But then, hours later, after he had been sent up to bed, the father would come groveling to his son, sobbing and begging for forgiveness. Not once, but repeatedly.[51] After the father left, weeping down the hall, Bethune felt sick and disgusted. His father's behavior was incomprehensible. Was the father wrong in punishing him? The father should know what was right or wrong; he was the one who made the rules; it was the father's will, and in that there was at least the compensation of sharing in his strength. But groveling, crying, begging

A Rotten Childhood

13

forgiveness – if that was anyone's role it belongs to the boy, not the father. Bethune was revolted. What his father had done was beyond impermissible. There arose in him a desire, not even fully grasped, to assume a certain provocativeness, a need to provoke the father to punishment, hoping that finally he would push him so far into anger that the groveling and unmanly weeping would stop. But nothing changed. Bethune began to feel, quite simply: *this father is not worthy of me*. In the end he felt nothing but contempt.

The contempt remained. He spoke of it, as he had spoken of his childhood in general, to Dr. Brown, who surmised that Bethune had "a little contempt for his father."[52] A little? No, something more than that. On 5 January 1929, Bethune wrote a letter to Frances Penney: "I spent Christmas with my family in Toronto. Shortly, Father and I had our usual hate together."[53]

But it was not yet, in his childhood, a matter of hate. Like love, hate takes time to grow, to blossom, and to bloom. Still, it cannot be said that the process had not yet begun: the contempt was there and the distance from contempt to hate was short enough.

The Reverend Malcolm was not blind. He noticed the contempt, and even the clumsy provocations, but he mistook them for pride. And pride was the road to perdition. He knew insolence and arrogance when he saw it. It was his duty, as both his father and his minister, to teach his son the virtues of humility. One day, perhaps incited by some defiant expression on his son's face as he strolled by, the Reverend seized the opportunity. It had been raining and the horse path to the stable had been churned to mud. Quickly, he threw out his arm and grabbed his son by the back of the neck. He marched him at a crouch to the dirt track and pushed his face down into the fresh mud, stinking of horse manure. "Eat it!" Bethune could hear his father commanding him from above, shouting into his ear. He bit into the mud, filled his mouth, and swallowed with difficulty through a throat constricted with pain and rage. His father's hand loosened and Bethune struggled to his feet. "You needed a lesson in humility," his father said, "I hope you won't need it again."[54] As soon as his father's back was turned, Bethune brushed at his face and his hand came away black with mud and filth. Trembling with the rage that rose up inside him, so violently that for a moment he truly did not know if it could be restrained, a single thought emerged: he hoped he would not see his father that night, kneeling by his bed, crying into his blankets, and pleading for forgiveness.

A strange lesson: his father humiliated him to teach him humility. And a mistaken lesson: what he took to be the strength of his son's pride was itself a fragility. Bethune's pride was nothing other than a defensive construct built *against* the originating wound of unlove. But if we are looking for the origin of what soon enough becomes "the usual hate" between son and father, it may well be here, between the tracks of the horse path, that the seed was planted. What cannot be loved will be hated. Before the summer of 1898 was out Bethune would no longer be his father's son.

At the age of eight Bethune rejected the name given to him by his father and mother.[55] This is a boy, a son, and in this sense the father reborn. The father has spoken: he shall be Henry. But he will not be Henry. He will return the first gift of his parents: his name. He who has had his face pushed into the dirt; will push his own father's face back into the mud: Keep your name. I don't want it. I won't have it. I reject it. And though he cannot have had words for it, and could not have spoken them if he did, in this rejection of the name is the rejection of the father himself. And yet, what name does he choose for substitute? The name of his grandfather: Norman. And, in accepting the grandfather's name he accepts the person of the grandfather into himself. He becomes the father of his father: I will be my father's father, and not my father's son. I am no longer your inferior; I am your superior. The tables are turned.

How are we to understand this change of names? Why does Henry become Norman? What is the meaning of this resurrection of the grandfather in his son's son, now living on inside him? We shall see immediately that there are powerful internal forces, powerful contradictions, at work beneath the surface. The change of name is an external manifestation which reveals beneath it Bethune's fundamental orientation to being.

If the rejection of the name given to him by his father is first of all a rejection of the father, and is intended to effect a reversal in the relations between father and son – albeit an *imaginary* reversal – it is also, and at the same time, a rejection of the mother. 'Henry' is, let us not forget, the name of the mother's father. When Bethune says, I will not be 'Henry,' he is hurling this name at the feet of the father. But it is, at the same time, a profound insult to the mother: I want nothing to do with you; do not imagine that I will ever be like your father, or will carry on any part of him, any part of *you* in my life. At this level the change of name is an ejection of both his father and his mother. This process of expulsion is necessarily doomed to failure. It is not so easy to exile their internal influence. For eight years Bethune has suffered. Now he has made a secret vow: I will never be their son; I will never be who they want me to be. He rejects them and, in rejecting the name they have given him, he tries to vomit up their being inside him. He is lacerated, resentful, hating without wanting to, damaged by their perpetual unlove. He has learned the nature of contempt and it sickens him. In truth, he would do anything to reverse the process of the last eight years. He does not want to hate, he does not want to feel that rage

A Rotten Childhood

15

that lies coiled inside him; like any child, he wants to be loved. In seeking a way forward, he is reaching for some way to break through the wall that separates him from his parents in the hopeless hope that he will discover the tenderness he believes he has lost in a past that never existed.

From this point of view, the secret vow is a fraud; the rejection is a bluff. More than that, it is a *provocation*. Not only does he fling his name in his father's face, he hammers the grandfather's medical nameplate to his bedroom door, like Luther challenging his forebears and announcing the birth of a new order – I am who I shall be, not what you have made me.[56] And what has his father made him? Sick with contempt. The provocation is nailed to the door for all to see. It is a sign to the father; perhaps this insult will be enough. For all his bravado, what this provocative child wants is a father who can be a real father to him, not this impatient and confusing fanatic, so that he can be his real son. If a masochistic impulse lies buried in this provocation, its sadistic edge would emerge whenever a loss of love threatened his tenuous pride.

But there is much more to Bethune's change of name. In this decision, everything that has happened to him in the past enters in to this moment, just as everything he will become in the future flows from it. The Reverend Malcolm and the unloving mother stand in dialectical opposition to the image of the grandfather. The parents ongoing influence on the young Bethune is primary; their presence is a daily reality, it is through them that Bethune has discovered the lostness and contempt they have bred in him. But ever since the loss of the grandfather, the first Dr. Bethune has become the source of any number of idealizing paternal tales.[57] Purged of all weaknesses, all selfishness or unkindness, the grandfather would appear to his grandson as the very example of what a man must be. For Bethune, his personal mythology would have many gods, but none more powerful than the grandfather, dying on the edge of his infancy, reborn as legend. The grandfather is a memory; but he is a *living* memory, and this memory can be his only ally. Now, by taking his name and making it his own, the grandfather is reborn within him through a conscious invocation. When Bethune fastens his grandfather's brass nameplate to his door it is not only a provocation, it is also, and on another interior level, a physical manifestation of his love for his grandfather, a sign of shared identity: To be my father would destroy me; to be my grandfather will save me. The grandfather was a doctor, a scientist, a professor, a man of books. Bethune's rejection of his parents and the internalization of his grandfather is therefore also a rejection of religion in favor of science. Evangelism is his parents' most central project, their chosen reason for being. Bethune's turn towards science is a turn away from their stifling ignorance toward the clean breath of freedom.

In making his grandfather's name his own, Bethune chooses sides: against his parents. And necessarily, because he is a child, the initial form this active opposition will take is play, and its focus will be the mother.

It began with the dissection of flies and chicken bones. It is unclear what instruments he used; possibly they are knives from his mother's kitchen. Certainly he would not have been given his grandfather's medical scalpels, and a boy's pocketknife would never have opened up a fly's anatomy. In any event, these dissections are not the work of a technician. Significantly, all we are told of these early experiments is that they leave a mess; and this is their hidden subtle function. Into the spotless home of a zealous missionary downgraded to the status of a Reverend's wife, shards of broken chicken bone and beheaded flies are thrown. Nor could any direct blame be laid at Bethune's feet. This was not open disobedience, nor even a child's thoughtlessness. No, the mess he leaves will necessarily be construed as of an entirely different order: it is the ghost of the grandfather's memory operating through the fingers of the child, the raw beginnings of the practice of medicine. As such, no matter how irritating, the young Bethune must be judged blameless. Soon decapitated flies were not enough. The house was suddenly pervaded with a stench that leaves the mother close to retching. Storming up the stairs, dragon wings unfolding, she traced the sickening odor to the attic. She flung open the door. Bethune was sitting with his back to her, cutting away the fetid flesh from a boiled cow's leg. A few feet away, the largest of her kitchen pots was still simmering on the old, unused, pot-bellied stove. Paralyzed between rage and disgust, a handkerchief crushed over her nose, she demanded to know what he was doing. Without turning, his voice flat and curtly reasonable, Bethune responded: "I'm getting the flesh off so I can examine the bones. They'll make good specimens." Later in the day, he disposed of the body parts and placed the bones along the backyard fence to dry.[58]

Is this proto-scientific activity itself a provocation? Certainly; and as an activity directed against the mother it is equally an act of sadism. We may observe here a hidden internal relationship, for Bethune, between his mother in childhood and his wife Frances; a relationship based on disappointment in love. We can see this clearly in the repetition of events; a repetition which comes near to a precise duplication. From the earliest days of their marriage, Bethune and Frances were unhappily in conflict with each other. He was frustrated and unsatisfied in their sexual relations, considering Frances to be almost pathologically frigid. Unable to leave her, the dependence and rage, rooted in infancy, is externalized in sadism; not the brutal sadism of physical violence, but the colder sadism of passive aggression: the same sadism he had aimed in childhood at the mother. In a letter

A Rotten Childhood   **17**

referring to their early lives together, Frances wrote: "Beth was always sterilizing instruments on the stove in our only saucepan."[59] No doubt Bethune
could have purchased another for the exclusive purpose of sterilizing instruments, but he chose not to, quite deliberately playing on Frances's phobias
and delicacies. Even more tellingly, during the first year of their second
marriage, as the reconciliation began to fall apart, Frances came home one
afternoon to find Bethune "sitting cross-legged on the floor, studying a
miniature skeleton." She asked him if he had remembered to buy meat for
dinner. Without expression, he told her it was in the refrigerator. Opening
the icebox door, and gasping in horror, "her gaze fell, not on the lamb chops
but on a *human intestine* he had brought home from the hospital."[60]

Bethune is no longer Bethune; the child of religious zealots, predestined
to a missionary vocation, has ceased to exist: he has given birth to himself
as his grandfather's son. No one understands this yet; least of all Bethune.
He grasps a corner of its meaning, but the full truth of his decision eludes
him. If his gaze focuses on the new horizon he has constructed for himself,
it escapes him toward an unknown future. "I am not Henry, I am Norman."
Perhaps it was just a game after all.[61] But it was not. The mother understood this more than the others; she had an uneasy feeling that her son had
begun to slide away from under her thumb. Not that this would prevent
her from trying to convert him; not then, not ever.

Whoever he was, whoever he might be, Bethune was dragged from one
flyspeck town to another across the backwoods of the Great Lakes.[62] The
Reverend Malcolm was always on the move: there were no end of souls to
save. And if Bethune was liked by others in the various communities of his
childhood,[63] he became "a complete alien in the family;" and "appalling to
the family."[64] Bethune was never at home in the tormenting households of
his youth. Miserable within the family circle, uprooted by the endless drift
across the northern shores, torn by inner contradictions, he was never more
alone. It was only on the banks of the great tumbling rivers and endless
lakes that he felt truly at ease, roaming where his steps took him. It was
there that he became increasingly comfortable and confident in his own
physicality; early on he had become well-muscled, "broad-shouldered and
well built."[65] If it was true that he developed a profound and lasting affection for nature, it was not simply because of the inherent beauty and power
of the northern wilderness, but because nature, so close at hand, provided
the only escape into the world and away from his mad and stifling family.
Physicality was freedom. There was nothing in the forests that evoked
contempt or hypocrisy; no dragons among the trees; nothing to tear at him.
Although he may have been alone, in the woods he was never *lost*.

And there was school; so often a refuge for those who are most unhappy at home. But even here the mother intervened. The family moved to Owen Sound for three years and, at fifteen, Bethune entered Owen Sound Collegiate.[66] One day, his mother discovered, to her outrage, a copy of Darwin's *Origin of Species* among his schoolbooks. In response, she stuffed, as usual, a series of evangelical tracts between the pages of his books. Bethune was disgusted; he crept into his parents' bedroom while they slept and slipped his Darwin beneath her pillow. In a mad fury, she flung open the door to the kitchen stove and viciously delivered the book to the oven's flames. She pled for Bethune's soul, no doubt loudly and to his face, telling him that he was lost, and that "she would pray night and day for him to find the road back to salvation."[67] Too late. Bethune had not believed a word of this since he was eight years old.

This is the end for Bethune. The very day after he graduates from Owen Sound, he is gone.[68] It is reported that his sister "spoke of his terrible temper, and that is why he left home early."[69] We do not need to search for the origin of this rage, we already know: seventeen years boxed in with these fanatical missionaries. What form, then, does this terrible anger take? Are there fistfights in the kitchen? We may consider this doubtful. More likely there are heated arguments, cruel but accurate words, a burning angst well beyond the common adolescent currency. Bethune's anger results from his parents' unceasing demand to truly control his life; to turn him into the Christian martyr he has no intention of becoming. Their constant annoying prayers, their insistence that he has set his feet on the road to perdition, their endless attempts to convert him to what he has already profoundly rejected, force to the surface what has been simmering inside him for longer than he can remember. Quite simply, he has had enough.

Bethune's rage may have taken many forms, but ultimately, here, at the end of his adolescence, and now that it is at last possible, it takes the form of *escape*. It is the parents intention to relocate the family to Toronto so that Bethune could proceed to university, as he was expected to do.[70] But he turns his back and heads off to the far northern Algoma district to work in the camps as a lumberjack.[71] He has escaped to the wilderness before, whenever the isolation and alienation from his family appeared too hard to bear. But this escape is more absolute; it is permanent, or appears to him as such. In any event, it marks the definitive end of his childhood. He spent over a year in the camps, from the summer of 1907 to the winter of 1908. He grew strong, learning to box and to fight, and was good at it.[72] He might have stayed there forever in Algoma, but the job came to an end, and there was nothing else available. Reluctantly, he returned to the family fold – now located in Toronto – and prepared for medical studies at the university.[73]

It has been said that manse life for so many sons of itinerant preachers

A Rotten Childhood   **19**

at the turn of the last century led to a surface sociability, while at the same time depriving them of lasting relationships outside the family.[74] This was never more true than for Bethune forced incessantly to move from town to town. Did he have any friends? Although he is said to have been a leader among a group of boys, and that "everyone liked him,"[75] there is no reference to a close and intimate best friend, nor indeed to any friends at all. Perhaps even more importantly, despite his later, quite false, reputation as a lover, even a libertine, there is no mention whatsoever of childhood sweethearts. If there were any young loves, no one has chosen to record it.

Equally, there are no recollections of any girlfriends at high school or at university. According to Bethune's sister Janet, he "never paid any attention to girls."[76] But he did dress up his sister, whom he called "Juna."[77] He bought her first evening dress and her first lipstick; he wanted her "to be beautiful;" he took her to parties and introduced her around as his "best girl friend."[78] Clearly, Bethune could not have passed off Juna as his girlfriend during his adolescent years; the towns where he grew up were too small and everyone would have known. Bethune did not return to his family until July 1909.[79] If he began to take Juna to parties late that summer, he almost certainly continued to do so during his first two semesters at university. It was only during this time that Bethune and Janet lived together for any extended period, with the family, near the university campus.[80] Janet soon put an end to the game. Bethune was nineteen, and possibly even twenty during these events, and he had apparently never enjoyed the company of any young woman at all. If his sister is to be believed, there was no one until Juna.

For many years he despised them all: mother, father, brother, and sister. He would continue to do so with the single exception of Juna. If he became closer to her during this time, it was precisely because he could *not* pay any attention to any other girls; that is to say, precisely because of a profound internal contradiction. It was not shyness or lack of confidence that prompted Bethune to dress up his sister for these evening gatherings. He wanted her to look beautiful so that his pretended "best girl" could demonstrate her elegance in front of the others; so that her beauty would reflect not only upon his taste but on his sexual prowess, itself a pretence. The truth is that Bethune was tragically and profoundly inhibited in his sexuality. He would remain alone; there would be no partners in passion for many years. If he was doubly wounded, not only in his infancy, but in the first stirrings of his Oedipal upsurge, in that singular childhood love affair, if he was rejected by a mother who can only be described as fundamentally castrative, should we wonder then at the repressed nature of Bethune's sexuality?

2

Nothing He Would Not Do

It is not our purpose to record in detail the more than twenty-five years that follow upon Bethune's entry into medical school at the University of Toronto, but to prepare ourselves for understanding who he is when Franco's coup erupts and Spain is threatened by fascism. We will need to pay particular attention to the fundamental contradiction within Bethune between the doctor and the artist; his relationship with women; his commitment to children; and his political evolution. In any event, from this point forward everything leads to a date: *24 October 1936,* when Bethune left for Madrid.

In 1914, the very day that war was declared, Bethune enlisted.[1] Like Algoma, the war was an escape; to stay would have meant another year under the parental roof. He was assigned to stretcher-bearer duty on the battlefields of France. Three months later, under heavy fire near Ypres, a German shell exploded nearby; shrapnel tore into Bethune's left leg.[2] After recovering, he was sent back to Toronto to complete his medical degree, re-enlisted in the navy, and was finally demobilized in England in February 1919.[3]

Bethune was a free man in London. He moved into a flat in Soho, and began his first internship at the Great Ormond Street Hospital for Sick Children.[4] Soho had become a fashionable place for radicals, writers, and artists, many of whom dropped by nightly to drink and to talk.[5] From that moment on he would be not only a doctor, but an artist. He was soon visiting art galleries, traveling to France and Portugal to buy paintings,[6] and frequenting the Ballets Russes where he was on speaking terms with the prima ballerina, the renowned Lydia Lopokova.[7] Still, at the age of thirty-one, he was reported to have said, reflecting the inhibitions that had been bred most deeply within him: "Women are very peculiar. They love me because they think I'm a boy, and hate me because I'm not a man."[8]

At about the same time, Bethune encountered Frances Penney, the woman whom he would love, and sometimes hate, and twice marry.[9] The daughter of a prominent Edinburgh family, Frances had all the advantages of established and inherited wealth. Overly sheltered, she was naïve to the point of absurdity. She had no knowledge of how children were conceived, and was both sickened and terrified by the thought of sexual relations.[10]

Nothing He Would Not Do

Certainly she was beautiful; and her social position and connection to wealth made her undeniably attractive. Even more, her naïveté, her feelings of inferiority, and especially her unquestionable virginity, meant that she would pose no threat to Bethune's own inhibited sexuality. After going to Edinburgh to take the examinations that would make him a Fellow of the prestigious Royal College of Surgeons, Bethune went to visit Frances. They were married in August 1923 in London. No relatives were in attendance. Frances wore black.[11]

From the first, their marriage was a disaster. Frances recalled that their wedding night "was a fizzle."[12] It appears that their sex lives were never normal. Even before the marriage Bethune had told Frances to see a doctor, apparently about her distaste for carnal relations.[13] In 1929, he wrote to her in Edinburgh – where she had retreated after the first divorce, and was preparing to return to Montreal for their second marriage – to see a doctor about her hymen since he "could not take this unnatural union any longer."[14] At one point he considered giving her drugs to eliminate her frigidity.[15]

After a honeymoon in Europe, during which Bethune spent some time in further medical studies in Paris and Vienna, they returned to London and then, mutually disillusioned, dissatisfied, and frustrated, but curiously devoted to each other, clinging to each other like the orphaned children each in some sense was, they sailed across the Atlantic.[16]

The following winter they arrived in Detroit, moving into an ancient apartment building on the corner of Selden and Cass; a deteriorated neighborhood where prostitutes worked the streets at night.[17] Minor posts at the Harper Hospital and the Detroit College of Medicine and Surgery barely paid the bills.[18] Prohibition was the law in America but Detroit, like all the big cities, ignored it. Speakeasies, where illegal liquor could be easily consumed, were increasingly popular, despite their connection to organized crime. Throughout the early months in Detroit, Bethune supplemented his income through whores and gangsters.

The prostitutes that worked Selden Street came easily to Bethune's office; and unlike so many of Bethune's early patients, they could pay well. But it was the gangsters who really paid handsomely. The most vicious group was the Purple Gang; reputedly named for the color of tainted meat. Their savagery was legendary: whoever opposed them was targeted for death. Violent gun battles took place under the very windows of Bethune's office.[19] Neither the Purple Gang nor their opponents could risk going to the hospital for the wounds they had sustained in gunfire. Bethune's name was known among the prostitutes and he never refused treatment to anyone; he was a doctor the Purple Gang could trust. According to A. R. E.

Coleman, Bethune "was called out several times to get bullets out of the gangsters who had been shooting each other up. My role was to illegally give the anesthetic for him."[20]

Coleman was not a doctor, he was an engineer with the Bell Telephone Company, from Montreal, who had been temporarily transferred to Detroit.[21] If he knew how to administer anesthetics it was only because Bethune had trained him. It is not clear how Bethune met Coleman, but they became close friends. Indeed their friendship soon involved Frances and led, eventually, over a space of ten years, to a bizarre triangular intimacy.

Gradually, Bethune became a recognized surgeon in Detroit, and he was able to attract a number of well-paying patients.[22] At the same time, he became aware that the class system in America meant that the unemployed, as well as the majority of working people, could not afford medical care. But his response to this endemic poverty was ambiguous. During the day he acted the part of the wealthy upper-class gentleman, but when night fell, he sought out the poor and indigent. On one of countless such occasions he went to the home of a Mexican migrant family that was living in an abandoned railroad boxcar on the edge of the city. The wife was pregnant and in labor. Under the thin glow of a kerosene lamp, Bethune delivered the infant, washed it, and handed it to its mother. The father, unable to find the English words to express his gratitude, gave Bethune a dollar bill. Bethune refused. The next morning he returned with diapers and a basket of food.[23]

Frances had had enough. In October 1925 she left Bethune for the first time. She went to visit a friend from her childhood, living in Nova Scotia.[24] Bethune, obsessed and alarmed and deeply threatened by her abandonment, wrote her within the week. Just as with his mother, he could neither love her nor leave her; nor could he bear not to be loved or to be left. Frances was apparently unmoved by Bethune's letter; from Nova Scotia she flew across to California to visit her brother, not returning until early in 1926.[25]

Nothing changed between them; the old dissatisfactions persisted. But at least there was now considerably more money: a lure for Frances as much as for Bethune, who bought himself a new car, and moved with Frances to a fashionable residential district.[26] Frances was kept well away from the medical office on Selden Street, but she was not kept away from Coleman, a cultivated and elegant Englishman who fascinated both Frances and Bethune equally. Frances was immediately attracted; she felt that Coleman was the first person she could talk to since she had left England. For the next six months, Coleman all but lived with them; when Bethune was occupied in the evenings, attending to the impoverished, Coleman took Frances to concerts. Frances was, for once, happy, and Bethune was grateful.[27]

Nothing He Would Not Do

But disease was everywhere among the poor and, exhausted from over-work, Bethune succumbed to tuberculosis.[28] He was eventually admitted to the Trudeau Sanatorium. Frances left him and returned to Scotland. By the time Bethune had recovered, Frances had filed for divorce.[29] Bethune's self-confidence was shattered; his obsession with Frances had led nowhere but to complete failure.

Bethune was released from the Trudeau in December 1927. The experience of tuberculosis profoundly changed his life. He no longer sought wealth and social position, and never would again. All that was finished. He would devote himself to thoracic surgery and the cure of tuberculosis. It was not merely that his own pneumothorax had so rapidly led to apparent recovery; there were thousands of lives that could be saved. Within a few hundred miles of Trudeau – in Boston and New York, in Detroit, Chicago, Toronto and Montreal, and in every city slum everywhere – thousands upon thousands were sickening and dying from a disease promoted by poverty and class inequality. He determined that he would give up trying to live within two worlds: attempting to build up wealth and fortune, while at the same time taking on the unwanted cases of the poor and destitute. He would devote himself entirely to the care of the sick, whatever might come.[30] At the age of thirty-eight, he would set a course for a new horizon, without home, without money, without family, without Frances, but with a new hope and a new purpose that would not be defeated.

Bethune moved to Montreal and began specializing in thoracic surgery at the Royal Victoria Hospital.[31] He developed a reputation as a brilliant, but controversial, surgeon.[32] He was fulfilling the promise he had made to himself at eight years of age when this future in which he was now living had been nothing but a glimmer on a far distant and inconceivable horizon. But he missed Frances; he was still obsessed with her. He begged her to return. She did. In November 1929, as the stock market crashed, they were married again.[33]

Perhaps inevitably, within a year Bethune's re-marriage to Frances started to unravel. She realized that he could not give her what she wanted: money, security, a life of concerts, dinner parties, the ballet, everything that Bethune had promised when they first met in 1921. But this man was dead; he had given up all that she believed she required. The threatened loss of Frances was too much for Bethune. His old demons rose again to torture him. His continuing affection for Frances was lacerated with the pain of renewed failure. He was lost without this woman and lost if he stayed with her. He responded with intermittent explosions of rage, and wounded pride, and drunkenness for many months.[34]

In April 1931, after eighteen months of marriage, Frances left Bethune and moved in with A. R. E. Coleman, for reasons that remain largely inexplicable. According to Frances, she was in Edinburgh when Bethune left the Trudeau Sanatorium, and that he "came to Montreal with A. R. E." and lived with Coleman.[35] From what evidence remains it is difficult to be certain when – or even why – Frances and Coleman became lovers. In a letter to Frances of 30 November 1931, Bethune wrote: "I have no desire to force you into marriage with R. E. Believe me, I will never force you to do anything . . . "[36] Clearly Frances and Coleman had been lovers for some months, but her central concern appears to be that Bethune will, somehow, *force* her to marry Coleman, apparently against her will. A month later, in a 31 December letter, Bethune wrote Frances: "If you remember, you begged me not to force you to marry R. E. and my reply that I would do nothing to put you in such a position against your own desires."[37]

Certainly it is very odd for Frances to imagine that Bethune could *force* her to marry Coleman; was she in such thrall to him that she seriously feared her will could be taken over by another? Despite leaving Bethune, and living with Coleman, she later claimed that she never really wanted to see Coleman again, but that she had "given her word . . . and when things are in a muddle one does what one says one will do."[38] Given her word? To whom: to Bethune or to Coleman? Whoever it might have been, she left Coleman repeatedly, and as often returned.[39] From April 1931 to the winter of 1932, she appears to have been deeply attracted to Coleman, and certainly sleeping with him, but at the same time her feelings were profoundly ambiguous. Frances and Coleman were lovers, but Bethune and Coleman were still close friends, as she was with Bethune. She remembered: "When we were alone, I would speak to Bethune about my troubles with A. R. E." Bethune was happy to listen and to offer advice; at one point he told her: "You move out of A. R. E.'s house, take a room, and A. R. E. and I will live together;"[40] an odd triangle in which Coleman seems rarely to have been consulted.

By March 1932 Bethune and Frances had finally determined to divorce.[41] A year later the divorce was officially granted and Bethune, Frances, and Coleman together toasted the event with a bottle of champagne.[42] The three continued to see each other, but Frances' alliance with Coleman was as difficult and contradictory as her relationship with Bethune had been. According to Frances, Coleman was "sensitive . . . and very capable"; he was "sane and conventional;" and they "might have been happy."[43] Eventually, she became pregnant by Coleman.[44] But they were as yet unmarried and Coleman was undecided about Frances and reluctant to have a child; he seems to have temporarily abandoned her. Frances turned to Bethune and insisted that he give her an abortion. He arrived and reluc-

Nothing He Would Not Do

tantly performed the procedure. According to Frances, she became immediately ill, but Bethune had to leave to attend to a patient at the hospital. She told him that she thought she was poisoned. Bethune said to her: "You can't die. Two men would get into trouble." When he returned, some hours later, he was, she said, frightened. In the meantime Frances had apparently recovered: they had a few drinks and went to the movies.[45]

Frances does not recall nor does she speculate on Bethune's response to her request for an abortion. She cannot have been unaware of his obsession with her; it is unlikely that he would have refused her anything. More to the point, she knew very well his intense desire to have children, indeed his fondness for all children, and it cannot have escaped her that she was asking him to abort the child that might have been theirs together and was in fact the child of his closest friend. If Bethune had often treated her with a degree of contempt, she apparently knew how to respond in kind.

After the abortion, Coleman returned to Frances and agreed to marriage.[46] Against any existing evidence, and quite illogically, Frances continued to maintain that she was only marrying Coleman because Bethune "told her to." According to Amy Russell, a childhood friend to whom she had written, "Frances hoped the church would forbid the marriage."[47] The church did not, and Frances became Frances Penney Coleman less than a year after her divorce from Bethune.

The strange triangle that developed between Bethune, Frances, and Coleman in 1925 ended ten years later in 1934. Bethune and Frances continued to see each other socially for some years, his obsession with her never entirely dying. And although Frances Penney's name is closely associated with that of Bethune, it is worth recalling that the time they spent living together was actually quite limited; more easily measured in months than in years. Frances was married to Coleman much longer: from 1933 until 1944 when she divorced him and returned to Scotland, addicted to some unnamed drug, living in various rooms, and descending into paranoia until her death in 1963.[48] As for Coleman, he joined the navy as a captain during the Second World War, and then nothing more was heard of him. There is a suggestion that he eventually retired to South America.[49]

Some months after Bethune's final divorce from Frances, and still disturbed from its devastating failure, he was introduced to Elizabeth Wallace, a woman with whom he fell deeply in love. She was separated from her husband and working in a department store to support her little girl. Like so many, her brother suffered from tuberculosis and had been taken into the sanatorium at Gravenhurst. Bethune came to see Wallace often. She wrote later:

I was twenty-eight. I soon was aware of peculiar sensations: a heightening of all my feelings, a strange new awareness such as I had never known. Whenever he was with me, I gathered from him a feeling of great strength and power, almost frightening at times. Then suddenly he told me he wanted to marry me.

Whenever they were together they spoke for hours. He told her about his childhood, and especially about his mother. There was nothing he would not tell her or do for her. The only obstacle that stood in their way was her husband; he refused to give Elizabeth a divorce. Bethune

was anxious; he wanted things done quickly. I was too bewildered to be aware of everything in his mind, but I sensed some sort of turmoil in him. . . . I didn't know what to do; in fact I did nothing, just watching him helplessly . . . seeing in him a great sensitivity, a great tenderness, and also violent explosions as I did nothing. Knowing him as I did I was amazed at his patience.

But nothing happened. The summer went by, half sweet, half sad, each wanting the other, the impossibility of it grinding them both down, Finally, realizing the situation was hopeless, Bethune left. First Frances, now Elizabeth. Was there no one for him?

Later, Wallace persuaded her husband to grant her a divorce. She thought, somehow, Bethune might return.

But then it was all over. A few times, desperately, I thought of going to him, of finding him again. . . . Perhaps he would come some day . . . He would rest and stay on, and all would be well again. What defeated hopes! Why should he come now? I hadn't given him what he really needed, what nobody seemed ever to give him – love.[50]

If Bethune's relations with women were so often unfulfilling, his concern for his patients was legendary. Wendell MacLeod, who knew Bethune well at the Royal Victoria Hospital and was close to him until he went to Spain, reported on his "warm and considerate manner with patients . . . This intensely personal concern for the patient's welfare is what I and others remember most clearly."[51] Bethune never ceased to advance new techniques, new methods, even new instruments to combat tuberculosis. In April 1932 he was elected to Associate Membership in the American Association for Thoracic Surgery; he became a full member in 1935, served on its Executive Council, and never missed a scientific meeting.[52]

Nothing He Would Not Do

In January 1933, Bethune left the Royal Victoria to lead the newly established tuberculosis service at the Sacré Coeur Hospital.[53] His permanent thoracic surgery team consisted of two young surgeons – Dr. Georges Deshaies and Dr. Gerard Rolland and the anesthetist Dr. Georges Cousineau.[54] Together they worked to reduce the high levels of mortality among their patients. Bethune instituted the use of epival, a liquid barbiturate that could be used as an anesthetic through intravenous injection; Cousineau became the first anesthetist to employ intravenous anesthesia anywhere in Canada. The procedure was a remarkable, but often overlooked, innovation at Bethune's Sacré Coeur surgery, and undoubtedly resulted in the survival of many lives that otherwise would have been lost.[55]

Deshaies admired Bethune from the first. It was his impression that Bethune was an extremely skillful surgeon, a revolutionary pioneer in thoracic surgery; as he put it, "Chest surgery at that time was a really new step in the treatment of pulmonary tuberculosis . . . a really great advancement . . . Bethune was always getting forward and forward in his treatment."[56]

By the end of his first year Bethune had introduced yet another innovation at Sacré Coeur: blood transfusions. In the early 1930s there were no blood banks, in the modern sense of the term, in any part of the world but the Soviet Union. Bethune's transfusions involved direct person-to-person blood flow; the patient and the donor lying on cots beside each other, the blood of the donor leaving his arm through a tube and then directly entering the arm of the patient; alternatively, and on occasion, blood was taken from the donor and refrigerated for a few hours before being transfused.[57]

Like MacLeod, what struck Deshaies most forcefully was Bethune's attitude toward the patients; there was nothing he would not do for them. As he put it: "His devotion to his patients was without limits." After surgery, "he used to go and see the patients more often than he was supposed to." Many times, if he was worried, he would come to a patient at night.[58] When Deshaies accompanied Bethune to the wards he would see the patients smile as soon as they saw him; it was evident that they were fond of him and he inspired them with confidence. Bethune was above all "kindness and consideration itself"[59] with his patients, but most especially with the children. "He was very attached to the children and could often be found on the ward in a rocking chair with a child on his knee."[60] At Sacré Coeur, as elsewhere, not all his patients lived and their loss tore at him, as Deshaies witnessed: "Of course, like any surgeon he lost patients, but I couldn't stay around when he lost a patient because he was so sorry . . . he would cry or be mad . . . at that time I preferred to be away from him."[61] Every corpse accused him: there was more he could have done. When he thought he had, at last, put those ancient demons asleep, they awoke, fluttering leather-like from the long ago past, their insidious and hectoring voices his own, but not his own: *You are not good enough; you are a failure; you will always be a failure; your sin is your pride.*

Bethune's creativity revealed itself not only in the advancement of medical technique; it was also expressed in painting. He had spent endless days in the art galleries of London. In 1931 he had joined art classes, but for the most part he worked on his own.[62] By far the best of his pictures is *Night Operating Theatre*. Reputedly painted as a challenge, Bethune maintained that he could paint a picture of sufficient quality that it would be accepted at the spring 1935 exhibition of the Montreal Museum of Fine Arts.[63] The artist Louis Muhlstock, who did not know Bethune until late 1935 or 1936, recalled only a single painting of his, "a water colour of one of those round-bellied Quebec stoves, with quite delicate colours."[64] But, most intriguingly, Bethune painted a series of murals about which we can know nothing. In the winter of 1934, his car often broke down and he was frequently late for work. It seemed best if he could spend the night near the hospital when an operation had been scheduled for the morning. Georges Cousineau found a landlady from among Bethune's patients, and a room was rented for him. When he arrived, he asked that all the pictures be removed. Within the first day, he began painting a sequence of large murals that eventually covered all the walls. The landlady was horrified. The nature of the murals remains unknown; they were painted over when Bethune left at the end of the season.[65]

Bethune's fascination with art was not limited to his own work; he had become a frequent visitor at salons and exhibitions. When Fritz Brandtner arrived in Montreal in 1934, Bethune was the first to buy one of his paintings.[66] He became acquainted with almost all the major *avant garde* artists gathering in the Montreal area, a distinguished list, many of whom became close friends. But perhaps most interesting, in this context, was John Lyman. According to Marian Scott, "The Lyman's evening functions were often referred to as the Lyman Salon and it was at one of them that I first met Bethune."[67] Charles Hill, a curator at the National Gallery of Canada, noted that Lyman founded a school of painters and other artists, including the architect Hazen Sise, who later served with Bethune in Spain, although it would appear that they never met at this time.[68]

If Bethune said often to others, "I am an artist," the reference, then, was most obviously and immediately to painting, but it was never to painting alone, it was to his sense of self, of who he was as a man. He was not, simply, a physician who painted; he was an artist in the operating theater, as much as he was an artist at the easel. If the project that he chose for himself at the age of eight was a decision for medicine, it at the same time bore within itself a rejection of hypocrisy, a resistance against falseness and superstition and forms without meaning. For Bethune, the very role of the artist lay in an almost surgical desire to smash through the dead weight of convention that seemed everywhere to oppress every natural impulse. If being an artist meant, to Bethune, creativity and commitment in medicine as much as in painting, it also meant a refusal to pretend that things are not as they are, a trajectory towards truth.

At the Sacré Coeur that truth was inescapably revealed. For Bethune, the Sacré Coeur was the discovery of that nation within a nation, "the Quebec of the québecois, the québecois as a people."[69] And these people were the poor of the poor; the patients that he saved returned home to squalor, relapsing into the very conditions that had sickened them to begin with. There was an intolerable contradiction at play: medical technique was advancing daily, but the conditions of poverty, in which the people were forced to live, negated every effort of the physicians who were pledged to safeguard their health.

In the summer of 1934 Bethune discovered a group of doctors who had begun to think about these matters. He had taken on an appointment at the Women's General Hospital and encountered a group of young doctors politically on the left; doctors who were concerned with the social and economic basis of the prevailing political malaise and about the rise of fascism. These were men Bethune could talk to and from whom he could learn. In particular, he was drawn to Hyman Shister, a cardiologist, and a member of the Communist Party, with whom he was soon in frequent and animated conversation. Shister was principled and forthright, with a "clear enquiring mind, much goodwill and a sweet disposition." They developed an increasing affection for each other based on a common understanding of the economic catastrophe in which so many now found themselves, and an intimation of the political struggles that lay ahead. Shister would become an invaluable comrade and in the days before his departure for Spain, it was with the Shisters that Bethune chose to stay.[70]

Driving home one day from the Sacré Coeur, Bethune came upon a demonstration of several thousand working people demanding "Milk For Our Children!" and "Jobs Not Breadlines!" Within minutes police officers, mounted on horseback, and stretching from one side of the street to the other, charged into the crowd and began beating them mercilessly with thick wooden truncheons. Bethune was outraged. He jumped out of his car and witnessed the worst of the attack – the senseless, brutal, hate-filled violence of the police. He opened his medical bag and began immediately to treat the wounded. And when he had done what he could for the first, he took the next one who needed him. And then the next and the next, until the sun fell and the streets were empty.[71]

He had seen it with his own eyes, and he could no longer unsee it: the response of the state to the starving and the destitute. It was no longer possible to simply treat the sick for free, to refuse to bill them, to comfort himself with the illusion of benevolence. The demonstration was a turning point for Bethune. Because he had come to see himself primarily as an artist, he had imagined that he was in some sense unique. And that therefore his gift to others, and first and foremost his medical gift, was a *generosity*. His relation to the working class was an act of sympathy, and not yet a relation of solidarity. Now something was alive in his mind; he could begin to feel it surface.

Some months earlier Bethune had encountered George Mooney who was working as executive director of the YMCA in Verdun, a working class district near Montreal's harbor front.[72] The day after the demonstration, he went to see Mooney. He outlined a plan to him; he would offer his services free of charge to the unemployed masses in the adjoining working-class districts of Verdun and Pointe St. Charles. Every Saturday he would arrive at noon, and using Mooney's office as his clinic he would treat every complaint that the people brought. The free clinic opened in July 1935, and for a year or more, until Bethune was preparing to leave for Spain, it continued.[73] The free clinic was a political act; Bethune's politics had moved further to the left, but he had not yet found a political home.

In August 1935 impelled by the desire to see Soviet medicine in practice, Bethune attended the International Physiological Congress in Leningrad, where the main speaker was the world-famous scientist Ivan Pavlov. For the next three weeks Bethune visited hospitals and sanatoria, examining Soviet methods of dealing with tuberculosis. Measures that he himself had considered essential to its elimination were being implemented. Every child was tested with tuberculin in an effort to detect the early onset of the disease; a series of halfway-house sanatoria had been established; tuberculosis clinics had devoted themselves to providing a wide range of diagnostic services, including the regular inspection of the bronchial passage with a bronchioscope. Not every clinic yet possessed such an instrument, but that made little difference to Bethune: they had recognized its necessity and they intended to universalize the service; the eradication of tuberculosis was a planned national effort.[74]

Within days of his return Bethune began a series of public speeches on his experiences in the Soviet Union. Membership of the Communist Party of Canada (CPC) had doubled since 1934 and was increasing daily. There

Nothing He Would Not Do

was much speculation about Russia at every level of society, and there were endless invitations for Bethune to speak.[75] At the Montreal Medico-Chirurgical Society he soon gave an intellectually staggering and rather beautiful speech comparing the Soviet revolution to the delivery of a human infant – the blood, the agony, the pain, and the mess that always accompanies a new life brought into the world; and at the same time he criticized the "sterility of soul" of those "who lack the imagination to see behind the blood the significance of birth."[76] It was inevitable, under the circumstances, that he would meet Louis Kon, Head of the Friends of the Soviet Union. In September 1935 he attended one of Bethune's speeches and made formal contact with him. Bethune was soon a frequent guest at the Kon household, meeting not only Louis, but his daughter Irene, with whom he became lasting friends.[77]

The recognition that the Soviet state – no matter how internally contradictory, and with no matter how many difficulties involved – was making the attempt to develop a society where the health of its citizens would eliminate the very conditions productive of every disease from tuberculosis to fascism, led Bethune to the doorstep of the Communist Party. In November 1935 he crossed that threshold and joined the Party.[78] But who was the man who then entered – a physician, a political militant, or an artist?

At the suggestion of the Party, Bethune threw his considerable energies into establishing the Montreal Group for the Security of the People's Health. He recruited Hyman Shister, Wendell MacLeod, and Libbie Park to form the core of a group that was soon to number a dozen others dedicated to bringing health care to the masses.[79] The Group met regularly over the winter of 1935 and, in the spring of 1936, Bethune appeared before the Montreal Medico-Chirurgical Society and delivered a paper entitled *Take the Private Profit Out of Medicine*. Not only did Bethune emphasize the terrible conditions under which hundreds of thousands lived in Quebec, and how those conditions undermined the people's health, but it directly attacked the wide-scale indifference of the medical establishment. As Bethune put it, health care was as necessary as food, but under the system of private medicine they were "selling bread at the price of jewels."[80]

In the summer of 1936, in the face of up-coming provincial elections, Bethune's group intensified their activities. They published a detailed Manifesto outlining a system of socialized medicine. The Manifesto was delivered to every political candidate and to the medical, dental, and nursing societies.[81] It hardly mattered; the fix was already in. Maurice Duplessis was elected to power – with the connivance of the Church and the conservative bourgeoisie – and established a quasi-fascist regime. The question of public health care was settled: there would be none. Pay or rot;

the working class could look to heaven for salvation, it was no business of the state.

It was discouraging, to be sure. But a lost battle did not mean a lost war. And although Bethune did not live to see it – it would be thirty years in coming – the plan that he first conceived, for socialized medicine and a health care system with equal access for all, became the medical policy of the nation.

But there was more to be done, more in fact that he had been doing, even while he worked with the health group. Every day at the Sacré Coeur he had seen the sad, sick children. They were unforgettable. What could he do for *them?* He had seen them everywhere, the children of the destitute, pale ghosts, not physically sick, or not necessarily so, but *sick of heart*. Bethune knew how joyless a childhood could be. And in every unhappy child Bethune saw himself; it was his own past, the hidden secret of his own childhood that he sought in these broken children; their sorrow was his own, and so their healing was a way, unacknowledged, of healing himself. Every child's life that he could save, or even brighten no matter how momentarily, was a torch to light the way into his own darkness.

Bethune established the Children's Creative Art Center in the spring of 1936 with aid of Fritz Brandtner and Marian Scott.[82] He traveled often to Toronto to seek the opinion of other artists, especially Paraskeva Clark with whom he developed a strong attachment.[83] The Center was fundamental both to Bethune's profoundly complex relation to children, and his identification of himself as an artist. The children who would come to the art center would be from the working-class districts, children whose sensibilities were being stunted by the poverty of their surroundings and deprived of the joy and happiness all children deserved.

The classes were free. There was no intention to teach the children to be artists; the Center was not an art school, but a place where poor children could be encouraged to explore their creativity. Wendell MacLeod observed that the children's pictures reflected not only what they had seen, but what they had felt: "anger, sadness, feeling crowded, or lonely, or frightened."[84] As Marian Scott later said, "Beth always had this very strong feeling that the children . . . who were having such a difficult life at the time, that if even for a short time each week they could come and . . . be free to draw and express their ideas or feelings, that this might even affect them later on when they faced hardships."[85]

The children responded to Bethune's care and attention. He showed them how to see and feel the world around them. Sylvia Ary, who later became a professional painter, recalled: "The children all loved him . . . he used to just talk to us, and always served us something for us to eat you

Nothing He Would Not Do

know, like milk and cookies. . . . I always got the impression about him that he was rather shy, and he certainly liked children, without being ostentatious about it. He was just wonderful to us."[86]

But, just as with the health group, the project that Bethune had nourished he would not see completed. Although the children were largely too young to understand, new monsters were afoot in the world: Hitler, Mussolini, Franco. In the quiet evenings, looking out from his window at the lights downhill in the harbor, listening to the lonesome sounds of fog horns over the water, he knew he would soon be leaving the children – *his* children, behind.

In the year before he left for Spain, Bethune had two significant romantic relationships with women: one hopeless, a second tragic and terrible.

Bethune had first met Marian Scott at one of Lyman's evening salons, but it was on board ship, while he traveled to Russia – and she to England – that he conceived an ardent love for her. He wrote to her endlessly, pledging his affection and imagining a shared life together. Scott was equally infatuated with Bethune; but still in love with her husband Frank. Much as he had with Elizabeth Wallace, Bethune ultimately realized they could never truly be lovers.[87] On 21 November, he wrote her a letter ending all possibility of a future affair, and at the same time providing a revealing analysis of himself and his relation to women. After a few introductory paragraphs, in which he wrote of his realization that she would never leave her husband Frank, he continued:

> Can you ever be free – perhaps not! Only through another who respects you as much as himself and who also anticipates the inevitable & is ruthless, kind & cruel. . . . F. [Frank Scott] can only keep you – as a free woman – by letting you go. I did this to Frances. . . . I didn't *need* any woman, or any man. That's what so shook Frances. She was seduced by Coleman's plea that he 'needed her.' She discovered too late that this is the universal plea of all weaklings. Their cry comes from a realization of their own structural weakness . . . It is made to the strong. And the strong are very susceptible to this cry. It is an appeal to their vanity. No human should ever make that cry to another. . . . But a straight glance, a firm hand – a plea – 'I love you, I want you' – is what a man or a woman should make to his mate. Otherwise he has merely shifted his position physiologically and anatomically and not spiritually – from the womb, from the breast, from the arms – back to arms & breast again – the eternal child – chronic infantilism. . . . But it is not treating a woman fairly to do so. It reduces them from the mate of a man to his nurse. . . . So I don't need you (except to bathe and bask in!). I want you as a man wants a woman. I like you too. I like you rather like I like

myself – with reservations! . . . You are the *first* woman in the world I have met about whom I have felt *no doubt* that we could live together, physically & mentally & spiritually mated. . . . I am glad now that we did not take each other physically. For me it would have meant that I would not have left you, as I am leaving you now . . . so sweetly! No. I should have behaved with most unseemly vigour, & lack of manners, shouts and clamours. . . . Yes. I understand you, my own, my darling. The great question – 'what do you do with your old loves'? . . . I am here if I can be of use to you at any time. And that's all one man can say to a woman. *Au revoir*.

We may extract from this psychologically acute letter, several significant themes. Libbie Park maintains that Bethune "had none of the stereotyped male attitudes, and did not speak of women in a derogatory sense. A woman was a person, her mind not the mind of a 'woman' but of a person. . . . He respected women and would not put up with hypocrisy or 'moralizing philistines,' be they men or women."[88] We can clearly see the evidence of such an attitude in this letter. In this he is genuinely a progressive. Still, there is, in Bethune, an unconscious dependency on women which he does not recognize, rooted in the unlove of his infantile years, and the inchoate rage that flowed from it. This dependency reveals itself in two forms, both of which emerge in the letter to Scott. "The great question – what do you do with old loves?" This question he answered in practice: he never abandoned them. When all hope of a life together had been forsaken, he continued an intimate friendship with Scott, discussing painting and politics, and enlisting her in his work with the children's art center. As for Frances, Bethune visited her frequently and accompanied her to various artistic and political functions.

This dependency on women, despite his overt claim that he needed no one, and his recognition that such a need would be somehow related to the mother, in a regression to "chronic infantilism," expressed itself not only in keeping his former lovers near, but in the outbursts of vulgarity and near pathological rage that accompanied the loss of love. Bethune himself was certainly aware of these bizarre reactions, as he suggests to Scott, even if the tone of this confession is somewhat minimizing: "I should have behaved with most unseemly vigour, & lack of manners, shouts and clamours."[89] Yes, all that and a good deal more.

At some point early in 1936 he entered into an ultimately horrendous relationship with Margaret Day. The details of this affair are difficult to recount with certainty, since the only existing account appears in an interview with Day taken when she was over eighty years old and had suffered from "recurrent sieges of depression"; indeed she appears always to have

Nothing He Would Not Do

been somewhat neurotic, and at some point to have undergone an extensive psychoanalysis.[90]

In 1933, at the age of twenty-four, Day was sent by her father to the Royal College of Music, in London. With the death of her father she found herself without money, returned to Montreal, and secured a position as a schoolteacher. Shortly thereafter her brother developed tuberculosis; he was treated at the Royal Victoria, and died there. Margaret, hovering on the brink of nervous collapse, began to read Marxism and was, falsely, "putting it about Montreal that she was a Communist." A wealthy friend from London agreed to lend Day sufficient funds to visit the Soviet Union, which she did, probably in the summer of 1935. Back again in Montreal she joined a Marxist study group, and discovered that Bethune would be giving a speech about his experiences in Russia. Day attended Bethune's talk and "fell in love with him in five minutes flat." At home, she wrote Bethune telling him that she was a virgin and "sick of it" and asking him to "go out" with her, if only one time. The next day she destroyed the letter.

Sometime later, Bethune appeared at her study group as a guest speaker. At the end of the evening she talked to him about her brother. According to Day, Bethune had previously performed an operation on her brother and had, in a gesture typical of his care for his patients, brought him some books while he was recovering. It was during Bethune's conversation with Day he learned that her brother had subsequently died.

Day and Bethune then went to his apartment, but at whose instigation she does not say, whereupon they made love. "I was looking for trouble," she said, "and I found it." In the morning, she told him about the letter she had written after his speech on Russia. "Why didn't you send it?" he asked, "We've wasted the past three months." Day was surprised and delighted: "My dream was only once. I wasn't aiming higher than that."

Day became pregnant some time in the late spring or early summer. She did not want the child. Bethune did. We know of his need for children, but it was a need that Margaret Day understood not at all. Bethune was certainly not in love with her, but offered to marry her. She refused and demanded an abortion: Bethune would have to do it. All the old wounds opened once more: the loss of his child, yet again! The child from Frances that should have been his and was Coleman's instead; lost, aborted, and now, after he had regained some fragile peace, it was all the same nightmare repeating itself, except this time it truly was his *own* child, wanted so desperately, and deprived of life by his own hands.

Day, who only a few months ago had looked up to Bethune as a kind and considerate physician and a radical champion of the oppressed, she now decided – or more likely decided sixty-three years later, during her interview – was entirely a different man: "He was a destroyer, he was not right in his mind, he was an alcoholic, twice divorced. I have seen him fall drunk on the bed at three a.m. when he had to operate at nine that morning."

Is it possible to credit her testimony? *Was he a destroyer?* What did he destroy? In the period simultaneous with his relationship with Day, he opened a Free Clinic for the impoverished in Verdun; he developed innovative new surgical and anesthetic techniques; he established the Montreal Group for the Security of the People's Health and wrote the "Manifesto" that would form the basis of a national Medicare system; and he created a free art center for children from the slums. *Was he not in his right mind?* Those who knew him well, and have written about him during this period noticed nothing of the kind; MacLeod tells us that he seemed at his most contented and that there appeared to be "integrative forces" at work in his personality.[91] Moreover, Day's implication that Bethune operated while drunk is entirely fraudulent. But then she never knew Bethune in any objective context; she only knew him as the man who, at her explicit request, took her virginity and destroyed the infant she was carrying. Did Bethune appear to her then, in the very specific and limited context of their personal relationship as *"a destroyer and not in his right mind?"* Even given the exaggeration, bitterness, and self-justification of Day's characterization, there can be little doubt that Bethune, denied forever the child that he so intensely desired, may well have raged at her, damning her with furious phrases and gestures, drunk to the point of incoherence. Bethune knew himself well enough to know that he would react in precisely this way; he had said as much to Marian Scott. Shouts and clamors to the point of madness, the rage at the unloving Dragon exploding in the face of Margaret Day. And yet, if Bethune appeared to Day as a "destroyer" and "not in his right mind," how is it possible that she could say to him, as late as August 1936: "I never regretted a moment of our affair"?

What do you do with old loves? As with every woman who had entered his life and then been lost to him, Bethune did not abandon Day. He came to see her again after Spain but by then there was nothing left between them.

By the early autumn of 1936 Bethune's affections for Frances Coleman and Marian Scott had resolved into deep and intimate friendships, but nothing more, and the agony of his affair with Margaret Day was finally over. His time was fully occupied with his surgical practice and with the various other projects that had become so important in his life; the children's art center taking on a particular significance in the wake of the unwanted abortion.

Bethune was hurt; Frances, Elizabeth, Marian, Margaret: there was no one for him. He was wounded, but he was not defeated. Soon he would carry

Nothing He Would Not Do

his scars into Spain, but he would keep them to himself. Wendell MacLeod reports that he was "optimistic about the future, even when he switched his focus from health planning to Spain," and that "there were at least two important companionships, separate, different and beautiful."[92] Clearly he did not know about Day, and he neglected to acknowledge the pain that these "companionships" ultimately caused him. But it would be untrue to imagine that Bethune left for Spain because his romance with Day had turned to nightmare; that he *fled* to Spain because nothing was left to him. He would have gone to Spain in any event; the entire trajectory of his social and political commitment led to Spain. And then, too, he had written to Marian Scott that he did not need anyone, no woman, no man; that "I am a solitary, loving privacy, my own satisfactory aloneness," and it was as much truth as self-deception.

3

Last Night Rose Low and Wild and Red

There is some difficulty in determining the precise sequence of events that took Bethune to Spain; there are conflicting accounts and reminiscences that cannot easily be reconciled. But it is worth recalling that the events of the summer and fall of 1936 took place under the overarching pattern of the call for popular unity announced by George Dimitrov through the Communist International. The threat of fascism had begun to take on global proportions; the probability of another world war was imminent; it was necessary for Communists to unite with social-democrats and a broad range of progressives in an anti-fascist front. In Canada, the Ninth Plenum of the Party, convened in November 1935, fully endorsed Dimitrov's position; the entire line of the Party was to be directed toward the development of working class unity; at the political level, this certainly involved a serious attempt to work closely with the CCF.[1] Events in Spain were becoming of paramount importance; it was increasingly evident that if fascism was to be arrested and defeated, Spain would be the battleground. If fascism were allowed to triumph there, a second world war would be all but inevitable. Despite endless provocations, murders, and assassinations, the 16 February 1936 Spanish elections resulted in a sweeping victory for the Popular Front and a democratic Republic was declared. But it was instantly threatened. In Moscow, the *Pravda* newspaper of 12 March reported that General José Sanjurjo – one of the central fascist leaders – had arrived in Nazi Germany and was engaged "in negotiations regarding assistance to counter-revolutionary military organizations in Spain which are preparing a new plot against the government. In particular Sanjurjo intends to acquire a large quantity of military equipment from German firms."[2] In Canada, the situation in Spain was on the agenda at every Party meeting and Marxist study group that Bethune attended. Like other Party members he viewed the rise of fascism with horror and distaste. To his friends he compared fascism to a disease, not unlike tuberculosis, spreading in the same ground of human poverty and misery, but posing a danger infinitely more difficult to eradicate.

Last Night Rose Low and Wild and Red

When Generalissimo Francisco Franco led a fascist assault from Spanish Morocco to mainland Spain on 17 July, declaring war on the legitimate Republican government, democratic and progressive workers in Canada, as in almost every nation, were outraged. The Communist Party newspaper, reflecting the Party's rapidly growing membership and increasing influence among non-Party workers and farmers, had recently achieved daily status and been renamed the *Daily Clarion*. Banner headlines and front-page stories on developments in Spain occupied the paper on every issue from 20 July to 29 July.[3] On 27 July Franco's fascists had taken Seville; four days later they were marching on Madrid.[4] On 4 August, the paper reported that two Popular Front officials, Charles Peisy and Jean Perron, visiting Montreal, had been attacked and beaten by a mob of local fascists associated with the Catholic Church.[5] On 5 and 7 August, the Party paper was calling for mass meetings and more visible action;[6] on 8 August it declared, "It is therefore our duty to organize meetings, collect funds, and in every possible way to assist the Spanish front-line fighters for democracy and against the rule of the fascist henchmen."[7] On 13 August, the Central Committee of the Communist Party, through the *Daily Clarion*, urged trade unionists, CCFers, and all progressive people to unite, organize, and engage in mass demonstrations.[8] On 17 August, the proto-fascist Duplessis government took power in Quebec.

At some point during these initial days of the Franco rebellion, responding to his Party's call to action, Bethune began to actively consider putting himself at the service of the Spanish people. The contagion of fascism was everywhere, raising its murderous head now even in the streets where he walked every day. But Spain was the focal point; it was there that the people were bleeding and the massacres had begun. In Badajoz, Franco's army dragged over two thousand of the town's people into the local bull ring and mowed them down; some of the men who had engaged in armed resistance were mutilated, or had their genitals cut off and a crude Christian cross sliced into their chests.[9] Late in 1935, at the Sacré Coeur, Bethune had operated on Fernand Dallaire, an air force chef. As with so many others, Dallaire maintained that Bethune was an extraordinary physician, and that "all the patients loved and trusted him." After Dallaire's recovery, Bethune took him, in late July or August, to a medical meeting at the Windsor Hotel, to present his case and describe the operation he had performed. After the meeting he confided to Dallaire that he intended to leave the hospital and go overseas to Spain. He explained his decision by asking him, "If you saw a crowd of injured people on one street corner and just one on another, where would you go to give help?" Dallaire answered him, as Bethune no doubt he expected he would, that "it would be better to go where the need was greatest."[10] With his friend George Mooney he was more explicit: "It's in Spain," he said, "that the real issues of our time are going to be fought out."[11] Everywhere he went, Spain was not far from his mind; there was no one with whom he did not discuss it. The artist Paraskeva Clark recalled, in her heavily-inflected and broken English, that on one of Bethune's frequent visits to Toronto that summer – most probably late in August after the Duplessis election had put an end to the most pressing work of the Montreal Group for the Security of the People's Health – "I remember we went out of town swimming at some hole, and yet around that night, I don't swim at all so I mean I was only around, it had something to with Spry, Graham Spry, which later of course turned out that Graham Spry was, that I would imagine was this Spain things, so he was coming out for, talking to various people."[12] In short, although Spry, the Chair of the Executive Committee of the Ontario division of the CCF, would later imply that he did not meet Bethune until the last days of September, it would appear that they were familiar with each other much earlier, and friendly enough that they would go swimming together. What they discussed about Spain we cannot know, but most surely Bethune would have spoken about his desire to employ his medical skills to benefit the Republican forces.

In any event, shortly after their meeting, on 30 August, Spry contacted other ranking members of the CCF and, according to a letter he sent to his future wife, "I talked over . . . the idea of organizing a committee to collect funds for an ambulance to be sent to Spain. I wrote to Mr. Dafoe, today, asking him what he thought of it, and how far he would put editorial support behind it. Tonight I am going to write some further letters, and see what happens."[13] Rose Potvin, Spry's official biographer, maintains that "his motive was to counter the publicity garnered by the Communists in urging Canadians to fight against fascism."[14] It was, of course, more than a matter of "publicity"; the Communist Party was enormously successful not only in raising public awareness, but in developing a series of mass meetings, demonstrations, and fund-raisers, and of bringing significant sectors of the working class and their allies into the anti-fascist struggle. Important as countering the Communist initiative was to Spry, there were other issues of equal importance. The Communists had called for a united front and they had demonstrated their willingness to do their part: throughout 1935 and 1936, the Communists had openly supported CCF candidates for public office, and publicly promised every degree of cooperation; Spry recognized, despite a certain personal reluctance, the political necessity of maintaining the united front. Finally, there was, without any doubt, a sincere desire on the part of the CCF to aid the legitimate Spanish government.

Four days later, on 2 September, Spry spoke at a united front public meeting at the Labor Lyceum in Toronto held under the auspices of the Jewish Anti-Fascist Conference. Spry noted that Hitler's Germany and Mussolini's Italy "were definitely involved in this struggle which threatens to involve the whole world. If we don't realize what is happening in Spain, when it comes to our own turn it will be our own fault." Spry announced the determination of the CCF to raise funds for the Popular Front government. Other speakers represented the League Against War and Fascism, the Anarchist Federation, the Jewish Workers Party, and the Amalgamated Clothing Workers. According to the *Daily Clarion*, Joseph Salsberg, speaking on behalf of the Communists, "stressed the menace of another world war due to fascist aggression, and referred to the development of fascist tendencies in Canada. . . . Tremendous applause greeted the final appeal of J. B. Salsberg for solid unity between the CCF and the Communist Party of Canada as the surest method of defeating fascism."[15]

Meanwhile, Communist Party leader Tim Buck and Central Committee member A. A. MacLeod were in Brussels, during the first week of September, attending the World Peace Congress. Immediately afterward, they were invited to Spain. Buck was briefed on the situation by José Diaz, who outlined the details of a Comintern plan to organize an International Brigade of volunteer fighters. MacLeod spoke with the President of Spain, Manuel Azaña, who told him that medical services and supplies were the Republic's greatest need.[16] MacLeod telegraphed Azaña's request to Party headquarters in Toronto. Bethune had already taken some steps on his own initiative to find a way to Spain. He had asked a friend, Percy Newman, for a loan of two hundred dollars, but Newman was unable to help. He wrote to the Canadian Red Cross Society to determine whether he might be useful to them should they be considering sending an ambulance to Spain, and received a letter from J. L. Biggar, the National Commissioner, saying, "the Society is not raising a Unit for Service in Spain and has not, I think, any intention whatever of doing so."[17] Bethune was, of course, a member of the Communist Party and as such he was under voluntary oath to act under Party discipline. He was extremely proud to be a member of the Party and under no circumstances would he have violated his oath. Therefore, if Newman had been able to lend him the money, or the Red Cross had been amenable to his plan, he would certainly have taken the matter up with the Party and sought its validation. When Azaña's request began to be actively discussed within Party circles, Bethune immediately approached the Quebec Committee of the Party. He volunteered to go to Spain in his capacity as a physician, and proposed that the Party organize a *Canadian Mobile Blood Transfusion Unit* to serve the Republican government forces fighting at the front.[18] The Party accepted the proposal, and most probably suggested to Bethune that he make contact with Spry since it was necessary, in the interests of the united front policy, that the CCF appear to be in charge of medical fund raising, and because they knew Spry was already organizing a committee for this purpose.

On 15 September, the Party made Azaña's appeal public. The *Toronto Star* reported on MacLeod's meeting in Madrid and the Spanish government's need for serums and medical supplies.[19] The same day, in Kitchener, Ontario, at a public united front meeting, a plan was approved to send a Canadian-staffed field hospital to Spain. Spry was the main speaker and announced that funds were expected to be raised across the country for doctors, nurses, ambulances, and surgical equipment.[20] On 22 September, the *Daily Clarion* revealed that funds were being collected for a full hospital unit, including portable equipment, that would function at the line of battle. "Full details of the plan are not yet known," the paper reported, "but it is expected that Graham Spry, member of the national executive committee of the Cooperative Commonwealth Federation, will make a complete announcement within a few days." It was also noted that *two weeks previously* Spry had begun to assemble a committee behind the project. The idea had been endorsed at a closed meeting consisting of trade union leaders, and ranking officials of the CCF, the Communist Party, the Jewish Anti-Fascist Conference and other organizations.[21] The very next day, Spry formally announced the launching of the project. He made it clear that the proposal did not originate with the CCF, but from a committee not representing any political party. This was more than a little disingenuous since the project was, in essence, a mutually agreed upon venture of the CCF and the Communist Party. The new announcement held that the proposed hospital would *not* operate at the front, as previously suggested, but would be a stationary unit. National fundraising was to begin without delay and had in fact already begun in Montreal.[22]

On 26 September Spry wrote a long article in the CCF newspaper, the *New Commonwealth*, under the front-page headline: *To Offer Field Hospital to Spain*. The national committee to oversee the establishment of finance, equipment, and transport was to be known as the Spanish Hospital and Medical Aid Committee. The committee was to "work in close association with the committees already set up in Toronto, Kitchener, Timmins, Montreal and other centres now raising funds." Spry noted that the Committee to Aid Spanish Democracy (CASD), representing trade unions, political parties, and other organizations had already raised over two thousand dollars. The CASD had been "contacting groups throughout Canada and will work in close collaboration with the hospital committee." As it happened, Spry's committee was dissolved within the month, and all work in the area was immediately transferred to the CASD. In keeping with Spry's political orientation the New Commonwealth article downplayed the originating efforts of trade unionists and progressive political organizations, and emphasized the need to "represent a wide section of Canadian opinion, including church, academic and professional representation;" in short, the political advancement of the petit-bourgeoisie over the working class. Significantly, Spry noted that "a representative of the committee has sailed for Spain and will contact the Spanish government and Red Cross immediately upon arrival." Spry did not reveal the representative's name but it was without doubt Henning Sorensen, who was soon to become a member of Bethune's blood transfusion unit in Madrid.[23] Writing to Spry many years later, Sorensen said, "We have met only once. That was in September 1936, the night before I left Montreal for Spain. You may remember you came to my apartment together with Frank Scott and Jacques Bieler. You had learned I was going to Spain and you came to ask me to act as an agent for a newly created Committee to Aid Spanish Democracy."[24]

Apparently, according to Spry, Bethune read the New Commonwealth article, telegraphed Spry to offer his services, and said that he would arrive in Toronto the next day.[25] Again, given the issue of Party discipline, Bethune would have been unlikely to take such a step without Party approval. But, most oddly, Spry was to write in a later letter:

> To my delight and alarm, Dr. Norman Bethune responded almost immediately. I was delighted that a man of his eminence should wish to be involved and alarmed because the Spanish Hospital and Medical Aid Committee was a figment of my imagination designed to stir interest in the Republic, with only a dim hope that it might eventually become a reality. When Bethune arrived in Toronto, I had to confess that there was neither an organization nor the money to send him to Spain. . . . The immediate problem was finding a way to pay for Bethune's trip to Spain. I remembered that Jane Smart . . . still had not cashed in the return portion of her steamship ticket to Europe. I rushed over to her flat . . . blurted out my request . . . she reappeared moments later with the steamship ticket in hand."[26]

What are we to make of this extraordinary letter? It is perfectly obvious that the Committee was in no sense a "figment of the imagination;" the organization had been established several weeks previously, it was already operating on the basis of existing committees throughout the country, and fundraising had already begun, with the pledged assurance and commitment of trade unions and political entities that substantial monies would be accumulated. Nor does it seem at all likely that the "immediate problem" would have been securing Bethune a steamship ticket, surely the most minor of costs compared to the price of extensive medical supplies. Indeed, the entire letter is baffling if taken at face value; its true purpose perhaps lying elsewhere.

The decision had been made: Bethune would travel to Spain under the sponsorship of the CASD. On the day that Bethune went to see Spry following the *New Commonwealth* story, fifteen hundred people filled Toronto's Massey Hall, under the CASD banner, to hear a speaker from the International Federation of Trades Unions speak about Spain; five hundred dollars was raised.[27] From Toronto, Bethune sent a telegram to Georges Deshaies at the Sacré Coeur saying that he was going to resign from the hospital and that he would explain when he came back to Montreal. Returning home, he wrote resignation letters to the various hospitals with which he was associated, giving them appropriate notice. At the Sacré Coeur he spoke to Deshaies, who recalled their conversation: "I am going to Spain," Bethune said, "because I feel there is some good to be done there." "Don't you believe," Deshaies responded, "that your duty is to stay here and look after the TB people?" Bethune replied: "No, because you are going to do that. I have to go to Spain."[28]

The situation in Quebec was becoming increasingly tense. Propaganda favoring Franco was being churned out by printing companies controlled by Duplessis and his pro-Nazi associates. The Catholic Church was condemning the legitimate Spanish government from the pulpit, spewing furious lies and deceptions, and whipping its youth wing into action. At the end of the first week of October, a mob of five hundred fascist hooligans ransacked the offices of *Clarté*, the French-language newspaper of the Communist Party.[29]

Bethune met with Party officials and together they discussed the details of his coming work in Spain. He visited his closest friends, Marian Scott, Libbie Park, Fritz Brandtner, Frances Coleman and many others, explaining what he was about to do and why he had to do it. He told Wendell MacLeod explicitly that he intended to establish a blood transfusion service in Spain.[30] Like anti-fascists everywhere, he recognized the threat to democracy and to human progress that Franco represented; and as a Communist, it was his duty to fight back. For the last time he watched the children at the art center, some laughing and chattering, some serious and quiet, as they stretched out on the floor, drawing and painting, the tubs of bright color all about them. That evening, after they had left, and he was alone, he looked out the broad living room window and saw the clouds parting to reveal the moon. He sat down at his table, took a blank sheet of paper and began to write a poem. It was the last he would ever write, save one more from the rubble of a hospital in Madrid.

Red Moon

And this same pallid moon tonight,
    Which rides so quietly, clear and high,
The mirror of our pale and troubled gaze,
    Raised to the cool Canadian sky,

Above the shattered Spanish mountain tops
    Last night, rose low and wild and red,
Reflecting back from her illumined shield,
    The blood bespattered faces of the dead.

To that pale disc, we raise our clenched fists
    And to those nameless dead our vows renew,
"Comrades, who fought for freedom and the future world,
    Who died for us, we will remember you."[31]

Bethune spent much of the last two weeks before his departure in Toronto. A. A. MacLeod had returned from Spain with three representatives of the Republican government: Marcelino Domingo, a former education minister; Isabella de Palencia, who had been a delegate to the League of Nations; and Luis Sarasola, a Franciscan priest, intending to take them on a speaking tour throughout the country. On 21 October a mass meeting was held at the Mutual Street Arena, in Toronto; eleven thousand attended to listen to the Spanish envoys and to Bethune himself, who appeared with them on the stage. The *Daily Clarion* reported: "arrangements are now being completed by Dr. Bethune to purchase medical supplies to carry with him into the war zones of Spain. He will take with him immediately the following supplies: surgical instruments, blood transfusion apparatus, 100,000 units of insulin, 1,000 units each of typhoid and smallpox vaccines, anti-toxin tetanique concentrated, and anti-gangrene serum." The CASD appealed for a further five thousand dollars to ensure that urgently needed supplies would follow Bethune to Spain. The Communist Party presented the meeting with a cheque for one thousand dollars, primarily collected through door-to-door canvassing conducted by the Party divisions of Manitoba and Ontario.[32] The next day, before returning to Montreal with MacLeod and the Spaniards, Bethune visited his friend, the painter Charles Comfort. Full of vigorous determination and high spirits, Bethune sketched out a half-humorous epitaph on a sheet of drawing paper: *Viva Espana. Long live the revolution! Born a bourgeois, Died a communist.*[33]

In Montreal the local fascists attacked again. With the Vatican fully supporting Franco, and the Spanish clergy largely working with the fascist invaders, Sarasola was under papal indictment for refusing to break with the legitimate government. In Montreal the Church denounced Sarasola in the press. Mobs of young fascists, carefully organized by the Church, patrolled the streets. They marched to City Hall and demanded the cancellation of the CASD meeting that had been scheduled to take place at the Mount Royal Arena. The chairman of the city executive committee appeared before them and ordered the police to ban the meeting, saying: "We will not allow Communism to take root here." The mob cheered. Frank Scott, a CCF sponsor of the meeting, went to Victoria Hall, in the neighboring suburb of Westmount, beyond the control of the Montreal police. The Hall's manager, fearful of repercussions, told Scott that the room had already been rented. With time running out and nowhere else to go, the sponsors acquired a small room in the Mount Royal Hotel that could hold no more than a hundred seats. Bethune, speaking from the platform, noted with anger that the mass meeting had been intended to raise money for vaccines and serums, and as a result of the police action thousands of Spanish children would die. Outside, the fascists paraded through the streets screaming, "Down with the Communists!" "Down with the Jews!" Halfway through the severely reduced meeting, in the middle of Isabella de Polencia's speech, the hotel management turned out the lights and informed the audience they would have to leave. Throughout the night, hundreds of fascists marched through the city smashing the windows of Jewish-owned stores. The police did nothing to prevent them; the following morning, 24 October, Duplessis showered the thugs with praise.[34] Bethune left Montreal with the accumulated medical supplies, American Express money orders, and a letter of introduction to the Spanish prime minister, and hurried to the harbor in Quebec City. Boarding the *Empress of Britain*, he was approached by a reporter from the *New York Times* who reminded him that Franco's forces were on the verge of taking Madrid, and asked him about his intentions. Bethune faced him, standing tall, erect, determined: "Whether or not Madrid falls before the invading forces," he said, "I will complete my mission."[35]

As Bethune headed out to sea the Archbishop of Quebec, Cardinal Villeneuve, celebrated the Feast of Christ the King. He called for all

Catholics to join in a crusade to exterminate communism, and denounced the Republican government as "a group comprised of new barbarians who have covered the lands of Spain with desolation and blood."[36] Hitler, Mussolini, Franco; thus were a new triumvirate of beasts raised to holy sanctification.

PART TWO

Capitalism Breeds Fascism the Way a Fly Breeds Maggots

4
The Double Pyramid

The problem of fascism is the problem of capitalism itself in its imperialist stage: that is to say, fascism has been inseparable from the capitalist system since the beginning of the twentieth century. Indeed, as we shall argue, fascism has its origins in nineteenth-century British imperialism. The bourgeoisie knows this very well: after all it is their own history. What the ruling class desires most is to deny its historical role in the development and support of fascism. Capitalism is not the opponent of fascism, it is its progenitor: capitalism breeds fascism the way a fly breeds maggots.

The bloody history of British colonial imperialism and its ideological pretensions were taken up by fascism, which was its true successor. It is not only the venomous ideology of the master race that will concern us; equally inherent in both imperialism and fascism is the assertion that the ruling class is biologically superior to the working class. Both the imperialists and their fascist successors pursued the identical policy of the ruthless suppression of the working class, and it is this, more than any other factor that led to the support of fascism by imperialism, and most especially British imperialism. The double pyramid of racial and class oppression forms the core of both imperialist and fascist state practice. We must now trace the development of this practice.

At the true heart of British imperialist ideology lay a contradiction between two equal falsehoods that formed an indissoluble unity – the assurance that they were a people specially chosen by God to dominate the world, and the certainty that they were biologically superior to non-white peoples. The ruling class held not only that the white "race" was superior to non-white races, but that the British people were superior to all other white people. At the same time, and on the same basis, the British ruling class thought themselves superior to the working classes whose labor daily provided for their wealth. Anointed by God, it was not only the privilege but the duty of the British ruling class to command; it was the duty of others to obey.

Although the working class was largely indifferent, at the beginning of the nineteenth century, to the idea of Empire, the wealthy classes soon began to work them over. The ideologists of imperialism passed up no opportunity to proclaim their racial uniqueness and superiority. According to the Colonial Secretary, Joseph Chamberlain, "that spirit . . . of enterprise distinguishing the Anglo-Saxon race has made us peculiarly fit to carry out the work of colonisation. . . . The Anglo-Saxon race is the greatest ruling race the world has ever known."[1] As Sir Charles Dilke put it: "the Saxon empire will rise triumphant from its long drawn out struggle with inferior races."[2]

The bourgeois newspapers were happy to act as a conduit for the ruling class ideology. The latter half of the nineteenth century saw a dramatic increase in mass circulation, and the bourgeoisie understood from the beginning that every page of newsprint under their control would act as a collective voice for their imperial aspirations. It was not difficult to ensure that the imperialist rubbish was parroted in every edition. Examples, of course, abound; in Africa: "The Zulu is a savage pure and simple, abjectly submissive to the loathsome superstitions of the witch finder and rain doctor, and with his life and belongings entirely at the will of a brutal tyrant."[3] For this ignorance, they were punished by the British army; ten thousand or more slaughtered defending their homes. In New Zealand: the Maori were "a hardy race of savages" who "ranged free,"[4] and were therefore ripe for colonization, massacre, and the usual invasion of the missionaries.

The racist implications of British imperialism resulted everywhere in invasion, armed intrusion, massacre and colonialist violence. "Empire *was* race," as James Morris has noted,[5] and this fundamental sentiment was expressed quite openly in Parliament as the following presumptuousness of Lord Palmerston to the Commons suggests: "These half-civilized Governments such as those of China, Portugal, Spanish America, all require a dressing down every eight or ten years to keep them in order. Their minds are too shallow to receive an impression that will last longer than some such period and warning is of little use."[6] Warning was apparently beside the point since it was always force of arms that guaranteed British expansionism and continued British profits: the "uselessness of rebelling against the white man"[7] was the lesson always to be taught, since "the white man is the master race and the black man must forever remain cheap labor and slaves."[8] Under the twin banners of white supremacy and the divine mandate, the British Empire took as its own the whole of India and Afghanistan, Australia and New Zealand, and Africa from Egypt through Sudan to the Southern Cape.

In 1865, following a small insurrection in Jamaica, in which a few white officials had been killed, governor Edward Eyre declared martial law and instituted a reign of mass murder. Suspected rebels, almost all of whom were innocent, were executed by the hundreds. A plan was adopted "which struck immense terror into these wretched men, far more than death": they were

The Double Pyramid   **53**

ordered to hang each other.[9] Britain's "civilizing mission" went only so far. Those who were so ungrateful as to reject colonization discovered the bloody violence that lay at its core. On every continent, and in every country, imperial expansionism put a bayonet to the throat of the indigenous population. Hopelessly outnumbered in any armed conflict, those whose territory had been invaded were blackmailed into submitting to the "elevating mission" of the British intruders, or they faced the inevitable slaughter and death. A British expeditionary force in Tibet encountered a small group of inhabitants who had gathered to resist the British army. The Tibetans were surrounded on all sides and within the space of two minutes as many as seven hundred were massacred. Three months later the dead still lay rotting where they had dropped. Since one hundred and sixty-eight of the wounded had been treated in a British field hospital, Edmund Candler, of the *Daily Mail* wrote: "I think the Tibetans were really impressed with our humanity."[10]

Those who survived were always impressed, though perhaps less with their new masters' peculiar sense of "humanity" than with their arrogance. Lord Curzon, who had secured India – that opulent and eminently profitable jewel in the Imperial crown – proclaimed the British sense of humanity without the least irony: "I do not see how Englishmen, contrasting India as it is with what is was or might have been, can fail to see that we came here in obedience to what I call a decree of Providence, for the lasting benefit of millions of the human race."[11] Whether at home or throughout the worldwide Empire it sought to impose, the British ruling class believed that "benevolent despotism is the best of all governments."[12] Of course it was the ruling class itself that defined what was benevolent. And most certainly that benevolence was not to be conferred upon those peoples whom the ruling class had decided were their biological inferiors and whose darker skin marked them forever as dispensable.

In 1803 the British claimed for the Empire the island of Tasmania, off the southern coast of Australia. The Tasmanians were not consulted. By the 1820s, the Tasmanians were driven from their seasonal hunting grounds; often they were hunted on horseback for sport, or captured and used as slaves. Sometimes the children were kept as pets; alternatively, they and their mothers might have their heads bashed to bits on some rocky outcropping while their fathers were tied up and used for target practice.[13]

The Reverend Thomas Atkins, after a visit to Tasmania, declared that it was God's law that "when savage tribes came into collision with civilized races of men, the savages disappeared."[14] Certainly that was the plan of the British government; the Tasmanians were simply in the way and so the entire population of Tasmanian people was to be removed elsewhere. The

Governor, Colonel George Arthur, led a line of twenty-five hundred soldiers and settlers across the island with the intention of flushing the Tasmanians, like game birds, from the countryside and driving them toward the southern peninsula. The operation was unsuccessful. New tactics were required. The government turned to George Robinson, an evangelical missionary, typically uneducated, grim, and dogmatic, and charged him with gathering the Tasmanians. Robinson learned the aboriginal language, made converts, and with their help rounded up group after group and brought them under government control. Eventually, the entire surviving body of Tasmanians was shipped from Hobart harbor to Flinders Island, sixty-five kilometers off Tasmania. The Tasmanians declined to survive. They grew thin, had no children, and drifted into chronic depression. A few years later, they were all dead. In the space of a single generation, British imperialism, gun in one hand, Bible in the other, eradicated an entire people in an act of conscious genocide. There was no outcry. The ideology of the English ruling class mandated that, as the correspondent of the Hobart *Mercury* noted: "the black shall everywhere give place to the white."[15]

The British ruling class imagined that they were, by blood and God's will, the master race: Empire was their destiny; leadership and possession their right. In an uneasy contradiction between a poorly understood Darwinism and an uncontested belief in God's unique favor, imperialist ideology held that the British were the most racially evolved people and that nature itself had somehow contrived with God to place them above an ignorant and benighted world. The ideology of British imperialism was based on the belief that as the Anglo-Saxon people, they had been especially touched by God as his chosen people, and that all other races were inferior to them. The notable index of inferiority was the color of the skin; the darker the skin, the more profound the inferiority. Nordic Europeans were, therefore, superior to Southern Europeans; the Spanish, Portuguese, and Sicilians were considered barely superior to olive-skinned Egyptians or Persians, who in turn were the racial superiors of Indians, Africans, or Malays, who were held to have a slender biological edge over indigenous Australians, Tasmanians, and Dyaks. The whole racial pyramid, with the English at the capstone, was offered as a justification and the primal purpose of Empire; it was always and everywhere instituted through white supremacy and armed force. God had mandated that his creation was to be opened to British exploitation, and at the point of a sword if necessary. As Karl Marx put it so trenchantly: "The profound hypocrisy and inherent barbarism of bourgeois civilization lies unveiled before our eyes, turning from its home, where it assumes respectable forms, to the colonies, where it goes naked."[16]

This naked form of bourgeois civilization in the colonies involved, as we

The Double Pyramid

have seen, racist ideology and institutionalized armed violence. The "respectable" form of barbarism practiced by the bourgeoisie at home was different in kind but not in quality. The "benevolence" and "elevation" pretended to by the imperialists in the colonies, was equally a fraud in the relations between the ruling class and the working class in England. Social oppression and economic exploitation took different forms at home than in the colonies, but they were nevertheless different forms of the same structure. The ruling classes necessary demand for profits – necessary for their own expansion and enrichment – led equally to debasement of the indigenous peoples in the colonies and to the degradation of the English working class.

Massacre and torture in the colonies found its equivalent in "social murder" in the great industrial cities of Britain.[17] The working class was, for the most part, crammed in to slums that lacked sewers, gutters, or even paved streets. Whole families lived in a single room no greater than twelve feet square, where it was dark and damp both day and night. These rooms often had no ventilation; the toilet was a hole in the floor. Whole families would sleep on a sack of feathers or wood chips crawling with vermin. For the privilege of living in these foul quarters, workers paid rents far in excess of their minimal value. These families were sick more often than they were well; starvation and near starvation was their common lot. What meals they took consisted of rotten vegetables and day-old fish. Vast numbers of infants died the day they were born; whole graveyards of children did not see their fifth birthday.

Disease was the common companion of the impoverished. In the worker's neighborhoods, dung heaps, rotten vegetables and animal carcasses were piled between the buildings. Lung diseases, and especially tuberculosis, were epidemic. Typhus and scarlet fever decimated the ranks of the working class. Pale, hungry, hollow-eyed, bones twisted and deformed from malnourishment, the British worker lived a life both short and brutal, and of no consequence whatever to the ruling classes who considered them, in every sense, as disposable as they were replaceable.

And yet it was out of these murderous conditions that the working class began to organize itself. In every slum and in every working district, men and women came together and formed trade unions, taught each other the rudiments of literacy, scribbled fiery manifestoes, and talked to each other about socialism. Debased, dehumanized, but dragging themselves out of the mud in which they had been thrown, the majority of British workers were as far from the eager grasp of the parsons as they were from the social imperatives of the industrial bourgeoisie.

Inevitably the ideology of British imperialism was apprehended and lived differently by different classes under different conditions. Given the class nature of British society, the ruling class found in imperialist ideology a justification for economic expansion and colonial domination; whereas the working class, whose interests lay elsewhere, primarily in the struggle for better wages and working conditions, remained largely unmoved by such justifications. If the ruling class maintained that imperialism's purpose was a "civilizing mission," the working class was more concerned with the uncivilized conditions under which it was forced daily to live. The class struggle in the heartland of British imperialism was of more immediate interest to the British working class than fables about imperialist glory. Nor had it escaped the working class that claims of British biological superiority applied largely to the ruling class itself, and at the workers' own expense. If imperialist ideology promoted the assertion that the British Anglo-Saxon "race" was superior to all other peoples, it simultaneously implied that within the superior British race the ruling class was biologically superior to the working class. There was therefore, and quite obviously, a double hierarchy: a hierarchy of race and a hierarchy of class. If imperialist ideology sanctioned racial subjugation in the colonies, it equally sanctioned class oppression at home.

Central to British imperialism was the claim that the Anglo-Saxon people were in possession of a divine mandate; that God had chosen the British to conquer and to rule. The divine mandate was simultaneously a biological mandate; that is to say, a racial mandate. Thanks to the pseudo-scientific theorizing of Sir Frances Galton and Herbert Spencer, the ruling class was able to maintain that genetic science and Darwinian natural selection had demonstrated the biological superiority of the English people, and that the English ruling class, in turn, was genetically superior to the working class. The divine mandate – an essentially feudal concept – was united with nineteenth century biological science into a powerful ideology of white racism, and justification for imperial rule. This conjuncture of religion and science held its own internal contradiction: certainly there were representatives of religion that suspected that Darwinism, no matter how construed, would explode and destroy religious pretensions and so therefore proclaimed that the divine mandate operated without any biological mediation; just as there were scientists who were moving in the opposite direction and elaborating a worldview that required no role whatsoever for divinity. Even so, as far as imperialist ideology was concerned, the fateful conjunction of the divine mandate with a biological imperative provided a political matrix that guaranteed the necessities of Empire.

History seldom moves in a direct line. Sometimes there are parallel developments; as often, what was born in one place and time jumps to

The Double Pyramid

another and continues along the historical course set by its predecessor. British imperialism has its own internal development, and one can follow its uneasy path into the present without difficulty; there is, after all, no lack of official historians connected to the state through the common bondage of a common education. Nevertheless, there is at the same time a collateral development just as firmly rooted in history and ideology, a legacy of British imperialism denied, dissembled, but nonetheless true and perfectly obvious. To put it quite simply, British imperialism precisely prefigures Nazism.

It is all there, as we have seen. And not merely in a minor key, or in embryo, but in full form. There is no irony, no pretence, in the British imperialists' claim to be the master race and the chosen people. Certainly on one level it is ideology, pure and simple; one can say it is a justificatory discourse aimed as much at themselves as at anyone else, a purely theoretical claim. But it is a theory joined to a practice and we have seen what that practice amounts to. The ideology of the master race is an ideology of Anglo-Saxon superiority, of Aryanism, of the inherent supremacy of the white race before whom all must kneel. Just as in fascism – which arose a mere twenty-five years after Victoria's Diamond Jubilee – the double pyramid of race and class operates as the basic structure of state practice. Significantly, economic expansionism through conquest – and ultimately the ground on which world domination is predicated – is in both cases the self-proclaimed necessity of what the German fascists later referred to as *lebensraum* – living space – which for those already inhabiting this penumbral area means submission or death.[18] We will, perhaps, be criticized here for mistaking means for ends. Surely the means employed by British imperialism, while doubtless unsavory, were aimed at different ends than that of Nazi-fascism; more benevolent ends? Undeniably, there is a unique iniquity in fascism that cannot be minimized. Still, the ends pronounced by British imperialism were more often than not an outright fraud and the ruling classes certainly convinced themselves that what they called "savages" were fit only to be slaves and laborers: when they resisted this definition they were massacred. There was, after all, the divine mandate and the imperatives of biological supremacy to be considered. Nor can we know with certainty what the outcome of nineteenth century British colonialism would have entailed had they been in possession of Zyklon-B instead of bayonets and rifles: in racial subjugation as in industry much depends on technique.

5
Men of Iron, Men of Gold

There is no question: British imperialism understands the class struggle. The dominance of the empire over the colonies is at the same time internally connected to the repression of the working class in England itself: the aspirations of the working class must be suppressed at all costs. The rise of the working class is, after all, as the ruling class understands it, deeply unnatural: it is an affront to the will of God; more important, it is a heresy against history. This ideology, born early on in the nineteenth century, had changed not at all a hundred years later in the 1930s.

For the British ruling class – schooled at Eton, Harrow, or Sandhurst – English political history begins with ancient Greece, just as English religious history begins with ancient Israel. This is a ruling class that imagines itself the heir to the builders of the Acropolis. In the schoolrooms which will give birth to what they believe will be endless generations of imperial masters, the study of ancient Greek has been the basis of all knowledge. The rain-soaked sports fields of the great schools of the ruling class are the sun-drenched olive groves of Olympia. Somewhere, lingering on the borderlands of unconscious desire, these young sons of the ruling class conceive their pale bodies to be the nude heroes of the classical statues their fathers have pillaged for English museums. Flawless, clean-limbed marble bodies, trained in logic and in battle, as disciplined as both the philosophers and athletes of ancient Attica – and by the same stringent methods. What is learned at Eton finds its inexorable expression in statecraft, in scholarship, in science, and in war. The English ruling class, falsely supposing a common heritage with Pericles and Solon, trace their political lineage to Plato. The birthplace of democracy, they never cease to proclaim, is the Academy of Athens.

But what is this democracy? It is a democracy in which the working class plays no part. Or, to be more precise, the part played by working class is to support the ruling class, to provide for the ruling class, to take up arms not for themselves, certainly, but for the benefit of the ruling class. Democracy – construed through a particular reading of Plato – is a private concern of the ruling class alone. The Republic of Plato is a conservative, even totalitarian, democracy. And the English ruling class knows this. It is what they

Men of Iron, Men of Gold

prefer. It is what they assume without question. The English ruling class has read their Plato; they have studied the ancient texts in the ancient language in which it was written. They know that for Plato, and therefore for themselves, there are two kinds of men, immutably: Men of Gold, and Men of Iron.[1]

Virtue, for Plato, is the acceptance of the social status bestowed on men by birth. The Men of Iron are workers. That is who they are, that is who they must be. The Men of Gold are rulers; politics is their privilege. The positions occupied by these two quite different forms of men are unequal. What Plato conceives of as a natural inequality between Men of Iron and Men of Gold is designed to promote the benefit of the state. A virtuous state is based on the recognition of the inherent superiority of the Men of Gold. Justice, insofar as it has any meaning in the Republic, is the maintenance of social stability based on the acceptance of innate inequality and everything that is entailed by such acceptance. The function of the Men of Gold, in their position as educators, as philosophers, is to teach that justice is inequality. The function of Men of Iron, in their position as recipients of justice, is to learn or to die.

The antidemocracy of Plato is the model of the antidemocracy of the British Empire. For the English ruling class democracy is what they say it is. Nothing more. They pride themselves on their democracy; it is an ideological weapon to throw in the face of those who do not consent to its rule. We are a democracy, the ruling class announces, and therefore we can do anything; therefore we have the *right* to do anything. Never mind that this democracy effectively excludes the working class, and consists solely in the jostling for state power among different factions within the ruling class. There are many veils that can be thrown over this particularly naked truth; the obscenity of ruling class democracy must be especially well disguised.

Imperialist democracy was never intended to apply to the working class: The Men of Iron must fend for themselves. The factories that produce the wealth, over which the ruling class will squabble democratically, are intended to be at the same time factories of servitude. Plato's justice of inequality is a lesson to be learned inside the factory gates. Outside, who cares? Let them struggle for whatever scraps of food they can find, let them contest for whatever few feet of shelter may be to hand. It is of no true concern to the ruling class; it has nothing to do with democracy.

Plato has taught the British ruling class what they would practice in any event: that men are not equal; that the Men of Iron should act in complete obedience to the law of the Men of Gold; that it is always wrong to disobey the state; that there is a hierarchy of authority, just as there is a hierarchy of peoples, and it is wrong to disobey it; that the mass of men can be brought to believe anything by the practice of repetition alone.[2] These profound lessons in antidemocracy continue to echo throughout capitalist, imperialist, and fascist circles; when war breaks out across the world in the 1930s, it will be a war against the working class, its institutions and political parties, and against those few states and governments that have begun to throw off the domination of the capitalist class; it will be a war against the future and in the service of the privileges of the past. In this war, the British and the American ruling classes will take the side of Franco, of Mussolini, and of Hitler; only much later, when it is to their benefit, will they turn against them, disowning fascism, their once-favored son, in the name of a democracy in which they have never believed.

6
The Frankenstein Project

The double pyramid, the core of imperialist ideology as it mutated into fascism, was based on a reductionist biology. Men of Iron, Men of Gold, were assigned their places in the social structure by nature: their very genes condemned them to rule or to kneel. But with the upsurge of scientism in the middle of the nineteenth century, the ruling classes began a program whose ultimate aim was the creation of a biologically perfected elite, a supreme white racial caste of world rulers. These new Men of Gold would be bred from the genetic lines of the most aristocratic, most financially dominant, and most Aryan families. For the imperialists and their fascist progeny, humanity would be perfected not by any revolutionary change in the social structure, but by the manipulation of human biology.

The entire purpose of this Frankenstein project was to solidify and make permanent the unequal relations propagated through the ideology of the double pyramid: the white race would endure and prevail, people of color would be driven further into enslavement or exterminated altogether; the ruling class would be raised to perfection, the working class shorn of its most decayed and deficient members and the remainder bred to toil and to serve.

In the middle of the nineteenth century, imperialist England's obsession with breeding began to express itself through the pseudoscience so beloved of its ruling classes — eugenics: the perfecting of the race through the inter-breeding of what they took to be the best biological strains, and the sterilization or murder of the lesser forms. Sir Frances Galton, the originator of eugenics, intended to ensure "the more suitable races or strains of blood a better chance of prevailing speedily over the less suitable." In terms that would, and later did, appeal to Hitler, Galton maintained that all "races" could be ranked, and that black Africans were entirely inferior to Europeans. Wealthy circles in Britain, the United States, Canada, and Germany funneled hundreds of thousands of dollars into the eugenics movement. Institutes were established, scientists recruited. Laws were implemented to prevent the procreation of "inferior families." In the United States, legislation was passed to restrict immigration to largely "Nordic" populations. Hitler, in *Mein Kampf*, wrote admiringly of the US Immigration Restriction

Act with its intended purpose of ranking "races" according to their genetic suitability. Throughout the 1930s, American and Nazi race scientists attended each other's conferences. American scientific journals were open in their praise of the Nazi racial state. Indeed, Nazi legislation on human sterilization was based largely on American laws and practices. Even after the Second World War had begun, American racial scientists continued to visit Nazi Germany in what amounted to nothing short of collaboration.[1]

In the United States, eugenics was extensively financed by the Carnegie Institute, the Rockefeller Foundation, and the Harriman fortune, and eugenic research was carried out at the universities of the wealthy: Harvard, Yale, Princeton, and Stanford. Millions of Americans were tracked through a card system in order to eliminate those belonging to certain bloodlines, and to deport or sterilize thousands of others. Nazi propaganda was imported, funds were sent to Germany to further Hitler's programs, and eugenics journals flourished. In both Germany and the United States, not to mention Great Britain, the ideal genetic strain was said to be blond-haired, blue-eyed, Nordic Aryans; other bloodlines were to be reduced; the "unfit" – the physically weak, and those suffering from mental retardation, mental illness, or carrying one of a number of physical diseases – were to be exterminated. Prominent American eugenicists argued for a network of "lethal chambers" – locally operated gas chambers – to be set up across the country. Although these execution chambers were never implemented in America, they were embraced by the Nazis: the first to be gassed, long before communist political prisoners and Jews, were the "unfit." In America, as in Canada, coercive sterilization was the preferred method. In California alone, sixty thousand men and women were involuntarily sterilized; thousands more in twenty-six other states. Sterilization would also become widespread in Nazi Germany, but it hardly would have been possible if the Rockefeller Foundation had not supplied hundreds of thousands of dollars to German race scientists throughout the 1920s and 1930s.[2] The double pyramid of racial and class superiority, the ideology that justified the genocide of colonized peoples and the oppression of the working class, first developed in imperialist England, reached its natural and logical conclusion in fascism. The elimination of the "unfit," the reduction of surplus members of the working class, the breeding of a new and superior form of the Men of Gold, this was the common program of fascism. In Nazi Germany it led equally to the gas chambers and to the *Lebensborn* project: the removal of blond-haired, blue-eyed children from Eastern Europe to Germany, and the establishment of stud farms where the most Aryan of young German officers were sent to breed with blond slaves. Galton would have been delighted.[3]

The Frankenstein Project

In Spain it was no different. It was the view of the wealthy landowners, the Church, the industrial bourgeoisie, and of Franco's fascist "Nationalists" with whom they conspired, that the working classes – the peasantry and the industrial proletariat – were not only economically, but *racially* inferior to themselves. It was a perfect instance of the double pyramid. According to Gonzalo Aguilera, the fourteenth Count of Alba de Yeltes, a landowner in Salamanca and an officer in Franco's army, the Spanish Civil War was "a race war, not merely a class war. You don't understand because you don't realize that there are two races in Spain – a slave race and a ruler race. . . . It is our duty to put them back in their places – yes, put chains on them again, if you like." The slave race were, in the eyes of the Men of Gold, not merely inferior Men of Iron, but little more than animals. "The Age of Reason indeed!" Aguilera said, "The Rights of Man! Does a pig have rights? The masses aren't fit to reason and to think." The fourteenth Count of Alba de Yeltes was not alone in his opinions; the fascist Governor of Burgos, Marcelino Gavilan Almuzarza, expressed identical sentiments: "We must get rid of all that drivel about the Rights of Man, humanitarianism, philanthropy and other Masonic clichés." Which is precisely what they did. So profoundly did they hold to the position that the peasantry were virtually subhuman that, during the fascist insurrection, "day laborers were slaughtered using the same technique as that employed with cattle."

For the Men of Gold, the working classes were unfit to govern themselves, let alone the State; they would need to be brought to heel. The methods were obvious: "We must restore the authority of the Church. Slaves need it to teach them how to behave. . . . In our state, people are going to have the liberty to keep their mouths shut." Repression for those allowed to survive and to work like slaves; for the rest, for the troublemakers, or for those who were foolish enough to think that they were neither pigs nor cattle, it would be extermination. "It's our program," Aguilera said, "to exterminate a third of the male population of Spain. That will clean up the country and rid us of the proletariat. It's sound economically, too. Never have any more unemployment in Spain, you understand." Captain Ignacio Rosales, a millionaire from Barcelona, was equally convinced that the proletariat had been infected by a quasi-biological strain of egalitarian ideas: "Of this taint in her bloodstream Spain must cleanse herself. She is purifying herself and will rise up from this trial new and strong. The streets of Madrid will run red with blood, but after – after – there will be no unemployment problem."

For Aguilera, the central problem was that, like animals, the working class was multiplying too fast. They would need to be culled by plague and disease, God's favored method. The Men of Gold had been too generous;

they had provided plumbing to the workers, and just as pigs should be shorn of the Rights of Man, the workers ought also to be deprived of plumbing. It was perfectly clear: "Sewers caused all our troubles. The masses in this country . . . are slave stock. They are good for nothing but slaves and only when they are used as slaves are they happy. But we, the decent people, made the mistake of giving them modern housing in the cities where we have our factories. We put sewers in these cities, sewers which extend right down to the workers' quarters. Not content with the work of God, we thus interfere with His Will. The result is that the slave stock increases. Had we no sewers in Madrid, Barcelona, Bilbao, all these Red leaders would have died in their infancy instead of exciting the rabble and causing good Spanish blood to flow. When the war is over we should destroy the sewers. The perfect birth control for Spain is the birth control God intended us to have. Sewers are a luxury to be reserved for those who deserve them, the leaders of Spain, not the slave stock."[4]

In the Anglo-American world: sterilization and the breeding of perfected bloodlines; Germany followed suit and added the gas chamber. For Spain the same results were planned through mass murder and the hand of God.

The secret of fascism is the collapse into the organic: this is its utopian moment. The New Man is to be developed through genetics, through racial breeding, through the creation of a new biology. Hence the biological determinism of fascism, its double hierarchy of race and class, its utterly insane biological experiments. But the ultimate purpose of this Frankenstein project is precisely nothing: it is an end in itself. Its function is the rule of the world in order to eliminate any possibility of disruption of the biological plan. Its program can be nothing but extermination in the service of inertia.

7
Imperialism Prefers Fascism

Fascism was much admired by the ruling classes of all the Western imperialist countries throughout the 1930s. With the bottom falling out of capitalism, the wealthy industrialists, financiers, and their government representatives, feared that the impoverished working class would rise up under the leadership of the Communists and assert its strength. Ruling circles in the Canadian state viewed with admiration the tactics of Mussolini and Hitler: their ability to control the working class with an efficient combination of propaganda and police repression. And they were determined to fully apply those lessons in Canada.

Prime Minister R. B. Bennett – whose authoritarian maneuvers and anti-working class policies certainly rivaled those of Mussolini – possessed a particularly vicious hatred of socialism and of the Communist Party. He made it known that he was prepared to crush the Communists under "the iron heel of ruthlessness."[1] During the five years of Bennett's reign, from 1930 to 1935, no less than twenty-eight thousand Communists, radicals, or those simply suspected of *becoming* radicals, were deported; usually secretly and without benefit of appeal. Bennett's government made every effort to hide the political purpose of such deportations. It was sufficient to claim that Communists and others had been charged with "unlawful assembly" or even "vagrancy." Those who had been detained in Canada as Communists and deported to Germany or central Europe were almost certain to be arrested by the Nazis and tortured to death in concentration camps – a chain of events of which the Bennett government was certainly well aware.[2]

Despite being a legal political party, Communist party members were denied almost every access to the machinery of elections. The party's offices were raided, furniture smashed, files stolen. In 1931, Bennett's government – replicating the practice of Mussolini, and later of Hitler – had the leadership of the Communist Party arrested and thrown into prison on the fraudulent charge of "seditious conspiracy." In doing so, Canada became the first of the Western imperialist powers to outlaw Communist organizations and to declare their property subject to state confiscation.[3]

In 1930 Bennett funneled some $18,000 to Adrien Arcand, an

outspoken Canadian Nazi, whose National Social Christian Party adopted the swastika as its emblem; in 1936 he donated a further $27,000 – significant funds in Depression-era dollars.[4] When Arcand's printing plant was destroyed by antifascists Bennett equipped him with new facilities, and later hired him as publicity director of his election campaign in Quebec.[5]

The fascist impulse did not manifest itself solely with Bennett and his Conservative Party, but was equally evident with his successor, the Liberal Prime Minister Mackenzie King. In 1937 the German Unity League – an umbrella group funded by the German government for Nazi organizations in Canada – held a mass meeting in Kitchener, Ontario. They requested the presence of the federal Minister of Trade and Commerce, William Euler, who was delighted to speak to the Nazi audience. He told the crowd that he was displeased with newspaper stories critical of Hitler's government, and thought that printing such stories ought to be made a criminal offence.[6] A year later, Mackenzie King, as Prime Minister of Canada, invited Erich Windels, the Nazi government's consul general in Ottawa, to an evening of entertainment at his house. According to the Prime Minister they all had "a most enjoyable evening." King was happy to have raised the spirits of Windels since, as he put it, the Nazis "had felt lonely and depressed at times." King found Windels to be pleasant company, and before the night was out they were cheerily singing songs together around the piano.[7]

Four years after the elections that brought Hitler to power, Mackenzie King visited the Nazi dictator and traveled across Germany. After an hour-long interview, King wrote that Hitler:

> smiled very pleasantly and indeed had a sort of appealing and affectionate look in his eyes, . . . really one who truly loves his fellow men and his country, and would make any sacrifice for their good. That he feels himself to be a deliverer of his people from tyranny.... His face is much more prepossessing than his pictures would give the impression of. It is not that of a fiery over-strained nature, but of a calm, passive man, deeply and thoughtfully in earnest...; his eyes impressed me most of all. There was a liquid quality about them which indicates keen perception and profound sympathy.[8]

After spending an afternoon with the Hitler Youth and an evening at the opera with a member of Hermann Goering's staff, King enthused, "There was a splendid order and efficiency about everything I saw." At the end of his visit, King gushed like a schoolgirl in his diary: "I can honestly say it was as enjoyable, informative and ever inspiring as any visit I have had anywhere."[9] While King was falling in love with the Nazi state and its

Imperialism Prefers Fascism

leadership, the Gestapo torturers were busy in their prisons, the concentration camps were filling up with Communists, socialists, Jews. Antisemitic legislation, and laws against all "non-Aryans" had been in place since 1933. Antisemitic posters, and the foul racial propaganda of *Der Sturmer* were displayed in almost every town and village. Mass public book-burnings were already four years past. The institutionalized brutality, and the killing, were already well underway. About this, King had nothing to say.

With the Nazi regime in Germany becoming ever more bloody and vicious, and its official propaganda making it clear that all "non-Aryans" were to be eliminated, the Jews of Europe sought refuge in Canada. But the Canadian state took steps to ensure that no Jews would be allowed entry. At the beginning of 1938, Jews were required to have at least five thousand dollars to enter Canada; by the end of the year the official figure had risen to twenty thousand: in practice, no amount of capital was sufficient. The consensus of the Mackenzie King government was that there would be no Jewish immigration, proclaiming notoriously that, "none was too many."[10] While the great majority of Europe's Jews were actively prevented from escaping fascism, and were all too soon to be murdered in the Nazi extermination camps, Mackenzie King wrote in his diary: "I believe the world will yet come to see a very great man – mystic in Hitler [who] will rank some day with Joan of Arc among the deliverers of his people."[11]

Canada, Britain, the United States: significant sectors of the ruling classes of all the Western powers looked toward fascism with approval, indeed even with enthusiasm.

Winston Churchill, a rabid anti-Communist who had tried to "strangle at its birth" the Soviet workers state,[12] was full of praise for fascism. In Rome, in 1927, he congratulated the fascists on their "triumphant struggle against the bestial appetites and passions of Leninism," maintaining that they had "rendered a service to the whole world." "Italy," he said, "has shown that there is a way of fighting the subversive forces," and that, "hereafter no great nation will go unprovided with an ultimate means of protection against the cancerous growth of Bolshevism."[13] This was no momentary lapse. Churchill's speeches throughout the 1930s were saturated with fascist ideals: "Elections" were to be "regarded as a misfortune" and an "inconvenience"; as in Nazi Germany, concentration camps, which Churchill termed "labour colonies," were to be established in Britain for insurgent workers.[14] Churchill not only approved of fascism's policy of crushing the working class, but was as thoroughly racist as either Mussolini or Hitler. As Secretary of State at the War Office, in 1919, two years after he had arranged an unprovoked aggression into Soviet Russia, he authorized the use of chemical weapons against the Kurdish population of Iraq. "I do not," he said, "understand this squeamishness about the use of gas . . . I am strongly in favor of using poisoned gas against uncivilized tribes to spread a lively terror."[15] At the Peel Commission of Inquiry, in 1937, he said:

> I do not agree that the dog in a manger has the final right to the manger even though he may have lain there for a very long time. I do not admit that right. I do not admit, for instance, that a great wrong has been done to the Red Indians of America or the black people of Australia. I do not admit that a wrong has been done to these people by the fact that a stronger race, a higher-grade race has come in and taken their place.[16]

Indeed, why would he? The Men of Gold apologize for nothing. Dogs in mangers, pigs, cattle; these zoological epithets express precisely how the lords of wealth view those whom they seek to exploit.

So attuned was British policy with fascism that, before invading Ethiopia in 1935, Mussolini asked Ramsay MacDonald, then Prime Minister of England, what Britain thought of this plan. Ludicrously, even somewhat insanely when it is considered what was at stake, MacDonald replied: "England is a lady. A lady's taste is for vigorous action by the male, but she likes things done discreetly – not in public. So be tactful and we shall have no objection."[17] A few months later, fascist Italy slaughtered Ethiopians in genocidal numbers. A ruthless bombing campaign was followed by the use of poison mustard gas in contravention of the 1926 Geneva Convention. The British government knew of these chemical attacks – they were openly reported in the newspapers – but it chose to remain silent. As many as three-quarters of a million Ethiopians were murdered during Italy's war of aggression and the succeeding five years of occupation. But MacDonald's open support for fascist genocide should not be surprising. The imperialist and colonialist powers, and England above all, held people of color in open contempt. Former Prime Minister Lloyd George, speaking in the House of Commons the year before MacDonald appeared in bonnet and crinolines before Il Duce, insisted "on the right to bomb niggers."[18] The racism engendered by British imperialism was in no contradiction with the racist practices of fascism. Ten months following Mussolini's invasion of Ethiopia, Franco and his fascist allies attacked the democratic government of Spain. Tact was apparently no longer an issue.

Hitler had hoped for some years to form an Aryan alliance of Britain and Germany; he had found support not only from Prime Minister Ramsay MacDonald, but from King Edward VIII himself.[19] Indeed, the King referred to such a union as "an urgent necessity," and assured Hitler that he would never interfere with his plans "re Jews or anything else."[20] As international events unfolded, however, it became necessary for the British elite to remove Edward. The cover story, invented for public consumption, was that the King was abdicating his throne out of love for Wallis Simpson whom he could not marry because of her status as a divorcée. Even after his abdication, and open war had begun, Edward knowingly disclosed to the Nazi government Allied plans relating to Hitler's potential invasion of Belgium.[21]

The situation was no different in the United States. The wealthy ruling circles, and the mass media they controlled, were as enthusiastic about fascism as were the British. According to Sumner Welles, an Assistant Secretary of State in the US government: "Business interests in every one of the democracies of Western Europe and of the New World welcomed Hitlerism . . . They saw in it an assurance that order and authority in Germany would safeguard big business interests there."[22]

Nor were American business interests content to see fascism established only in Europe. William E. Dodd, US Ambassador to Germany in the 1930s noted: "A clique of US industrialists is hell-bent to bring a fascist state to supplant our democratic government and is working closely with the fascist regimes in Germany and Italy. I have had plenty of opportunity in my post in Berlin to witness how close some of our American ruling families are to the Nazi regime.... A prominent executive of one of the largest financial corporations, told me point blank that he would be ready to take definite action to bring fascism into America."[23]

Throughout the period of Hitler's consolidation of power, the news media of the ruling classes openly called for fascism. An editorial in the *Nation's Business*, the magazine of the US Chamber of Commerce, declared: "Many thoughtful people believe that our form of government must be changed to something resembling the fascist form;" and that "Many big businessmen think well of fascism and secretly hope for it."[24] The *New York Herald* was even more expansive:

The hour has struck for a fascist party to be born in the United States. Someone will give the signal. It may be the clean youth and imagination of a Charles Lindbergh calling upon men of good will to join him in a party of law and order. It may be the sagacity and experience of a Henry Ford summoning men to match the organization of the underworld with a more potent organization. In every part of the country, men are waiting for that call.[25]

How the Men of Gold admired Hitler! He would crush the working class, destroy socialism, and make the world safe for profit.

But the American financial and industrial elite did more than merely admire fascism; they actively supported Mussolini and Hitler. The Chase Bank, IBM, International Telephone and Telegraph (ITT), General Motors, the Ford Motor Company, Standard Oil, DuPont, the Texas Oil Company, and many other corporate powers, were fully complicit in Nazism; their history is now well known.

Standard Oil of New Jersey not only shipped fuel to the Nazis, they supplied them with tetraethyl lead, a necessary additive in aviation gasoline, furnished oil to Italian and German vessels through Central and South America, and in Nicaragua served the fascist cause by distributing pro-Nazi propaganda. ITT engaged in improving Hitler's communications systems, and built parts for the aircraft that bombed British and American ground troops. The Texas Oil Company fueled German U-boats, sent financial aid to Nazi corporations operating out of South America, and provided its Nazi friends with plans to American navy yards and army forts. DuPont helped finance the Nazi Party through its business dealings with Opel Motors and the I.G. Farben chemical plants.[26] Indeed, Irénée DuPont – in a moment of Frankensteinian euphoria – called in a speech to the American Chemical Society on 7 September 1926, for the creation of a master race of supermen to be brought about by the injection of certain special drugs into young white boys.[27]

General Motors, through its German subsidiary, produced trucks, bombers, and torpedoes, and funneled thirty million dollars into I. G. Farben factories. The Ford Motor Company provided military trucks, armored cars, and tires to the Nazis.[28] Henry Ford had admired Hitler from the first; he was a vocal antisemite, and used his newspaper, the *Dearborn Independent* – distributed nationally through Ford automobile dealerships – to publish *The International Jew*: an on-going series of antisemitic diatribes much loved by Hitler; he had stacks of the book-length edition of the text on a table outside his office.[29] Ford in turn, sent substantial funds to finance the Third Reich. In 1938 the Nazi government awarded Ford the Grand Cross of the Supreme Order of the German Eagle, a swastika-emblazoned decoration created by Hitler as the highest honor to be bestowed on a distinguished foreigner.[30]

For many in the ruling circles of the Anglo-American world the eventual war against Hitler, Mussolini, and Hirohito was never an anti-fascist war; it was and remained a war of inter-imperialist rivalry. These circles that – scant years before – were conspiring to support and expand fascism, underwent no fundamental change of opinion when war broke out. It was only the struggle of the Soviet Union against fascism, the armed resistance of Communist-led partisans throughout Europe, and the anti-fascist sentiment of a great many working class men and women across the world – those, in fact, who did the actual fighting – that gave the war its final and redeeming anti-fascist character.

8

The Butchers' Revolt

The Spanish people had had enough of being treated like pigs and cattle. In 1931, their country was still enmired in medievalism. The working classes had begun to demand change, but under the general and all-pervasive repression of the oligarchy they possessed no access to power. The middle class, facing financial difficulties with the deepening of the Depression, required a new form of regime. Zamora, their political representative, formed a Liberal-Republican coalition; Largo Caballero, representing the Socialist Party, joined with Zamora. The monarchy, in the person of Alfonso XIII, was convinced to leave Spain, never to return, and a republic was established. It did not last long. The republic was opposed by the four ruling circles that had supported the monarchy: the wealthy landowners, the industrial bourgeoisie, the Catholic Church, and the army.[1]

Ineffective, reformist, and everywhere opposed by the ruling circles, the liberal republic tottered and fell, and was replaced by the reactionary right-wing government of Alexandre Lerroux and Gil Robles in 1934 and 1935. Gil Robles, leader of the Clerical Party of Catholic Action ruled on behalf of the Catholic Church, an enormously wealthy institution that sat like a giant bloated spider feeding on the body of Spain. "Our need," he announced, "is for complete power. Democracy for us is not an end in itself, but the medium to launch us in conquest of a new state. The moment is coming. The Parliament will either submit, or we will see that it disappears!"[2] What little progress had been achieved was reversed; the minor reforms instituted by the Zamora government were rescinded. But it was obvious to all that the Spanish working people had begun to rise, to organize themselves as a class, and would not be restrained for much longer. Gil Robles opened negotiations with Mussolini who promised to supply the government with funds, soldiers, military equipment, and airplanes should they be required.[3] German Nazis were permitted complete liberty to establish dozens of *Landesgruppe*, centers of the NSDAP-AO – the German Nazi Party "foreign organization" – throughout Spain, whose purpose was to insert German propaganda in the press, circulate Nazi films, engage in espionage, make contact with the Spanish army generals and recruit agents from among the officer class. Spanish reactionaries were sent to be trained in

The Butchers' Revolt   **73**

Germany, and Gil Robles personally attended the first Nazi Congress in Nuremberg.[4]

The overt and violent repression instituted by the Lerroux–Gil Robles government – the murders, the assassinations, the mass slaughter of striking miners in Asturias, the increasing support for fascism – led to the rapid growth of the opposition: the left-wing of the Socialist Party and the Communist Party of Spain whose influence was rising throughout the trade unions, the peasant cooperatives, the intellectuals, and the youth. On 2 June 1935, the Communist Party proposed the formation of a Popular Front of all left, progressive, and liberal forces.[5] While the leadership of the other parties were at first cautious, the working class itself, both peasants and industrial workers, was enthusiastic. Popular Front committees sprang up across the country. By the end of the year there was open cooperation between virtually every political party from the center to the left. Gil Robles, Lerroux, and the Right were losing control; internal quarrels and financial scandals brought down their government. New elections were called for 16 February 1936, and an interim prime minister, Portela Valladares, installed. In mid-January the Popular Front pact was signed: by mutual agreement of all, only the various liberal Republican parties – the Left Republicans headed by Azaña, the Republican Union, and the Catalan Esquerra – would form the government, while elected Socialist and Communist deputies would support the government's minimum program for social change. Meanwhile, General Franco and the fascist Falange were already plotting a coup, in conjunction with Nazi Germany and Fascist Italy, to take over the country and proclaim a "Nationalist" state.

On 16 February the people brought democracy and the Popular Front to power. The road to victory was absolute unity of the Left. But the Right was not about to countenance anything so dangerous as democracy. At four in the morning, the day after the elections, Gil Robles went to Valladares offering full support of the Right should he wish to assume dictatorial power; at seven o'clock General Franco made him the same offer; at noon, a fascist assault squad opened fire on a demonstration of women marching through Madrid.[6] The Communists and the Left-Socialists understood that a full-scale fascist rebellion was imminent; the Republican parties did not. The fascist general José Sanjurjo flew to Berlin. Germany and Italy prepared the destruction of Spain.

From every church the Catholic priesthood inveighed against the Popular Front; they loathed and hated a government that was committed to the re-distribution of land, the workers' right to strike, the right of divorce, and especially secular education and the separation of church and state. They supported fascism from its inception, while always posing as a victim of persecution. Its hierarchy drove around the streets in limousines while peasants starved. The Church owned vast tracts of land, factories, power plants, hotels, and department stores: their wealth was endless, their power oppressive. During the war they invented endless tales of the mass rape of nuns. But the truth was otherwise: when the fascist army invaded a village, it was the Catholic priest who gave them a list of Republicans, or Communists, or trade unionists, or simply villagers who refused to go to church. It was the priests who would wave flashlights in the dark to direct the fascist bombers to their targets. Throughout the war, the Vatican supplied Franco's fascist and Falangist butchers with nearly two million lire a day.[7]

With the inevitably of a fascist revolt daily more likely, the working people filled the ranks of the left parties. The Communist Party had thirty thousand members in February; by July there were over a hundred thousand. In April, Socialist Youth, an organ of the Socialist Party, merged their two hundred thousand members with the fifty thousand of the Communist Youth. Within the Socialist Party, the majority of its members sided with its own left-wing, the leadership of Largo Caballero, and later his successor, Juan Negrín. It would be these two Parties, working primarily outside the government but in full support of it, which would form the true resistance to fascism. The parties of the left, despite their now massive size, refused to take over the government: their commitment to the political necessity of the Popular Front was total. For the Communists, the Popular Front constituted a new terrain which — if and when fascism was defeated — would lead to a new form of popular democracy, a form in which new institutions would emerge; a new situation in which the progressive unification of all the popular forces would lead to a new and democratic socialism. The left forces, now united, consistently offered their resources to President Azaña to halt the growth of fascism, but the government refused, just as it ignored the warnings of the major labor unions. Instead of organizing the people to resist, the Republican leadership allowed, through inaction and false confidence, the fascist menace to develop. The financial bourgeoisie, backing Franco, exported capital; wealthy landowners burnt crops; fascist gangs bombed Socialist meetings, machine-gunned newspaper editors, attempted to assassinate both Azaña and Caballero. Within the army, officers posted notices in the barracks claiming, falsely, that law and order no longer existed in Spain. The menace was real. Through constant political and economic disruptions the fascists attempted to build popular discord and to justify their planned insurrection. But the people remained loyal to the Popular Front: they could not be moved in their support for a people's democracy.

In July 1936 the coup that the ruling class had been preparing for many

The Butchers' Revolt

months was approaching zero hour. Plans had been made to imprison and execute the leaders of all political parties and trade unions in the first days of the revolt. Contact and secure communication lines were opened between Army Generals, Monarchists, the Falangist leaders and other ranking members of the conspiracy. Military maneuvers had been agreed upon. A state of war would be proclaimed; there would be simultaneous military risings throughout the country; four columns would converge on Madrid. General Franco was at camp in the Canary Islands, west of Spanish Morocco, ready to move.

On 11 July a British plane left England from Croydon airport. On board were the pilot, Captain Bebb; Luis Bolin, a fascist plotter; and Major Hugh Pollard of the British secret service. It landed in Lisbon so Bolin could meet with Sanjurjo, and then flew on to the Canary Islands: its mission to transport Franco to Morocco so that the revolt could begin.[8]

At 6:30 on the morning of 17 July, an agent of the rebel plotters entered the telegraph office in Bayonnes, France, and sent a series of coded telegrams: the signal for the fascist insurrection across Spain to rise.[9]

The fascist revolt broke out, as meticulously planned, in every province of the country. Not surprisingly, it was not received without resistance. Thousands of people poured into the streets of every major city in Spain, declaring their loyalty to the Republican government and begging it to give them arms. In Madrid, a delegation of the left went to the prime minister with a single message: arm the people. But the government, in a foolish and naïve attempt to quell the revolt, offered a representative of the insurgent Generals the post of Minister of War, with two other cabinet posts reserved for his collaborators. The fascists refused; there was to be no compromise. The government, belatedly, issued an order to the governors of every district to distribute arms to the people, to the unions, and to the workers' organizations.

But it was too late. The fascist revolt was already well under way. In the south – in Seville, Cadiz, Cordoba, Granada – the army declared war against its own people. But with what few weapons they had, the Communists, the Socialists, and the trade unionists formed into militias, threw up barricades, and declared a general strike. They were joined by the remnants of the army that had remained loyal to government. In Seville, terribly outnumbered, the working class fought and held out for two days. And then the fascist reinforcements arrived through the port of Cadiz – Franco's Foreign Legion and the Moorish *Regulares* from Morocco. By 25 July, Seville was taken. There were thousands of dead and the workers' militia resistance was massacred. The bodies of men, women, and children were heaped in great piles, arms and legs entangled; there were nine thousand dead. In every city and every town across the south the situation repeated itself. The working people, organizing into militias, threw up barricades and defended the Republic; they held back the fascists as long as they could. Thousands were shot, thousands died. In Granada, five thousand were murdered and their corpses thrown into the ravines of Viznar. General Queipo de Llano took to the radio; his message to those who would resist: "We will kill you like dogs!"[10] But the people did resist. In Malaga, Almeria, Huelva, and Jaen, the militias and loyal factions of the army held firm. But the first major defeat of the fascist coup was not on land, but at sea. The officers of the Spanish fleet stood with Franco. But the sailors were socialists and republicans. In almost every cruiser, battleship, and submarine, the sailors defended the Republic through organized mutiny: they arrested their officers and made for safe harbor.

In the eight days since the beginning of the rebellion, the fascists encountered armed resistance everywhere, except Navarre – and even there they shot seven thousand. Every union, every political party of the left, had formed their own armed militias. In the Basque provinces, the fascist revolt was contained and then defeated. In Asturias and Galicia the workers mounted a magnificent defense but were slaughtered by the thousands. But in Madrid, in an action of heroic proportions, the people's militias, armed by loyal military forces, fought and defeated the fascists; they encircled the rebel barracks, stormed them, and overwhelmed the occupants. The rebellion in the capital was forcefully eliminated. With arms won from the defeated garrisons, the people's militias pushed back fascist troops at Guadalajara, and in organized units defended the Sierras to the south. And as in Madrid, the entire people of Barcelona, of every political grouping, rose against the fascist revolt and brought it down. For eight days the Spanish people – workers and peasants, Communists, Socialists, Anarchists, Republicans – stood united in defense of their government, of the Popular Front, of democracy, of freedom itself, and they defeated fascism. On the night of 18 July, Dolores Ibarruri – the Communist deputy known everywhere as La Pasionaria – had given the cry of combat from Radio Madrid: *No Pasaran! They Shall Not Pass!* The people had taken up the slogan, they had fought by it, and, for the moment, they had won by it.

After eight days, despite a campaign of ferocious slaughter and unparalleled sadism, the fascists controlled only the colony of Morocco, sections of southern Andalucia, and the northern regions of Navarre, Leon, and Galicia. The capital, and the major industrial, political, economic, and cultural centers remained under Republican control, and these were the areas where the organized working class was most powerful; the areas controlled by the fascists were primarily agricultural and under the

The Butchers' Revolt

strongest domination of the wealthy landowners and the Catholic church. And while it was true that the government had largely lost the army, the air force remained loyal, as did the fleet. Perhaps even more importantly, the Republic was defended by the overwhelming majority of the people and their newly formed militias. There was no doubt that within a few months – perhaps even a few weeks – the zones dominated by the fascists could have been liberated and Spain re-unified.

But Franco had already prepared for the possibility that the original *coup d'etat* would not be entirely successful. He had friends he could turn to: the fascist revolt had been organized in conjunction with Berlin and Rome. On 22 July, Nazi agents in Spanish Morocco flew to Berlin, with Franco's representative, bearing a letter for Hitler: air transport was required. Hitler responded; gigantic JU 52s were dispatched. Simultaneous representation was made to Mussolini; squadrons of bombers were flown into position. German bombers soon followed. Within a week, bombs were landing all over Spain. Fighter planes arrived, and with them anti-aircraft guns, battleships, destroyers. It was no longer a question of Spanish fascists, cloaked under the name of "Nationalists," in revolt against the legitimate Republican government. In short, it was no longer a "Civil War," if indeed it ever had been. After the first brief eight days the war in Spain was an international aggression, a combined Falangist–German–Italian attack on a sovereign state. To refer to the events in Spain from 1936 to 1939 as the "Spanish Civil War" is to obfuscate its true nature. Elements of the Spanish oligarchy had collaborated with international Nazi-Fascism to transform Spain into a fascist state. Two post-war letters from Franco to Hitler make the issue entirely clear: Franco to Hitler 22 September 1940: "I reply with the assurance of my unchangeable and sincere adherence to you personally, to the German people, and to the cause for which you fight. I hope, in defense of this cause, to be able to renew the old bonds of comradeship between our armies." Franco to Hitler 26 February 1941:

> I consider as you do that the destiny of history has united you with myself and with the Duce in an indissoluble way. . . . You must have no doubt about my absolute loyalty to this political concept, and to the realization of the union of our national destinies with those of Germany and Italy . . . I need no confirmation of my faith in the triumph of your cause, and I repeat that I shall always be a loyal follower of it.[11]

So loyal, in fact that in the same year Franco had a list created of the names and addresses of every Jew in the country and handed it to Heinrich Himmler so that they might be deported and exterminated.[12]

By October 1936, four months after the inception of Franco's revolt, armed intervention in Spain reached massive proportions. Nazi units of the crack Condor Legion arrived with two hundred and fifty aircraft, one hundred bombers, and a hundred and fifty fighters; six hundred and fifty other aircraft were supplied, as well as two hundred tanks, and seven hundred units of heavy artillery. Rome supplied one thousand tanks, one thousand aircraft, seventeen thousand bombs, two submarines, four destroyers, and a quarter of a million rifles. One hundred and fifty thousand Italian fascist soldiers and fifty thousand German Nazi troops fought on Spanish soil. The Portuguese dictator, Salazar, offered his airfields to the Germans and Italians, and supplied twenty thousand ground troops to Franco. As Benito Mussolini was later to say, "The great unity of the Axis includes Nazis, Fascists, and Spanish Falangistas. There is no longer any distinction between Fascism, Nazism, and Falangismo."[13]

It was impossible for democratic Spain to survive. It is to the immense credit of the Popular Front, of the elected Republican government, and of the Spanish people, that they were able to resist the fascist assault as long as they did. For three years and more they fought back. At the very center of the resistance were the Spanish Communists. As early as July they formed the famous Fifth Regiment; about half its members were Communists, the others Socialists, liberal republicans, and antifascists with no political affiliation. The Fifth Regiment – led by Vittorio Vidali, using the *nom de guerre*, "Carlos Contreras" – was the most disciplined, organized, and effective fighting force at every front. They strove to unify the various militias springing up around the country, each from their own labor union or political group. In the spring of 1937, when the militias and other armed groupings were finally unified into the Army of the Republic, the Fifth Regiment was at its core. And yet it was obvious that with the combined might of Nazi Germany and Fascist Italy bearing down upon it, the Republic would be drowned in its own blood unless it could purchase arms outside its own borders, as every legitimate government everywhere had always been permitted to do. When it made that necessary request, the imperialist powers conspired to refuse it.

9

Imperialist Betrayal

At the very outbreak of the fascist assault, the governments of Great Britain, the United States, France, and Canada declared a policy of neutrality – of "non-intervention" – and placed an embargo on any weapons sales to Spain. But their neutrality was a pretence. Covertly they supported Franco: a fascist defeat of democratic Spain would provide an exemplary lesson to the increasingly restive working class at home. The Men of Gold would never countenance a government of the Men of Iron. The firestorm of brutality that was unleashed against the elected Spanish government eventually cost at least a million lives, and the blood of the dead rested as much in the hands of the Western imperialist powers as it did in the hands of Franco.

The position of the British government was resolutely on the side of fascist aggression, as the statements of its leadership made exquisitely clear. As Sir Anthony Eden, head of the Foreign Office put it: "Britain prefers a rebel victory to a Republican victory." Chatfield, the First Lord of the British Admiralty, echoed the statement, saying: "Franco is a great patriot." Sir Henry Chilton, the British ambassador to Spain, made the matter entirely explicit: "I am awaiting the time when they finally send enough German planes to finish the war."[1] Not content with mere posturing, Britain had actively collaborated with the fascists from the beginning: Captain Bebb's flight was mere prelude. In mid-August, Franco's Air Minister, Kindelan, paid a visit to the authorities in British Gibraltar: a peculiar mission since, at least officially, the British government recognized only the elected Republic. Immediately afterward, a British warship, the *Queen Elizabeth*, sailed into the fascist held harbor of Algeciras, near Cadiz, quite deliberately preventing the loyal Republican fleet from shelling the port. Gibraltar, too, was a convenient location for the British to supply Franco with needed ammunition.[2] Significantly, the British fleet helped Franco transfer troops from Morocco to the Spanish mainland, not only encouraging the revolt but aiding in its implementation. Later they block-aded much of the Spanish coast. They sold the fascists aircraft and other munitions by funneling them through Portugal.[3] And in mid-October 1936, according to a report of the Nazi *chargé d'affaires* in Spain, a British naval commander had supplied the Nazis with information on Russian arms shipments which, he wrote, they "certainly would not do without instructions."[4] Instructions, that is to say, from the highest echelons of the British government.

The United States, officially neutral, was no less eager than the British government to encourage a fascist victory. Within hours of the Franco uprising, Standard Oil was ordering five of its tankers to sail to a port occupied by the fascists and to unload their gasoline. On 23 July 1936, a mere five days after the Nationalist uprising, the US Secretary of State gave orders to desist from fuelling any ships of the Republican navy. Throughout the rebellion, US companies supplied Franco's allies with motor oil and aviation gasoline: the Nazi German and Italian Fascist warplanes that bombed and strafed the Spanish people were powered by American fuel. The Nazi planes that leveled Guernica with incendiary bombs, and that mowed down hundreds of defenseless refugees on the road from Malaga, were powered by American gasoline. Almost two million metric tonnes of fuel were delivered to Franco, much of it by the Texaco corporation alone. At the same time, General Motors, Ford, and Studebaker sold twelve thousand trucks to Franco's Nationalists – more than three times the number of trucks delivered by Germany and Italy combined; neither gasoline nor trucks were sold to the legitimate Republican government. At least sixty thousand airplane bombs were sold by the United States to Nazi Germany in 1938 with the tacit understanding that they would be transferred for use in Spain.[5] Neutrality was a farce, non-intervention a façade behind which the leading financial circles of the imperialist powers sought to ensure that fascism would destroy popular democratic power in Spain. The four horsemen of oppression that trampled Spain – the industrial bourgeoisie, the wealthy landowners, the church, and the army – had stables throughout the western world. Politically, the imperialist powers intended to cement an unofficial pact with Germany; to convince the Nazis that they bore them no ill will, and that they would not stand in their way in a war against the Soviet Union and against socialism in whatever form it might take no matter how popular.

Less than a week after the telegraph office had broadcast the coded message to the insurgent fascist generals, the British were determined to give them a free hand. They put pressure on the French government to deny arms shipments to the legitimate government, and set about assembling the "Non-Intervention" Committee: its entire purpose was to bring about the destruction of the Popular Front and hand Spain to Franco. As the English Liberal, Lloyd George, remarked: "If Democracy is defeated in this battle; if Fascism is triumphant, His Majesty's Government can claim the victory for themselves."[6] In order to deny other nations the right to provide arms to the Republic, it was necessary for the Committee to pretend that Germany and Italy were not actively intervening on Spanish soil. Britain, of course, knew absolutely and without question what was going on; they had spies everywhere: not that they needed them; they had only to open any newspaper printed in London. But the hypocrisy of the British government was unbounded. Repeatedly they announced through the Committee that: "*no proof exists of Italo-German violation.*"[7] If England had chosen to play the role of the discreet milady, fanning her painted cheeks while Mussolini committed genocide in Ethiopia, she had no role left to play now other than whore to Franco.

Throughout August, September, and October 1936, the Soviet Union brought to the Committee's attention what they already knew: Germany, Italy, and Portugal were systematically violating the non-intervention accord. The British, of course, chose to deny every evidence. In Spain, Franco was advancing with four columns to the very doorways of Madrid, with Nazi bombers leading the way. On 6 October, and again on the 12th, the 23rd, and the 28th, the Soviets demanded that the Committee recognize the obvious. The Committee refused. The Soviets then made their position clear: that since Germany and Italy had so obviously flouted the Committee's accords, they no longer considered themselves bound by the fraudulent principle of non-intervention. They were correct to do so. No evidence would ever satisfy the British. Indeed, as late as the summer of 1937, when a German warship bombed the defenseless civilians of Malaga in front of the whole world; and Mussolini published the names of the ten generals who had led the Italian army on Santander, the British still announced that there was *no proof whatever* of foreign intervention on the side of Franco.[8]

True to their word, the Soviet Union began to arm the Spanish Republic: much to their honor, outside of a minor, but heartfelt, contribution from Mexico, they were the only government in the world to do so. Could it have been otherwise? Certainly. Long before the Soviet Union came to their aid, the Republican government had begged every one of the Western powers for arms, and they had been turned down flat. Perhaps unfortunately, the Soviet military contribution to Spain was initially limited. In the course of the entire conflict no more than five hundred or, at most, one thousand ground troops were sent. Material aid involved approximately two hundred and fifty aircraft, seven hundred tanks, seven hundred cannon, fourteen hundred trucks, twenty-seven anti-aircraft guns, and thirty thousand tons of ammunition. Much more was intended, and much more was in fact sent, but an unknown number of Soviet ships bound for Spain were torpedoed by Italian and German submarines throughout the Mediterranean, and, in the last years of the war, 1938 and 1939, some four hundred aircraft, five hundred pieces of heavy artillery, and ten thousand machine guns were sent to French ports for trans-shipment to Spain; they were never delivered.[9]

The apologists for imperialism have never failed to pretend that the conflict in Spain was a war between fascism and communism. But this was never true. At no time were there ever more than two Communist Party members in the Republican government. And at no time did the Communist Party of Spain ever advocate an armed revolt against the government. Nor did the Soviet Union at any time seek the Spanish's government's overthrow, or tie any of its aid to a policy of subversion. Indeed, the truth is entirely otherwise. We have already noted that for the Spanish Communists, the Popular Front constituted a model in embryo of the form in which the working class might come to power and usher in a new and democratic socialism. There is no denying that the Popular Front government was an experiment in pluralism and democracy. Throughout the full length of the war, there was, on the Republican side, a legal government, a functioning parliament, political parties, autonomous trade unions, a free press, and freedom to assemble and to dissent: there were forms of direct democracy at all levels; all of it maintaining itself under the most adverse conditions. The Communist Party saw these institutions as an advance toward a democratic socialist state that would involve a multi-party system, a parliament, and full freedom and liberty for parties in opposition. Perhaps surprisingly, the government of the Soviet Union agreed with these thoroughly democratic policies. A 21 December 1936 letter to the Spanish prime minister Caballero, signed by Stalin, Molotov, and Voroshilov, reads in part:

> We have considered, and we continue to consider, that it is our duty, to the extent that we can, to come to the aid of the Spanish government, which heads the struggle of all the working people, of the whole of Spanish democracy, against the military-fascist clique which is in the service of the international fascist forces. The Spanish Revolution is opening up roads that are different in many respects from the road traveled by Russia. This is determined by the difference in conditions in the social, historical, and geographical spheres, the demands of the international situation, which are not the same as those which confronted the Russian Revolution. It is very possible that the parliamentary road may turn out to be a more effective procedure for revolutionary development in Spain than it was in Russia.[10]

In short, the war in Spain was, despite enormous complexity, between the democratic Republican government on the one side, and the fascist triumvirate of Franco, Hitler, and Mussolini – supported diplomatically, politically, and materially by London and Washington – on the other. The true nature of the war was sufficiently clear that large sections of the working class around the world, including, but by no means limited to, those organized in their respective communist parties, actively developed forms and methods in which they could stand with the Spanish government. Committees to aid Spain were established and food, clothing, money, and medical aid began to pour into Madrid; individuals arrived prepared to take up arms on behalf of the Republic. Paris became the headquarters of the International Committee for Co-ordinating Aid to Spain, and the International Medical Center, uniting antifascist doctors of the most diverse political convictions. Paris, too, became the main portal for the International Brigades bound for Spain. In September 1936 Maurice Thorez, leader of the Communist Party of France, had flown to Moscow and argued for the establishment of the Brigades.[11] Largely through the imagination and organizational skill of the Communist Parties around the world, somewhere between forty and sixty thousand men and women from almost every country of Europe and the Americas, as well as Africa and China, volunteered to fight for the Spanish Republic. The majority of the members of the International Brigades were Communists; many others were social-democrats, liberals, or those without political affiliation. Volunteers from Canada, the United States, and Britain were forced to leave their countries illegally, defying laws deliberately designed to prevent their participation.[12] It made no difference; they came anyway; they fought and they died for Spain, for democracy, and to prevent the coming of the world war so clearly arriving upon the horizon; almost seventeen hundred from Canada, organized into the Mackenzie-Papineau Battalion; over three thousand from the United States, organized into the Abraham Lincoln Battalion; some two thousand from Britain, organized into the British Battalion.[13] The men and women of the International Brigades wrote with their blood a legend in the history of human solidarity; they were the fighting expression of the hundreds of thousands, the millions, of working people who responded to Spain's agony in whatever way they could.

The people of the imperialist nations stood with the Republic; their leaders supported fascism. Two months after the Nazi warplanes had obliterated Guernica and annihilated its occupants, Canadian Prime Minister Mackenzie King was in Berlin falling in love with Hitler. The final betrayal was Munich. After two and half years of an overwhelming assault and destruction at the hands of Franco and his Nazi-Fascist allies, the only real hope for the Republic was that the now truly massive pressure of the working people in the imperialist countries would finally force their governments to reverse their policy of fraudulent non-intervention and permit the sale and transfer of arms to the legitimate Spanish government. It was in this context that the Republic examined the developing crisis in Czechoslovakia. Hitler was demanding that the Prague government cede a significant portion of its territory – the Sudetenland – to Germany. The Czechs were adamant that they would not; they were determined to fight. But to successfully resist would mean that their treaties with the western powers would have to be honored, and arms would need to be supplied. For the Spanish, the situation came down to this: if Britain permitted Czechoslovakia to purchase arms, *they would no longer have any legitimacy in refusing Spain the same right*; moreover, if a new front against fascism was opened in Czechoslovakia, German troops and air power would be transferred from Spain, and the Republic could prevail; if Britain refused Czechoslovakia the right to resist, Spain's position would become increasingly untenable and fascism would triumph. The situation was entirely clear.

Alvarez del Vayo, the Foreign Minister of Spain, appeared before the League of Nations to argue his case. Lord Halifax was determined that there would be "no more nonsense to delay Franco's victory . . . Del Vayo made a dignified speech before the Council, and Halifax, to show his colors, got up in the midst of it and ostentatiously strode out."[14]

On 21 September 1938, Spain played its last card. Prime Minister Negrín formally announced, before a full session of the League of Nations, the government's decision to withdraw and repatriate the foreign volunteers of the International Brigades in the hopeless hope that this would encourage the imperialist powers to demand the withdrawal of German and Italian troops. No such demand was forthcoming.

On 29 September, Britain, France, Germany, and Italy signed the Munich Pact simultaneously betraying both Czechoslovakia and Spain.

On 23 December, three hundred and fifty thousand fascist troops launched a final offensive against what remained of the Republic. Catalonia fell. Half a million Spaniards, women, children, the elderly, and the wounded fled in exodus across the Pyrenees into France. The last units of the Republican Army, almost without arms, fought a hundred rear-guard battles to allow the refugees a path of escape.

On 22 February 1939, Franco paraded through Barcelona for three hours, preceded by a contingent of his Moorish bodyguards, the whole procession led by troops of the Italian Legionary Army.

On 27 February, Britain and France recognized the fascist government of Franco. The Republican government refused to surrender. Negrín believed, accurately as it turned out, that if the Republic could survive for

Imperialist Betrayal

only another six months the international situation would alter significantly to Spain's benefit. But the six months was not granted to him.

On 28 March, Franco's troops entered Madrid and democracy died in Spain. Hitler and Mussolini rejoiced. From the Vatican, the Pope sent a telegram to Franco congratulating him on his "Catholic victory."

10

They Killed My Soul

Fascism demands human sacrifices: it is a project of social necrophilia, its goals so repellant to human freedom that it is everywhere resisted and only made possible by mass murder. In this respect, Nationalist Spain was no different than Nazi Germany. Wherever Franco's forces advanced thousands were arrested and disappeared; they were thrown alive from cliffs into the sea; or thrown from high bridges on to stony creek beds below; or thrown down wells or open mineshafts; others were summarily executed and buried in mass graves. Tens of thousands were murdered, primarily Republicans and supporters of the Popular Front government: a thousand corpses dumped into unmarked pits in Oviedo and Gijon in the north, Teruel in the east, Seville in the south, thirty-five hundred near Merida in the southwest; there are hundreds of anonymous graves across Spain. In Porrino the bodies of those who had resisted fascism were buried in a pit beneath the foot of the local church "so everyone would walk on them, forever desecrating them."[1] Two hundred thousand defenders of the Republic were executed by Franco in the course of the war. Nor did the killing end with the fascist victory; the butchery continued: in the five years between 1939 and 1944, a million men and women were herded into concentration camps and two hundred thousand more were assassinated.[2]

This slaughter did not go uncontested. For some years after the collapse of the Republic, the Communist Party led guerrilla units against Franco throughout several areas of the country. On 17 July 1943, in the city of Oviedo, the fascists ordered thousands into the streets to celebrate the eighth anniversary of Franco's revolt. German Nazi officers stood in the reviewing stand side by side with Franco's generals. The German national anthem was played; fascist salutes were raised. At the same moment sixty kilometers away in San Esteban de Pravia, antifascist guerrillas forced open the jails and released every anti-Franco political prisoner; they unlocked the arsenal and carried away the rifles, the submachine guns, the ammunition, in trucks and wagons; three hundred and fourteen men from the town left home and joined the guerrillas.[3] Over the next several years, military barracks and supply and communications centers were raided, military trains were attacked and derailed; guerrilla warfare intensified in

They Killed My Soul   **87**

the countryside, and daring operations were carried out in several towns. But ultimately the situation was hopeless. Every action was met by the most savage terror on the part of the regime and fierce persecution and torture of those it captured. The frontiers were effectively closed, and new munitions, supplies, and combatants could no longer enter the country. Where the Popular Front had failed, it was impossible for guerrilla warfare to succeed.[4]

Both during and after the war, children of the murdered were stolen, taken to homes run by the fascist state's "social aid" department. Decades later, after Franco's death in 1975, the stolen began to speak. Francisca Aguirre: "The people from social aid rounded us up and told us we were filth, the children of vile reds, assassins, atheists, criminals, and that we didn't deserve anything." Uxeno Alvarez: "We had to be like them, like the victors. They stole my childhood, they killed my soul in 1936." Emilia Giron's son was removed from her in 1941 because she was a communist and therefore unfit to raise him. "They took my child to baptize him," she said, "but they never brought him back." Thousands of the children had their names changed in registry offices; many were adopted by Franco's supporters – the infants never knew, their older brothers and sisters often soon forgot the families into which they were born – many were sent to convents and monasteries. Children who had been sent into safety in France or Britain by their Republican parents were brought back to Spain through a systematic campaign of subterfuge. International agents of the Falange repatriated the children without their parents' knowledge, often forging papers to pretend they had their family's permission. The sisters Florencia and Maria Calvo were stolen from France and separated from each other. When Florencia arrived in Spain she asked the nun, into whose care she had been delivered, where her sister was. "They must have thrown her from the train," she was told. It was not true. Sixty years later she found Maria. But by then the intended damage had been done: the families of the Left had been smashed, splintered apart, parents slaughtered, children separated, opposition to the fascist state suppressed.[5]

Less than a year after the Second World War concluded – a war allegedly fought against fascism – the official representatives of Great Britain and the United States voiced their opinion, before the Security Council of the United Nations, that Franco's fascist regime was not a threat to peace and voted not to pursue the issue of its criminal nature.[6] Before long, Spain was admitted to full status in the United Nations under the guidance and sponsorship of the Western democracies. They had supported Franco's revolt from its inception; they had declared his regime legitimate even *before* the Republican government had fallen, and they saw no purpose in abandoning him now. There would be no war crimes trials for Franco and his henchman. The hand of friendship, once hidden, would now be extended openly.

PART THREE

Life's Blood

II
The Plan

Bethune left Quebec on 24 October 1936. Six days later he walked into the Spanish Embassy in Paris and presented the ambassador, Luis Araquistain, with his bona fides: the letter of introduction to the Spanish Prime Minister, and a letter from the CASD identifying him as its representative. He also gave the ambassador $1000 to be used by the Spanish medical authorities as they saw fit. Bethune was handed a safe conduct pass for entry into Spain and took a flight to Madrid. He was accompanied by the celebrated novelist André Malraux, who had organized the First International Air Squadron – a volunteer air force in defense of the Republic.[1]

Bethune arrived in Madrid on 3 November. It was a city under fire. The Spanish capital had been under intense bombing by German aircraft for five days: Nazi officers had ordered a necrophilious experiment to determine the effects of massive aerial bombardment on a civilian population. At the same time, four columns of Franco's fascist Nationalist troops, under the leadership of General Emilio Mola, were advancing with strength toward the city and forcing back the Republican defenders. The core of Mola's army consisted of troops from the Spanish Foreign Legion and Moroccan *Regulares* of the colonial army. They had been trained in terror. The citizens of Madrid no doubt recalled when an entire battalion of the Legion had awaited inspection with the severed heads of local Moroccan tribesman stuck on their bayonets.[2] As the fascist army had moved toward Madrid, they had massacred, mutilated, castrated, decapitated and raped anyone even suspected of leftist sympathies.[3] Mola was on the doorstep of Madrid: within the city there was a secret organization of fascist spies and sympathizers, a "Fifth Column," which, Mola implied, would be decisive in the Nationalist victory.[4] From the airport, Bethune went immediately to the Gran Via Hotel and rented a room. He had with him the various serums, vaccines, anti-toxins and, most significantly, *the blood transfusion equipment*, that he had brought from Montreal. The Gran Via Hotel was a location much favored by foreign correspondents since it was directly across the street from the Telefonica building, the central communications center, and home to the city's press offices. The choice of hotel was no accident: Bethune had made plans to meet there with

Henning Sorensen who had entered the country as a journalist several weeks previously.[5]

The next day, finding that Sorensen was not in his room, Bethune went to El Bar Chicote, a café attached to the hotel, to pass the time and wait for his arrival. He struck up a conversation with the proprietor, who spoke some English, and the Austrian journalist Ilsa Kulcsar;[6] an unfortunate choice since she was under some suspicion of being a Trotskyist spy.[7] The café was filled with armed militiamen, and one young man among them, Bethune noticed, seemed to be paying close attention to him. He left the café with Ilsa and began walking down the street discussing the situation in Madrid. They returned to the hotel, Ilsa went off to work, and Bethune returned to the café. When he left a second time, the suspicious *miliciano* followed him. Bethune stopped in front of a store window and, as he later recalled, "this lad came up to me jabbering in great excitement. He put his hand in his pocket and I knew what that meant even if I couldn't understand his words – I have seen enough tough guys in the States to realize that he had a gun in that pocket." An interesting remark; doubtless a recollection of his early activities with the Purple Gang in Detroit.

Bethune went back to the hotel, followed by the armed man. In the lobby Bethune, the concierge, and the *miliciano* began to argue with each other. The concierge explained that the young man thought Bethune was a fascist spy because he was well-dressed, held himself with an apparent military bearing, and wore a mustache. Besides, he had heard him use the word "fascist" – the only English word he recognized. Bethune left them, still arguing, and went up to his room. The *miliciano* insisted that the concierge phone the authorities. A few minutes later the police knocked on his door, five guards with rifles and an inspector with a briefcase who told Bethune he was under suspicion and would have to show him his papers. The militiaman was with them. Bethune surrendered his passport and safe-conduct pass. Satisfied, the inspector returned the documents and left with his entourage.

At that moment, Sorensen arrived at the hotel and asked the concierge for Bethune's room number. The concierge gave it to him, but warned him not to go up since the police were in his room. Sorensen ignored him and bounded up the stairs. When Bethune let him in, the room was empty. They exchanged greetings. Before Sorensen could ask for an explanation of the concierge's warning, Bethune handed him a letter he had brought for him from Montreal. Evidently the police inspector and the *miliciano* were hiding outside and had been listening at the door. They forced their way in and the inspector grabbed the letter. "I must read it," he said. It was nothing but a love letter. Annoyed, and feeling somewhat foolish, he assured the young

The Plan

militiaman that Bethune and Sorensen were not spies, and left the room. Bethune shaved his mustache; an improvement since Sorensen thought "he looked more like a police officer on leave than anything else."[8]

An amusing incident? Certainly Bethune thought so, and later, with Allen May, he wrote it as such for the *Daily Clarion*. But it spoke to the political tensions in Madrid, and on his second day in Spain a police report would no doubt have noted his interrogation as a potential spy.

In the days that followed, Sorensen, who spoke fluent Spanish, as well as French and Danish, accompanied Bethune to examine the military hospitals.[9] Several dozen had been improvised across the city in the wake of the fascist putsch: in the center of Madrid, near the Prado Museum, two luxury hotels, the Ritz and the Palace, had been converted for that purpose.[10] One of the few remaining pre-war hospitals, the ultramodern Hospital Obrero – the Workers' Hospital – located in the working-class district of Cuatro Caminos, was now lacking in antibiotics, anesthetics, and personnel, but was filled with wounded militiamen. Not long before Bethune's arrival, Sister Amalia, a Catholic nun and fascist agent, poisoned the hospital food and killed some one hundred patients.[11]

Bethune met with many of the Spanish doctors and discussed the medical situation. Privately, he noted the totally inadequate facilities for blood transfusion, and he knew that the people of Madrid were dying because of blood shortage.[12] The Spanish medical service proposed that he join the surgical staff at one of the military hospitals, but he declined on the grounds that the number of surgeons at the hospitals seemed sufficient, and more importantly that had he accepted, he would "simply go into a hospital as a surgeon and that would be the end of the '*Canadian Unit*'": there would then be no specifically Canadian presence in Spain.[13]

Bethune and Sorensen then traveled south to Albacete, intending to survey the medical problems and requirements at the administrative headquarters of the International Brigades. All around the city, the little villages were housing the training bases of the various national units and battalions that were arriving daily. The logistical problems involved with the influx of so many volunteers from so many different countries created a certain degree of necessary confusion. After two wasted days, they were finally introduced to Dr. Pierre Rouquès, the harried French doctor in charge of the base. Bethune bristled at the doctor's apparent inability to deal with the situation, and decided to return to Madrid. "I couldn't work with the bastard," he told Sorensen, "he doesn't know what he's doing."[14]

Meanwhile, the battle for Madrid intensified. The city would certainly have fallen to the fascists if had not been for the timely intervention of the International Brigades. Among the first units of the Brigades to arrive in

Spain was the Thaelmann Battalion of the 11th Brigade, named for Ernst Thaelmann, the outstanding leader of the German Communist Party, arrested by the Gestapo in 1933 and later shot, and his body burned, in the Buchenwald concentration camp. Composed initially of German antifascist political émigrés living in Spain, they saw battle at Huesca as early as 24 July 1936, and fought on the Aragon front for two months beginning at the end of August. Later, anti-Nazis from Germany itself, desperately escaping the Hitler regime, joined the Battalion at the administrative center of the International Brigades, in Albacete, a town to the southwest of Valencia. Altogether, five thousand German antifascist volunteers fought against Franco, most of them integrated into the newly formed 11th Brigade along with French, Polish, and Italian antifascists. On 1 November, the troops of the 11th, headed by the Thaelmann Battalion, were readied to move north from Albacete to the defense of Madrid.[15]

On 7 November, the Caballero government, knowing that a major fascist assault on Madrid was imminent, moved undercover of dark to Valencia on the Mediterranean coast. As the government was preparing to evacuate, the volunteers of the 11th Brigade moved into the city, marching through the streets in formation and singing revolutionary songs in half-a-dozen different languages, to the wild cheers and applause of the citizens. The next day, at sunrise, twenty thousand of Franco's troops, under the protection of an advance Nazi bombardment, attacked Madrid. The 11th Brigade engaged the enemy with a fierce determination, assisting the highly-disciplined Spanish Communist Fifth Regiment and other people's militias in holding their ground against the massive assault of the enemy. The battle lasted several days, moving from street to street, building to building. The 11th Brigade lost nearly half its men fighting on the front lines but the fascists were repulsed and Madrid was saved.[16]

Franco's forces had penetrated to the perimeters of the Casa de Campo and the adjoining University City districts, western suburbs of Madrid: it became one of the major fronts in the war. Fighting was constant. Directly behind this line were the survivors of the embattled Thaelmann Battalion. Bethune had determined to contact General Emilio Kleber, the military leader of the International Brigades, and offer his services. At Bethune's insistence, he and Sorensen went directly to the front, in search of Kleber. They took cover in a building occupied by the worn-out and exhausted soldiers of the Thaelmann, their trenches and foxholes not more than three kilometers from the Gran Via Hotel.[17] Through Sorensen's translating abilities, Bethune talked to the men, paying particular attention to the wounded and their needs. He had brought a motion picture camera with him which, according to Sorensen, "whenever he raised the camera to his

The Plan   **95**

eye looked rather like a sub-machine gun at a distance, and he was quietly tipped off that he was liable to get shot if he persisted."[18] When fascist soldiers began another round of sniping at the building, the Brigaders answered back, firing through the windows and then ducking down quickly to avoid being killed. To Sorensen's amazement, Bethune refused to take cover and walked quickly from window to window, observing the enemy while bullets flew towards him, seemingly confident that he could not be hit.[19]

When the firing stopped, Bethune found Dr. Kisch, chief surgeon of the Brigades, and General Kleber in a nearby bunker. Kleber, whose real name was Manfred Stern, was born in the Romanian region of the former Austro-Hungarian Empire, and had reputedly spent some years in Canada; certainly he spoke English. Bethune, Kisch, and Kleber spent some hours in friendly conversation discussing both the military and the medical situation and their shared certainty that Madrid would hold out against Franco. Kleber initially suggested that Bethune assume the position of chief surgeon at the front, a possibility that Bethune said he would need some time to consider. Again, it was the same problem that had arisen when the Spanish medical service had requested he enter their surgical staff: to do so would mean the absence of a specifically Canadian medical unit. A few days later, Kleber told Bethune that he had acted precipitously and had to rescind the offer, since "he could not interfere with the authority of his medical officer, Dr. Fraenkel."[20] It is doubtful that Bethune ever seriously considered acting as a surgeon. His skills in general surgery had lapsed; he had done nothing but thoracic surgery for some years as he himself recognized; less than a year later, before he left for China he would submit himself to a necessary retraining. Besides, he had other plans.

Leaving Madrid once again, Bethune and Sorensen then proceeded by train to Valencia, the new political capital, in part to purchase at Rouquès suggestion, an ambulance for the International Brigades.[21] The train was slow-moving and Bethune and Sorensen were sitting facing each other with a small folding table between them. They were silent for a while, and then Bethune said, "Henning, I think I've got an idea."[22] Bethune revealed to Sorensen the mandate which had brought him to Spain. The Committee to Aid Spanish Democracy had authorized the establishment of a Canadian hospital unit, but the form which it was to take had been left to Bethune's discretion. It will be recalled that before he left Canada he had already proposed to the Quebec Committee of the Communist Party that he organize a mobile blood transfusion service; the proposal had been accepted and, as he had told Wendell MacLeod, that was precisely the assignment he intended to carry out. He had observed the situation in Madrid's military hospitals, at the front, and in Albacete, and nothing he had seen had changed his mind; on the contrary, a blood transfusion service was precisely what was needed. At the Sacré Coeur he had previously had some experience with transfusions; he was one of the first surgeons in Canada to employ a hospital blood service. Bethune read widely in the medical literature, and issues involving blood transfusion were increasingly common in the 1920s and 1930s. As a Communist, he may well have paid particular attention to the quite startling advances made in blood transfusion and blood banking at the Soviet State Institute of Blood Transfusion, as we shall see. It is certainly not unlikely that Bethune was familiar with the Soviet Institute's work; his own practice in Spain would be much the same, with the single and most important exception that he would take blood directly to the front lines, under fire and in battlefield conditions, to infuse the wounded when they needed it most and when there was the greatest chance of saving their lives. By the time they reached Valencia, Bethune had fully outlined his plan to Sorensen who had become the first recruit to the Canadian Blood Transfusion Service.

Sorensen was something more, and quite other, than merely a journalist who had found himself accompanying Bethune around the circuit of Spanish hospitals. It will be recalled that Bethune joined the Communist Party in November 1935, and was shortly afterwards assigned to the Sun Life club of the Party, a "closed" club consisting of professionals, most of whom worked at the Sun Life Assurance Company building, and whose membership was kept secret. A 23 December 1942 secret police document reveals that Sorensen worked at the Sun Life from 13 August 1929 to 19 September 1936, and that an informant asserted: "it was common knowledge" that Sorensen associated with persons known for their "communistic activities," and had "made statements to indicate that he was communistically inclined." The police report further noted: "it would appear that his field of activities was amongst the workers of the Sun Life Assurance Company to whom he showed his radical inclinations."[23] This information is certainly intriguing: was Sorensen, like Bethune, a secret member of the Communist Party? Were Bethune and Sorensen in fact in the same Party club, the Sun Life club, and therefore known to each other long before they separately left for Spain? It is of further interest, in this regard, that Norman Lee, the Quebec chair of the Committee to Aid Spanish Democracy, not only also worked at the Sun Life, but was a member of the Party and of the same Party club to which Bethune belonged.[24] That Sorensen was a secret member of the Communist Party of Canada seems undeniable; certainly in Madrid he joined the Communist Party of Spain.[25]

Arriving in Valencia, Bethune and Sorensen went to the head office of

The Plan   **97**

the Socorro Rojo Internacional (SRI), the Spanish branch of the International Red Aid, an organization founded in Moscow in 1922 to conduct campaigns in support of Communist prisoners, and to provide material and medical support to workers and their families. In Spain, the SRI collected and distributed food, provided shelter for orphaned children, and established soup kitchens and refugee camps in the Republican zones; they had also become largely responsible for the majority of the medical services. The SRI officials were initially cautious. The novelty of Bethune's plan seemed to require scientific experimentation and confirmation, tasks more than difficult under conditions of war. Bethune argued that it was precisely because of the war that a mobile blood transfusion service was required; the lives of the defenders of the Republic must be saved. In the end, the officials were won over. They were impressed by the force of Bethune's plan and assured him of a laboratory and facilities in Madrid. The only problem was financing. Bethune satisfied them that all the necessary funds to equip the service would be raised in Canada.[26]

Returning to Madrid, Bethune sent a cable to CASD headquarters in Toronto outlining his intentions and the commitments he had made to the SRI, and said he was on his way to Paris to gather the necessary equipment. The Committee agreed without hesitation, and funding was sent through American Express money orders. With Sorensen, Bethune flew to Paris on 21 November; he had been in Spain for eighteen days.[27]

Once in Paris, Bethune began to search for the medical and transportation equipment he would require. Despite Sorensen's fluency in French, there were some difficulties, allegedly involving "linguistic problems," and much that Bethune required could not be discovered in France.[28] Bethune left Sorensen in Paris, presumably to continue searching out supplies, and continued on to London.

Bethune arrived in England on 24 November and purchased a wood-paneled Ford station wagon to act as an ambulance for the mobile blood service.[29] In order to avoid paying expensive duty on the vehicle, during the intended return journey through France, he contacted the French Embassy, which advised him that the Canadian government would need to assure them that he was indeed a physician engaged in humanitarian work. Bethune went to the Canadian High Commissioner in London, Vincent Massey – later the Governor General of Canada – who sent a cable to the Department of External Affairs, in Ottawa, for instructions.[30] There then followed a flurry of diplomatic telegrams and internal memos. On 27 November the Minister for External Affairs received a memo from a department investigator reporting that: "Dr. Bethune's medical mission to Madrid was dispatched by the 'Committee to Aid Spanish Democracy' . . . This is understood to be a Communist organization under the chairmanship of Reverend Benjamin Spence. And it has been said that Tim Buck is associated with it in some way."[31] The Canadian government knew, of course, that the CASD was not a specifically communist organization, but since the Government had already allied itself with the British position favoring Franco, they had no intention of aiding in any way medical relief to the legitimate government of Spain. The next day, not yet having received instructions, Massey further informed Ottawa that Sorensen would be accompanying Bethune.[32] Since there had already been diplomatic concerns about Sorensen in October — when he had reported his presence to the British Embassy in Madrid as a foreign correspondent — Massey's information to Ottawa was less than helpful.[33] The department investigator sent a second memo to the Minister who was apparently still considering the matter: "I think this changes the complexion of the request. Sorensen is not a medical man, but a journalist and Danish subject, and — it would appear from the earlier correspondence — is likely to have political activities in mind."[34] Later that day, 28 November, Massey received a final telegram reeking of hypocrisy and false concern and turning down Bethune's request:

> While Government has full sympathy with any efforts to relieve sufferers on either side of the present Spanish conflict, it would not be possible in view of what appears to be the political complexion of this mission as indicated by your second telegram and by other circumstances to sponsor it by making a formal request such as indicated.[35]

In a final effort, Bethune pressed Lester Pearson, First Secretary in the Department of External Affairs — and later to be the fourteenth Prime Minister of Canada — presently attached to Massey's office in London, for a "letter of introduction." Pearson complied, but the letter turned out later to be ineffective.[36]

While in London, Bethune was staying at the home of Clunie Dale, the brother of his former platonic lover, Marian Scott. Dale was a friend of Hazen Sise, a Montreal architect, who had moved to London. Interestingly, like Marian Scott and Bethune, Sise had frequented the artist John Lyman's evening artistic salons in Montreal, but apparently he had never encountered Bethune.[37] On the wet Sunday afternoon of 29 November, Sise was spending a lazy day in his Chelsea studio apartment, casually looking through some books he had recently bought. The telephone rang: it was Dale, calling to tell him that Bethune, a doctor on leave from Madrid, was at his house and perhaps he would like to meet him.[38]

Sise's politics were distinctly on the left; he was a socialist, but not a communist. Certainly he loathed fascism and all that it stood for; he was "determined that somehow it must be stopped, and when the Spanish war broke out this seemed to be a great turning point in history and seemed to offer a possibility of stopping fascism . . . the Nazis, and the Italian Fascists and the Spanish Fascists." The previous year he had been in Paris, and witnessed the traditional Bastille Day parade. He had been much moved to see the last survivor of the Paris Commune leading the march. Later in the day he had seen the hundreds of thousands gathered to watch Leon Blum take the oath of allegiance to the French Popular Front. But in the wealthy district, in the Champs Elysées, men from the Jockey Club were giving the fascist salute. He knew, as Bethune knew, that if fascism could be halted in Spain, it could halt the undergrowth of fascism in France, in Britain, and throughout the imperialist world: if it could not be halted the whole world would be at war.

Sise was immediately eager to meet Bethune. He already had two tickets for a massive popular meeting in aid of Spanish democracy at the Albert Hall that evening. He invited Clunie Dale and Bethune to come over for dinner and to attend the meeting afterward. Clunie was otherwise occupied, but Bethune arrived at Sise's house at six o'clock, a "ramrod erect figure" wearing a trenchcoat. They went into the studio and Bethune "immediately started launching into a description of what Madrid was like under the siege, what the incredible emotion was of a people's army in resistance, the whole citizenry of Madrid manning the barricades, and the emotion of the first of the International Brigades marching into the line at University City." He had only been talking for a few minutes when Sise said, "I wish I could go back with you."

They went out to dinner, where Bethune continued to discuss the Spanish situation, and then to the Albert Hall. During the course of the meeting, Sise thought why not; why not go? Leaving Albert Hall, Sise put it to Bethune formally, asking if he could take him with him, and whether he could be of any use to the unit. "I'm quite serious about this," Sise said. "I'd like to go back with you." Bethune told him he would have to check with the CASD to inquire whether he had the authority to take on recruits. The next day he cabled Sorensen asking him to come to London, and commented about Sise: "We'll be lucky to get him; his father is one of the fifty most important men in Canada;" a remark which Sorensen found to be insufficiently communist.[39] Bethune then cabled the CASD and, after receiving their permission to take on new recruits – such permission apparently not being required for Sorensen – he telephoned Sise, to tell him the good news. He pointed out to Sise that he would not have to stay in Spain if he changed his mind, but to be ready to leave in four days.

Sise put his affairs in order and found an architect to take over his current commission. He was suddenly gripped by fear: he had heard of the pleasure Franco's men took in torturing their prisoners. He went to see a friend who was a doctor and asked him for morphine. The doctor gave him, as Sise put it, "enough ampoules to kill a dozen people." He would later carry the morphine with him wherever he went in Spain.[40]

Bethune divided the rest of his time between gathering the necessary medical supplies and equipment during the day and reading material on the latest techniques of blood transfusion during the night. Sise recognized what had no doubt already occurred to Bethune : the power of blood. As Sise put it many years later:

> The giving of blood had an enormous emotional punch to it, particularly for Spaniards but also for people all over the world. Blood is a tremendously powerful symbol, in all our literature and history, and the replenishing of blood is therefore something that raises enormous emotions, and it's very true to say that in terms of aiding the Spanish Republic the attention and sympathy that was generated through the publicity given to our work there on blood transfusion was as important politically as the medical help we gave.

And it was not at all lost on either Bethune or Sise that the giving of blood for the wounded, in terms of a specifically Canadian unit, would make it that much easier to raise funds in Canada not only for the transfusion service, but on behalf of Republican Spain in general.

With Sorensen's arrival in London the newly formed blood transfusion unit made last minute preparations to leave for Madrid. Wednesday 2 December was spent purchasing the final equipment for the Ford ambulance. Sise spoke with his friend Claud Cockburn who had previously indicated that he might travel with them to Madrid, but had now made other arrangements. Sise's friendship with Cockburn lends further evidence of Sise's political sympathies. Cockburn was a member of the Communist Party of Great Britain, and had been asked by its leader, Harry Pollitt, to act as their newspaper correspondent in Spain. Bethune, Sorensen, and Sise, crossed the English Channel at Folkestone – the Ford station wagon piled to the roof with medical supplies and a kerosene-powered refrigerator – and arrived in Boulogne, France, on the morning of 3 December, driving south through the deepening dark. In Paris the next day, Bethune traded his motion picture camera for a Leica and a light meter. Sorensen had signs painted for the side of the Ford reading, in French: *"Service-Canadien a Madrid de Transfusion de Sang."* Sise obtained safe-conduct passes from the

The Plan

Spanish Embassy. He suggested purchasing gas masks, a proposition that Bethune initially opposed on the grounds that it would be uncomradely since no one else in Madrid appeared to have them, but Sise convinced him that if the troops were issued masks, there would be none left over and that their own efficiency would then be prejudiced. Surprisingly, gas masks were difficult to find; Parisians had recently been buying them in large numbers, anticipating a possible fascist assault. On Saturday 5 December, they attached Sorensen's signs to the ambulance; a crowd of workers cheered them with the antifascist clenched-fist salute as they left Paris. For the next two days they traveled south through driving rain and snowstorms. The weather cleared as they passed through southern France, and everywhere on the road they would meet knots of workers who turned from their labors and, just as in Paris, raised their clenched fists in the air as they drove by. On Tuesday, 8 December they approached the Pyrenees Mountains and the border with Spain.

They passed through the French border guards and a contingent of Spanish militia, crossed the mountains and drove down into the vineyards of Catalonia. Further south, on the way to Barcelona, there were increasing numbers of *milicianos*, sand-bagged barricades, and the flags of the major unions, the Confederación Nacional del Trabajo (CNT) and the Unión General de Trabajadores (UGT). At Barcelona they took the ambulance to a garage to be re-painted. When it was finished the next day, the painters, in a gesture of solidarity, refused payment. Bethune, Sorensen, and Sise continued down the road south towards Valencia passing towns where the militia were training in the public squares and nearly everyone was armed. In Valencia, they reported immediately to the Socorro Rojo office where Bethune outlined his plans for the blood transfusion service in detail; arrangements were finalized; papers were signed, the Ford ambulance inspected. There would be a blood transfusion headquarters in Madrid. Bethune was ecstatic; the work he had planned would soon become a concrete reality: the wounded would be saved; the dying returned to life: Madrid would become the tomb of fascism.

From Valencia they headed inland, rising up onto the great central plateau of Spain, and drove along the high road through the open, austere landscape almost devoid of trees, villages spread out in great distances from each other, clinging to the sides of the hills, surrounded by olive fields. At last they crested a final rise and Madrid was laid out below them, the smoke of bombed and burning buildings rising into the crisp winter air. They drove down into the city and made their way to the Gran Via Hotel.

12

Based on Blood: A New Type of Human Relationship

Madrid was cold but teeming with people. The constant fascist attacks had taken their toll. There were long lines of men and women waiting for food or fuel. On some streets buildings had been bombed to rubble, on others there was tangled, skeletal wreckage open to the sky where families had once lived; barricades and machine gun nests had been set up. In the Puerta del Sol, in the center of the city, Sise happened to notice Claud Cockburn, and pointed him out to Bethune and Sorensen. Cockburn looked a little dirty and unshaven, but he was happy and enthusiastic. He had spent the night with the International Brigades south of Madrid, and had adopted the name "Frank Pitcairn" as his *nom de guerre*. He would soon be one of many frequent visitors at the Canadian Blood Transfusion Institute.[1]

Bethune's group had lunch at the café in the basement of the Gran Via Hotel that was, as always, crowded with militiamen and reporters. While waiting for a five o'clock appointment with the SRI in Madrid, they drove out to the trenches at University City and talked with the soldiers.[2]

The chief physician at the SRI was entirely accommodating and efficient. The Blood Transfusion Institute – whose official name would be the *Servicio Hispano-Canadiense de Transfusion de Sangre* – was to be housed in an extensive fifteen room apartment directly below the SRI offices at 36 Principe de Vergara. It was the perfect location: the broad tree-lined boulevard was located in the Barrio de Salamanca, the wealthiest district of the city – and so was never bombed by Franco or the Nazi air squadrons – and its intimate proximity to the SRI facilitated administrative and medical collaboration.[3] The apartment, however, was presently being used as refugee housing; while the SRI saw to their removal to other quarters, Bethune and his colleagues helped them to pack. The premises had previously been occupied by the Chilean Embassy, and a lawyer for the German Embassy who had, at some point, fled in a great hurry. He had left behind, hidden in a "strange long cupboard in the side of the living room," rather a large number of documents revealing the true extent of Nazi collaboration with

Based on Blood

103

Franco's rebellion. Claud Cockburn, who read German, spent several hours going through these papers and verifying their incriminating nature. The documents were then packed into an oversized laundry basket, and Bethune dispatched Sise to Valencia where he was to turn the papers over to Alvarez del Vayo, the Foreign Minister.[4]

The work proceeded quickly: Bethune threw himself into action. As Hazen Sise recalled: "He would pass from thought to action without any gap whatsoever."[5] Within the space of a day or two the transfusion equipment was installed – refrigerators, the autoclave, incubators, the distilled water apparatus – all of the equipment run by kerosene and designed to be fully mobile for transportation to the various hospitals in and around Madrid and to the casualty clearing centers at the front lines of the war zones. In addition to the larger apparatus, there were vacuum bottles, blood flasks, drip bottles, three complete direct blood transfusion sets, microscopes, chest instruments, hurricane lamps, gas masks, two thousand sets of blood serum for testing donor blood groups, and sodium citrate for blood preservation. Besides the rooms dedicated to the storage of equipment, there was a room devoted to receiving donors and recording their personal information and a three-bed transfusion room for taking their blood; other rooms were allocated as bedrooms, a library, and a common room. Seconded to the Institute were two Spanish medical students, a Spanish biologist, a cook, two maids, a laundry man, and a military armed guard.[6] They were soon joined by four Spanish doctors: Valentin de la Loma, Andrés Sanz, Vicente Goyanes, and Antonio Culebras.[7]

Almost immediately there were visitors, reporters, foreign correspondents, and volunteer staff. Celia Greenspan, the wife of George Marion, a correspondent for *New Masses*, was the first American woman to volunteer in Spain. A Communist Party member since 1935, she approached Bethune and informed him of her qualifications as a nurse and laboratory technician. Bethune was delighted and asked her to set up and organize the laboratory, and to train Spanish women in the process.[8] The prominent British evolutionary biologist and Marxist J. B. S. Haldane was soon living at the Institute.[9] Indeed, Bethune opened his door to anyone who could be of service, and most especially to foreign journalists who could report the exciting and innovative mobile Blood Transfusion Unit to the world's eyes. Bethune recognized from the start the tremendous propaganda value of the blood service. Blood for the wounded soldiers of democracy; blood to save thousands of lives: such a service would have an immense appeal to people around the world already concerned about Spain, and vastly increase the awareness of those who were as yet unaware of the true nature of the conflict. Publicity for the Blood Transfusion Unit would at the same time translate into donations of money and food and clothing, all desperately needed by the Spanish government.

The blood transfusion service was predicated on the obvious necessity of having a sufficient number of blood donors. Would the people of Madrid come to give their blood? Bethune was nervous: this was the only aspect of the situation he could not control.[10] On 19 December appeals for blood donors were transmitted through the radio. But by whom? Possibly by Sorensen, since he was fluent in Spanish, but far more likely by a member of the SRI. It may have been Tina Modotti, known in Spain as "Maria." Modotti had been born in Italy, but had lived for many years in Mexico. There she had become an internationally famous photographer associated with the *avant guarde* movement and an intimate friend of the muralist Diego Rivera, and had joined the Communist Party. Under attack in Mexico by anticommunist forces, she escaped to Moscow with her lover, Vittorio Vidali. When the war in Spain broke out, Modotti and Vidali came to Madrid: she to work for the SRI in a senior position; he to lead the SRI and, as "Carlos Contreras," to function as political commander and organizer of the Communist Fifth Regiment. Modotti lived in the building next to Bethune, and had her office in the floor above him. Since much of Modotti's work for the SRI involved both medical aid and publicity, it is entirely possible that it was she who made the radio appeals. Later, she helped Bethune with blood transfusions in Madrid and in the surrounding countryside; during the evacuation of refugees from Malaga, she was with him.[11]

On the morning after the first radio broadcast for donors, Bethune looked out of the window. The tension left him. The donors were there. Not just a handful, but, as Sise recalled, "this long, long line of people right around the corner of the block. . . . It was a very moving thing. . . . It was a very exciting moment. We never had any trouble the whole time we were there. Blood donors would flock to us. Something which appealed to the Spaniards very deeply emotionally, the replenishing of blood at the Front."[12] One by one the donors entered the Institute. At first, only the donor's name, address, blood type, and medical record were registered; donors were asked whether they had ever suffered from syphilis or hepatitis. Then, several days later, the donors were notified to return: 500cc of blood was taken and stored in a bottle containing the sodium citrate preservative. The bottle was labeled and stored in a refrigerator. After the blood was taken, a can of beef, paid for out of the CASD funds, was given to every donor, along with a small glass of brandy. Many of the donors, primarily members of the working class, were in a semi-starved condition and Bethune ensured that they were given extra rations.[13] As to be expected, there were minor problems, but they were soon solved. Donors no longer

Based on Blood

needed to be asked about many of the diseases they might have had; Greenspan developed the necessary tests. And not all the equipment operated as expected; the first batch of refrigerated blood had frozen solid and Bethune had to replace the kerosene-powered fridge with another fueled by butane.[14]

As we shall shortly see, the Blood Transfusion Unit soon began to expand its services well beyond Madrid and to the shifting war zones across the country. It was always Bethune's intention, and perhaps his greatest innovation, to bring blood as close to the front lines as possible; he saved countless lives by reversing the usual order: instead of taking the wounded to the blood, he took the blood to the wounded. The more rapidly a wounded soldier could be operated on, the more likely he would survive. This was the essence of the Blood Transfusion Unit – its *mobility*. Certainly Bethune recognized, where others had not, the role of hemorrhage in wound shock, and he was the first to conceive of a blood supply system based on mass-scale, free civilian donations of blood that could be rapidly delivered to the front. Bethune's contribution to military medicine is uncontestable: he pioneered the use of whole blood in combat areas, he created the first mobile military blood bank and, even more importantly, he developed the first *unified blood transfusion service* in medical and military history. Perhaps ironically, mobile blood services similar to his own were shortly to be used in the world war that he and other antifascists had striven to prevent by coming to the aid of Spanish democracy.

But Bethune's other great innovation, perhaps less known, certainly less commented upon, was not so much the military aspect of the transfusion service, but its uniquely *human* aspect: on every bottle of donated blood he had not only the blood group and the date written, but the name and address of the donor so that the soldier into whom the blood would be transfused would know who had saved his life. There was none of the usual anonymity, none of the usual separation: here, two people were brought together by the mediation of blood. What's more, Bethune kept a large ledger book in the transfusion room. After the donor's blood was taken, he would explain: "In this book the donor's name is entered, and later, on the same line, the name of the wounded soldier into whose arm the blood will flow. *A new kind of human relationship is begun on this page*, a new kind of friendship begins, strengthened by blood." On many occasions, Bethune would take the donor to the recipient, to meet, to become known to each other, so that each donor could understand, quite vividly, the true and human contribution their blood had brought to the restoration of the comrades who would defend them.[15]

Donor, recipient, the financial support of the CASD: for Bethune each was part of the same circle; each part of the necessary network of propaganda. Just as donors and recipients strengthened each other's resolve, so too were Canadian workers, as they were made aware of Bethune's activities, encouraged to strengthen the blood unit through sustained fund-raising. The mobile blood transfusion service was the gift of life that the working class of Canada gave willingly to the Spanish Republic; it was their concrete response to that most vile of fascist slogans – *Viva la Muerte! Long Live Death!*

If it was certainly true that Bethune understood the propaganda value of the Canadian Blood Transfusion Service, it was equally true that the Spanish government recognized the necessity of employing English-speaking journalists, scientists, and other sympathetic sources in broadcasting the real situation in Spain to audiences in Britain and North America. With the fraudulent Non-Intervention Pact making legitimate arms purchases impossible, it was of supreme importance to rouse popular support in English-speaking countries to put pressure on their governments to reverse their positions and dissolve the Pact. Although the imperialist governments never did, of course, abandon the Pact, the Spanish government could not then have known that. When the government short-wave radio station, EAQ, invited Bethune to speak he readily agreed, contributing five broadcasts between 24 December 1936 and 5 January 1937. During the same period, Hazen Sise broadcasted three times, as did Haldane, who had taken to living at the Institute, and was engaged in experimentation with gas masks, and advising various organizations on defense against potential poison gas attacks.[16] The broadcasts were delivered at two in the morning from a small room in the cellar of a building near the Gran Via; its windows fortified with mattress against the sound of bomb blasts.[17]

Bethune was an experienced speaker and a frequently brilliant orator. His short-wave broadcasts demonstrate not only his propagandistic talents, but his firm commitment to communism. In his first communication he spoke of the international character of the Spanish conflict, and of the Popular Front government as a revolutionary force:

The revolution of the workers against the economic, religious and intellectual slavery happened to have occurred this year in Spain. It might just as well have happened in a dozen other countries but that you had the courage, the dignity and the audacity to face your problems with more open eyes, firmer lips and stouter hearts than the workers of the rest of the world. What Spain does today, what you Spaniards do tomorrow, will decide the future of the world for the next one hundred years. If you are defeated the world will fall back into the new dark ages of Fascism – if you

Based on Blood   **107**

are successful, as we are confident you will be successful, we will go forward into the glories of the new golden age of economic and political democracy. Remember we Canadian workers are with you. We have come here as into the opening battle of the world revolution. Your fight is our fight. Your victory is our victory. Ask us how we can help you. You will find us ready to respond.[18]

Other broadcasts focused primarily on the medical needs both of the people of Madrid and of the International Brigades; the type of injuries they had sustained – the prevalence of serious brain wounds due to the refusal of the imperialist powers to permit the legitimate government to purchase steel helmets – the form of care they were receiving and would need to receive as the war progressed. But perhaps Bethune's most beautiful and stirring broadcast spoke of Madrid itself and the resilience of its citizens in the face of constant fascist bombardment. The full text, from 2 January 1937, is reproduced below:

Madrid: Peaceful Amid War
Madrid is, paradoxically enough, the most peaceful city in Europe.

It is a city at equilibrium within itself, a city without intense class antagonisms and discords that are called disorder in any other city. That is due to its homogenous society – the workers, the small shop-keepers and the petit-bourgeois all moulded into one class with one idea – winning the war against the Fascist aggressor.

So, as in a family or clan in which there is internal peace although the family or clan may be fighting against its external enemies. No police are needed to maintain the law. Every member, every citizen, is under the strict necessity of order – self-imposed and conscious.

Private property is respected – confiscated property belonging to the people at large, is equally respected. On large magnificent mansions, which once belonged to the so-called nobility, one may see signs such as these: 'Citizens, this property belongs to you, respect it.' Note the wording of the sign – not 'Belongs to the State' – the State as an institution superior to and above the people, but 'belongs to you' – belongs to me. So, if you or I damage it, we are damaging our own property.

There is absolutely no looting. This is clear from one manifest fact – the things which are looted in a war are first of all articles of necessity such as clothing or food. Later come the luxuries – jewels, fur coats, etc. Now the people of Madrid are wearing the same clothes as they wore before the rebellion in spite of the large quantities of fine clothes left by fleeing Fascists and members of the so-called upper classes.

Buying of necessities and clothing is brisk in the shops. I was in a large departmental store today and saw a woman of the so-called middle classes buy a tricycle for her boy of 10 and a large doll for her daughter of 5.

We were heavily bombed from the air today about 12 noon. Twelve huge Italian tri-motored bombers came over the city and bombed not positions of military importance, but a poor quarter of the city called Cuatro Caminos. This is a district some miles behind the front line, inhabited by the poorest people living in one or two storey mud and brick dwellings. The massacred victims were mainly women, children and old people.

Standing in a doorway as these huge machines flew slowly overhead, each one heavily loaded with bombs, I glanced up and down the streets. People hurried to 'refugiois;' a hush fell over the city – it was a hunted animal crouched down in the grass, quiet and apprehensive. There is no escape, so be still. Then in the dead silence of the streets the songs of birds came startlingly clear in the bright winter air.

What is the object of these bombings of lowly civilian habitations? Is it to produce panic in the city? Because, if so, it is a completely cruel, useless and wanton endeavour. This people cannot be terrified. They are being treated by the Fascists as if they were soldiers bearing offensive arms. This is murder of defenceless civilians.

No one can realize what utter helplessness one feels when these huge death-ships are overhead. It is practically useless to go into a building – even a ten-storey building. The bombs tear through the roof, through every floor in the building and explode in the basement, bringing down concrete buildings as if they were made of matchwood.

It is not much safer to be in the basement of the lower floors, than in the upper stories. One takes shelter in doorways to be out of the way of falling masonry, huge pieces of façade and stone work. If the building you happen to be in is hit, you will be killed or wounded. One place is really as good as another.

After the bombs fall – and you can see them falling like great black pears – there is a thunderous roar. Clouds of dust and explosive fumes fill the air, whole sides of houses fall into the street. From heaps of huddled clothes on the cobblestones blood begins to flow – these were once women and children.

Many are buried alive in the ruins. One hears their cries – they cannot be reached. Burst water and gas mains add to the danger. Ambulances arrive. The blackened and crumpled bodies of the still-alive are carried away.

Now observe the faces of, not the dead, but those who still live. Because it is the wished-for effect on them which is the motive for these massacres,

Based on Blood

not just the killing of a few hundred innocent civilians and the destruction of property, but the terrorizing of hundreds of thousands who escaped this death. They stand and watch or work themselves at the rescue. Their lips are set and cold. They don't shout or gesticulate. They look at each other sorrowfully, and when they talk of the fascist assassins, their faces express fortitude, dignity and contempt.

These people have endured from the arrogance of wealth, the greed of the church, the poverty and oppression of centuries. This is just one more blow, one more lash of the whip. They have stood these blows, these lashes before and they will stand them to the end. They cannot be shaken.[19]

The reference to the fascist bombing of the working-class district of Cuatro Caminos in this broadcast occasioned the last poem Bethune was ever known to have written. The air attack had destroyed the *Hospital Obrero* – the Workers' Hospital – one of Madrid's most important medical facilities. Bethune visited the burnt out remains and the surrounding area. His anguish and fury were reflected in a poem, *I Come From Cuatro Caminos*, which, compared to the poetry he wrote in Montreal, is far from his best. It is notable too that, even in the midst of war, and under the hectic conditions of establishing the blood transfusion service, Bethune continued his self-identification as an artist, the consequences of which would later become problematic. What's more, four lines of the poem indicate his ongoing concern for children that, toward the end of his time in Spain, would come to equal his commitment to the blood transfusion service:

My eyes are overflowing,
And clouded with blood.
The blood of a little fair one,
Whom I saw destroyed on the ground.[20]

On Christmas Eve, 1936, Bethune again visited the soldiers in the trenches to the west of the city. Returning home, he wrote an open letter to physicians in Canada urging that they join him in Spain and "come to the relief of human suffering" regardless of their political opinions. Late that night, he took the microphone again and gave another broadcast through EAQ.[21]

On Christmas day, Bethune, Sise, and Sorensen traveled fifty kilometers northwest from Madrid to the Sierra de Guadarrama, partly to test their truck's refrigeration system for potential transfusions at a distance. They visited the imposing granite palace and monastery of the Escorial. As they stood admiring its austere architecture, they could hear the distant sound of Franco's guns shelling Madrid, the on-going murder of innocent non-combatants. Shortly afterwards, they were driven to the front line trenches of the Guadarrama in an armored car, the fascists firing at them from forty meters away. The trenches themselves were not continuous, but concentrated in fortified posts, "the dug-out areas strong, roomy, and comfortable." Each post was equipped with a library and a school under the command of a political commissar. As Sise explained:

> It seems that the Spanish people, having been forced to defend themselves in a war not of their making, are determined to make the war the occasion for the economic, social and spiritual regeneration of Spain. So they fight with textbooks as well as machine guns. From one post we visited, within earshot of the enemy, the political commissar gives the Fascists a mighty lecture through a megaphone. As a result, there is a steady trickle of Fascist deserters coming over on dark nights. As one young officer explained to me with a justifiable pride in his voice, "the Fascists shoot their prisoners but we send them to school and make real men of them."[22]

The schools and libraries in the trenches fulfilled a dual function: they sought to eliminate the appalling degree of illiteracy in Spain – the fault of the Church which had previously exercised complete control of the educational system – while at the same time strengthening the soldiers intellectual understanding of the cause which already, as Sise said, "through their hearts had led them to heroic deeds."

Later in the evening the young soldiers held a party, with guitars playing, and singing and dancing. "Bethune," Sise recalled, "enjoyed this tremendously, this camaraderie. He got a great thrill out of those kids." The next day they went further into the mountains, near the Navacerrada Pass, and found a Republican ski battalion operating in the snow fields on the high ridges. Distant Madrid was far below, half-hidden in the mists. Borrowing skis, Bethune and the others skied across the hills, half expecting to feel fascist bullets firing out towards them across the cold, keen air.[23]

Sise does not indicate whether anyone accompanied them to the Guadarrama mountains, but possibly Vera Elkan was present; she later reported spending the night near the Escorial during precisely this time period.[24] A photojournalist from South Africa, based in London, Elkan met Bethune through Haldane, with whom she had shared a "rather horrid" hostel. Haldane told her he had already arranged to stay with Bethune and said to her, "Come with me, they'll take you too." Elkan lived at the Blood Transfusion Institute for some time. As for Bethune, she later remembered him fondly. "I saw him every day," she said,

Based on Blood

I spoke to him every day, we ate together . . . He was very nice, very calm, very quiet, very stern . . . very dedicated . . . He had a constant supply of Canadian whiskey, which was a very good thing . . . we came home absolutely frozen, we had to unfreeze our hands in order to pick up a glass and drink some whiskey and get a bit warmer. And the only thing we had to eat was lentil soup . . . bread which had to be hit with a hammer because it had gone so hard and old, and butter which was all streaky.[25]

According to Sorensen, when Bethune first met Elkan he said, "Give me your hand, look me in the eye, you know you're a very nice person." She replied: "May I sleep with you tonight?"[26] It is unlikely that this casual encounter turned into a serious romance. Elkan was in Spain for only two months – December 1936 and January 1937 – primarily photographing the International Brigades for fundraising purposes. After she met Bethune, she took a number of pictures of the Blood Transfusion Institute, and traveled with him not only to the Madrid hospitals, delivering blood, but to the various fighting fronts, and to Albacete and to Valenica, where Bethune assisted Dr. Douglas Jolly of New Zealand in the removal of a bullet, without anesthetic, from the hip of a patient. Certainly Vera Elkan was with Bethune at a field hospital near the front lines on 1 January 1937. On that night, Bethune spoke in a radio broadcast of having observed a fight between a single Republican aircraft and five German and Italian bombers. The Spanish airplane and one of the Nazi aircraft plunged to the ground in flames. Bethune had walked across the field to the wreckage and removed an identifying plate from the engine of the German plane: physical proof of armed Nazi support to Franco, and incontrovertible evidence to counter the ludicrous claims of the Non-Intervention committee. Elkan took at least four photographs of Bethune and members of the International Brigades with the debris of the downed German plane.[27]

So rapidly did Bethune work that toward the end of December he was able to report to Ben Spence, the chair of the CASD:

We are now completely organized and settled in for work. . . . Through the press and daily over the local radio we broadcast appeals for blood donors. As a result we have thousands of volunteers and are busy grouping them and card indexing them. We have now 800 and in a few days will have over 1,000. There are about 56 hospitals in the city. We have surveyed the entire situation and have a list of them containing the information as to size, capacity, addresses, under what organization, telephone, chief surgeon, type of service, etc. . . . We collect the blood every day from a selected group of donor types I, II, III, IV. We are running about

1 gallon daily just now. This is stored in our refrigerator. On call from the hospital the blood flasks are transferred to heated vacuum bottles and carried in knapsacks . . . So on arrival we're ready to start work at once. We go to the man and decide what he needs – either blood or physiological serum, or glucose, or a combination of these. If blood is needed on account of acute exsanguination we 'group' him at once with our serum. This is done by a prick of the finger, a glass stick and serum and takes 2 minutes, then after grouping we give him the blood of the type needed . . . If in doubt we can always give IV as this is called the 'Universal' donor. We are not sure how long the citrated blood will keep good in our refrigerators but we are experimenting and hope for several weeks. We have plans to branch out and give the service up in the Guadarrama Mountains . . . [28]

The Blood Transfusion Unit began collecting blood from donors shortly after Christmas and transporting it to the hospitals.[29] At first, they rarely took blood more than twenty-five kilometers from the city: the front line of the war passed through Madrid itself. Fascist bombing and shelling occurred as frequently at night as it did during the day; Bethune could be called to the front at any time. A field hospital would telephone. If they were sleeping, Bethune, Sise, Sorensen, and their armed guard would be dressed within minutes and, with bottles of blood taken freshly from the refrigerator, they would drive through the pitch dark streets, answering the passwords at the barricades, the sounds of machine-gun fire and rifle shots ringing out through the night. With a flashlight in hand, Bethune would find the door to the hospital operating room, most often in the relative safety of a basement.

Bethune gave his first transfusion in the early hours of 3 January in the village of Fuencarral to the north of Madrid. The palace of a local duke had been converted into a hospital; its chapel turned into an operating room. Where the altar had stood, there was now an operating table. A soldier lay on the table. Bethune could barely feel a pulse. The man's femoral artery had been ruptured by a fascist bullet; he was bleeding heavily and in a state of shock. Bethune put aside the bottled blood he had brought with him. There was no time to test the wounded soldier's blood type. He asked Sorensen, who had accompanied him, to donate his blood through the direct arm-to-arm method; his blood was Type IV – the universal type. Within minutes the soldier was restored to life.[30]

Many of the soldiers with whom Bethune was confronted were suffering from both shock and extreme loss of blood. Frequently, under conditions of extreme exsanguination, he was forced to inject novocaine in the elbow, cut into the flesh to find a vein, insert a small glass canula, tie it into the vein and run the blood through gravity into the body.[31] Bethune described one evening's work in which he gave blood to a member of the International Brigades and to a Spanish student: he was often much moved by these encounters:

> After I had given a transfusion to a French soldier who had lost his arm, he raised the other to me as I left the room in the Casualty Clearing Station, and with his raised clenched fist exclaimed 'Viva la Revolution.' The next boy to him was a Spaniard – a medical student, shot through the liver and the stomach. When I had given him a transfusion and asked him how he felt – he said 'It is nothing' – Nada! He recovered. So did the Frenchman.[32]

Hazen Sise similarly recalled standing with Bethune and observing the typical reactions of the soldiers, dying of shock, as they received transfusion:

> The wounded man would be very pale, sweating and in a sort of comatose condition, and then you would get that vein in the arm and start pumping blood into him and the change was miraculous. You'd see the man come around and it was the greatest reward you could ever ask; you would literally pluck them from the jaws of death, see the color rise in their faces and they'd start paying attention . . . They became alive right in front of your eyes within the space of a several minutes. It was extraordinary.[33]

Along with Sise and Sorensen, Haldane often accompanied Bethune in the few weeks he was in Spain. He noted that the hospital he most frequently attended had been set up by the International Brigades, a field hospital occupying an abandoned school building a few kilometers behind the front:

> Ambulances with wounded were constantly arriving from the line. The slighter cases were sent on to Madrid, the dangerous cases kept for several days. There were a great many abdominal wounds. These had to be dealt with at once . . . One man had fourteen distinct holes in his intestine, all of which had to be sewn up. Such an operation leads to considerable shock. And both for shock and loss of blood the best treatment is transfusion of blood, and plenty of it . . . When we began the patient reminded me of one of the great Spanish paintings of the dead Christ. As the blood entered his veins, his face changed from dead white to pale pink. As Dr. Bethune sewed up the vein . . . he tried to speak but he was still too feeble. But as

we left him he braced himself, raised his clenched fist to his forehead, and gave us the red front salute."[34]

At some point in the latter half of December 1936 – the precise date is not known – Bethune encountered Kajsa Hellin Rothman; later, in January, they became lovers. Born in Karlstad, Sweden, in 1903, she moved to Paris after completing school, supporting herself as a nanny and by writing newspaper articles. At twenty-two she joined a competitive dance troupe traveling across Europe and North Africa, but in Cairo, the organizers absconded with the troupe's prize money, and she moved to Romania where, for a further two years, she again worked as a nanny. By 1934 she had moved to Barcelona, where she was employed by a travel agency. Details of Rothman's life in Barcelona are unclear. The Great Depression had undermined the Spanish economy as deeply as that of any European country, and it may be that the travel agency simply floundered and failed. In any event, by July 1936, Rothman appears to have become unemployed: she was reduced to marathon dancing – a form of couples dancing in which the truly impoverished shuffled across the dance floor day and night, day after day, until only a single couple remained on their feet and were awarded a meager prize. Rothman was in the twelfth day of a marathon dance when the Fascist revolt was declared. Despite having no medical training, she immediately volunteered with the Red Cross and was apparently assigned to an anarchist militia unit, the *Columna de Hierro* – the "Pillar of Iron."[35]

For reasons which are, again, unclear, Kajsa Rothman left Barcelona and the anarchist unit, and went to Madrid where she joined the Scottish Ambulance Unit in late September or the beginning of October. The Scottish Ambulance unit was run by the puritanical and politically ambiguous Fernanda Jacobsen described as "an incredible woman, small and square, with a huge bottom. She always dresses in a kilt, thick woolen stockings, brogues, a khaki jacket of military cut with thistles all over it, huge leather gauntlet gloves, a cape also with thistles, and, the crowning glory, a little black Scottish hat edged with tartan and with a large silver badge on it."[36] Jacobsen diverted food intended for the Republic to fascist sympathizers who had taken refuge in the British Embassy, and helped smuggle Franco supporters out of the country. Later, Jacobsen would claim that Rothman was expelled from the Scottish Unit for "immorality," but it is equally possible that Rothman left on her own volition, as other members of the unit eventually did, disgusted by Jacobsen's pro-fascist activities. Whatever the circumstances of the departure, Rothman was briefly detained by Spanish government authorities, but soon released. Shortly thereafter she met Bethune and began to work at the Blood Transfusion

Based on Blood

Institute headquarters as a secretary, greeting and registering blood donors in the reception room.[37]

Bethune developed an intense affection for Rothman. She has been variously described as "a big, blond Swede whose striking appearance and warm nature had made her a well-known figure in Madrid"; and as a "handsome giantess with red-gold flowing hair."[38] How soon Bethune fell in love with her it is difficult to say. Quite possibly they slept together very early on. Certainly there was more to the affair, from Bethune's point of view, than simply Kajsa's stunning beauty. He was *happy* with her, in a way he had not been with any woman since Elizabeth Wallace. And Rothman, even if she may not have been in love with Bethune, was devoted to him; she took care of him and made sure he took care of himself. Always helpful, always ready to do whatever needed to be done, always there to talk to and to listen; she was his companion as much as his lover. It is possible to say that, in a certain sense she *mothered* him – she took the place, unconsciously – of the mother he had always wished he had: this was his constant need and Rothman could be and was, for a time, that woman.

But all of the intense activity of the early weeks in Madrid – establishing the Blood Transfusion Unit, collecting blood, distributing the blood to the hospitals, talking with the boys in the trenches, visiting the front lines with Vera Elkan, clambering through the fields to retrieve evidence of Nazi collaboration with Franco, the evening radio broadcasts, finding love with Kasja Rothman – was brought to a strange hiatus by the events of 4 January 1937. Henning Sorensen, motivated by suspicion, and possibly resentment, had informed a senior official at the Socorro Rojo that there were large numbers of foreigners constantly gathering at the Blood Transfusion Institute; the official informed the police. On 4 January, the police raided the Institute. A full list of those who were detained appears to be unavailable, but everyone present in the building was taken into custody including Bethune, Sise, and Sorensen himself. The SRI took responsibility for the Canadian team and ensured their immediate release. Among others, the prominent Norwegian antifascist journalist, Lise Lindbaek, was detained and released. Haldane was taken to the War Office and subsequently released. Kajsa Rothman was not set free until sometime later, after being interrogated and her police records checked. Commander Herrmann Hartung, an Austrian, who worked as a Press Censor with the Foreign Propaganda service was arrested; quite possibly a spy, he somehow avoided execution and survived the war. Bethune was familiar with Hartung since it was through him that he had mailed letters intended for Ben Spence of the CASD, and others intended for a variety of foreign press offices – letters that Hartung never sent. Other individuals that congregated at the

Institute included Claud Cockburn, Vera Elkan, and probably the reporters and correspondents who often accompanied her: Philip Jordan of the *News Chronicle*, Herbert Matthews of the *New York Times*, Tom Wintringham of the *Daily Worker*, and certainly George Marion[39]

We may ask ourselves why there were so many people unconnected to the Blood Transfusion Unit gathering at the Institute. The answer is both two-fold and quite simple. Firstly, it will be recalled that when Bethune lived in Montreal he never locked his door; his apartment was always open to visitors, artists, writers, and political activists who were welcome to eat and drink, to read and to discuss, whether he was present or not; he did not change this habit of generosity in Spain, at least not initially. Secondly, as we have already noted, Bethune understood the immense value of propaganda, as apparently Sorensen did not. While Bethune, Sise, and Haldane lent themselves to the government short-wave service, Sorensen, despite his fluency in a number of languages, never did. It was important to Bethune to court the foreign correspondents who had descended on Madrid in such large numbers and to invite them to the Institute; any reporting on the Blood Transfusion Institute benefited not only the Institute but the Republican government; apparently Sorensen did not grasp this elemental point.

But there are more serious issues involved. Sorensen went behind Bethune's back and, in terms of the chain of command, over his head, with his baseless complaints and suspicions. While it is true that Sorensen's official function was to act as liaison officer with the SRI and the Spanish doctors, the question remains: why did he do what he did? The obvious answer is to save the Blood Transfusion Unit. But to save it *for* whom and *from* whom? To save it for the Spanish people, clearly, but from what? And here the only answer can be to save it from what Sorensen falsely perceived as Bethune's incompetence, from his inability to lead the unit effectively, to be able to recognize the difference between a comrade and a spy. In short, to save the Canadian unit from *its single and sole Canadian physician and the unit's recognized leader*. It is notable that Sorensen did not take his discomfort and suspicions to Bethune himself. In an interview given over thirty years later, Sorensen repeated twice that he found the other Canadians in the unit "naïve about spies" and that he suspected Kajsa "was a spy and stole money from the Institute."[40] And yet, as far as can be determined, he was mistaken: the only probable spy was Hartung; Kajsa Rothman was not. And so the circle of trust within the Institute became irrevocably broken, *even if it was not immediately recognized as such*. We shall see that conflicts, jealousies, mutual suspicions, eventually destroyed the Institute, and that Sorensen's role in this did not diminish; quite the contrary. But these repercussions were in fact *not* immediately evident, although it is difficult to believe that Bethune, with his always fragile sense of self-valorization, did not harbor from this point forward, a true resentment towards Sorensen.

Nevertheless, despite the events of 4 January, the short-wave broadcasts continued as they had before. Haldane apparently spoke on the very night of 4 January, Bethune on the 5th, Haldane again on the 6th and 13th. Sise, on 12 January, spoke most movingly of how the Socorro Rojo had raised enough money to distribute Christmas presents to the children of Madrid on the traditional Twelfth Night of 6 January, despite the presence of constant fascist shelling.[41] On the other hand, there may be some significance to the fact that these were the last of the radio broadcasts, and that some of them may have been previously taped; it is unlikely, after all, that Haldane would have spoken on 4 January, and there are indications that he had left Spain and returned to London prior to his broadcast of 13 January.[42] Whether the broadcasts were discontinued on the initiative of the government, or of Bethune's team, or whether they were simply no longer required, it is impossible now to say, but none of these broadcasts gave any inkling that Bethune or the others were in any way unsettled by being detained. Nor does Bethune's letter to Spence on 11 January give any direct reference to the police raid other than the postscript which reads: "I nearly forgot to mention the reason you received so little news of me in December was I gave letters to the Foreign Propaganda Chief who was arrested a week ago as a suspected spy. None were sent out! . . . There are too many fascist spies here."[43] This latter comment suggesting that Bethune was not as naïve as Sorensen thought.

The work of the Blood Transfusion Unit did not falter. Donors continued to arrive; blood continued to be distributed. But still, the worm was in the apple and the sequence of events set into motion by Sorensen's startling and unfounded lack of trust in Bethune would poison the Institute within a few short weeks and bring it to the edge of self-destruction.

13

I Would Not Be Anywhere Else

The siege of Madrid came in waves. Mola's deadly troops had been stalled. On 6 November, Franco announced that he would enter the city and take mass the next day. He did not. With the strength and courage of the Communist Fifth Regiment in the lead, and the unwavering support of the International Brigades, Madrid held out until the very end: 28 March 1939, when the arrests, and the firing squads, and the mass murder began.

On 11 January, Bethune reported to Spence that Madrid was under the heaviest attack since November. Fresh German-Nazi troops had led a fierce ground assault, but were being successfully repelled by Republican machine guns and the shock troops of the International Brigades. Even so, the city was under constant air bombardment and artillery shelling; fifth columnists engaged in intermittent sniping from windows and rooftops: thousands of non-combatants had been killed. After the bombing, what remained of the bodies was removed and the streets hosed clean of blood. Workmen took shovels and dug into the bombed-out buildings and brought out the dead bodies, many of them children; their small corpses horrified Bethune and drew both his deepest indignation and most profound sympathy:[1] all children were always his children; every wounded child always himself. Still, Bethune wrote, "Madrid is the centre of gravity of the world and I wouldn't be anywhere else."[2]

In the midst of this renewed assault, Bethune did an interview at the Telephonica building with Frederick Griffin, of the *Toronto Star*. Sise recalled that on this, or perhaps on a similar occasion, he and Bethune had gone on a number of errands, and that Bethune appeared to be "carefully timing our trip from one shop to another so we would arrive at the Telephonica building at four o'clock. Madrid was shelled at that time with typical German thoroughness, punctually, sharp at four o'clock every after-noon. So his idea was obviously to get inside the target at the moment it was going to be shelled and that's exactly what happened." Sise attributes this to Bethune's "complete contempt for danger," and his belief that "Bethune really got a kick out of being in dangerous situations." While there is some truth to Sise's observations, he appears to have forgotten that the Telephonica was one of the safest locations in Madrid. It was immensely sturdy and well-constructed, and despite its height – it was the tallest building in Madrid – and its function as the central communications center in the city, both of which made it an obvious target for fascist attack, there were very few casualties among its occupants during the entire period of the war.[3]

The Griffin interview was taken, then, as high explosive shells hit the Telephonica. Bethune spoke enthusiastically about the blood transfusion service, barely pausing to remark, after a direct hit caused the building to shudder: "he's got the range all right." Central to his concerns was the issue of malnutrition. "One thing we've got to watch in testing our donors," he said:

> is any sign of diminishing nutrition or of falling hemoglobin as a result of people not getting enough food . . . if this siege goes on and if the food situation should grow worse, such a nutritional drop is inevitable and the hemoglobin in the blood will suffer. Then we might have difficulty getting blood, for we would have to be careful not to rob impoverished blood of precious hemoglobin.

On the related issue of blood preservation, Bethune observed that he did not know how long donated blood could be kept, but "we have an idea that we can keep such blood very much longer than has yet been thought possible. We may find out some very interesting things in this work." The ultimate solution would be to develop a completely artificial blood; to extract the red blood cells and add them to a chemically prepared serum. "That," Bethune said, "is the problem we would like to solve."[4]

It is evident that Bethune saw the Blood Transfusion Institute as more than a vehicle for the vitally necessary transportation of blood to the wounded at the front; it was intended to solve, or at least to begin to solve, the many mysteries of blood – its cellular and intracellular nature, what caused it to decay, how long it could be preserved; some weeks later he would begin to probe into whether the blood from human cadavers could revive the living. Already in early January, Bethune had moved from the more difficult gravity method of blood transfusion, where blood was poured into a canula sewn into to vein, to the simpler, easier, and less painful method employing needles and a syringe pump. In mid-December Bethune had been faced with the problem of determining whether a donor's blood was infected with syphilis. Initially, he found a private laboratory able to provide the standard Wasserman test. However, the doctor who applied the test reported a number of positive reactions so far below the known national estimate that Bethune terminated his services; a police investigation indicated that the doctor was a fascist sympathizer. By the time of the Griffin interview, a new laboratory had been located.[5]

Despite Bethune's absolute commitment to the antifascist struggle, both in its political and military aspects, as well as in its specific expression in the Blood Transfusion Institute, he was not free of the contradictions that remained within him following his joining the Communist Party more than a year previously: that is to say, the contradiction between the solidarity of the communist militant – a solidarity of equality – and the "generosity from above" of the individualist artist. Nor did he become free of the complex structures of his personality, deriving from primal unlove, simply by coming to Spain's defense. Sise, having in truth only known Bethune a matter of weeks, referred to him, with a certain degree of exaggeration, as "a sybarite," who "loved good living and saw no contradiction between doing good work for humanity and enjoying the pleasures of this world."[6] But the contradiction existed nonetheless. In London, while locating the supplies he would need for blood transfusion, he took the time to purchase an expensive set of monogrammed silk shirts – with funds provided by the CASD.[7] On the few occasions when he went to Paris on Institute business, he would attend a championship tennis game with Ted Farah, a Canadian reporter, or dine at the best restaurants, ordering champagne with Louis Huot, another reporter, but in Madrid he could eat little more than lentils for days on end without complaint.[8] He could be rude and even arrogant. Always impatient to get the work done – the transfusions, the interviews, the radio broadcasts, the organization of the Institute – he would explode quickly into irritation or anger, and as quickly calm down and apologize; often Sise or Sorensen would have to soothe the offended party. In a Madrid bank, anxious to be on his way, Bethune asked Sorensen, as his interpreter, to demand that the teller serve him first, before the other people who were waiting in line. Afterwards, Sorensen remonstrated with Bethune saying, quite correctly, "a Party member should not behave that way;"(a further indication of Sorensen's own secret Party status).[9] At the same time, Bethune was fully and consciously aware of himself as a Communist, proud of his Party membership; in a café he could suddenly launch into a disquisition on the potential of socialism, often enough to those who understood the issues as well or better than he did: Haldane, for example, would listen politely and then respond with a certain irony, "Yes, teacher."[10] Without unduly simplifying, it is possible to say that in work, Bethune was a Communist and expected others to work with the same dedication; when he was not working he became the bourgeois artist: it was a serious contradiction, and the direction of its eventual resolution would lead through the complex ramifications set it motion by Sorensen's role in the 4 January police raid, and wend its way through to Bethune's final days in Spain.

At some point early in January, the Institute began to expand. Two Spanish doctors had been attached, probably by the SRI, to the personnel already working there: Vicente Goyanes and Antonio Culebras joined Sanz and de la Loma. Bethune saw in this collaboration between Canadians and Spanish a living example of the Popular Front policy that had sent him to Spain, and a necessary expression of Marxist internationalism. He was as eager to establish working connections with the Spanish medical system, as he was to maintain the identity of the Canadian unit. Impressed with the results he had already achieved in Madrid, Bethune approached the SRI with a plan to establish a unified system that would deliver blood to every fighting front in Republican Spain: wherever men were fighting back the fascists, blood transfusion would be immediately available. The SRI was sympathetic, but suggested to him that a plan of such scope would need to be authorized by the Sanidad Militar (the military health authority) in Valencia.[11]

On the afternoon of 11 January, Bethune left with Sorensen for Valencia in the Ford station wagon; Kajsa Rothman was needed at the Institute, and it was with much regret that he left his lover behind. At Valencia, Bethune met with Colonel Cerrada, the head of the Sanidad Militar. Sorensen translated while Bethune reiterated the plan he had outlined to the SRI. Cerrada was in full agreement. The plan made sense; every soldier was needed, none that could be saved should be lost. Bethune assured Cerrada that the CASD would cover the costs, but Cerrada made the point that no unified blood service would be possible without the cooperation of Dr. Frederic Duran-Jorda.[12]

In Barcelona, Duran-Jorda had established a blood bank system at the outset of the war, using the latest discoveries of, among others, Soviet physicians. It was operating at a relatively high technological level: donor blood was introduced into glass ampoules under gas pressure, and each ampoule was packaged with a sterilized needle and all the other necessary equipment for immediate transfusion. Moreover, the blood from six different donors of the same blood group was pooled into a single bottle, leading to less danger of adverse reactions on the part of the recipient. Duran-Jorda's blood bank had been limited to Barcelona and the surrounding area, a zone that was militarily quiescent for the major part of the war; its chief virtue was not, therefore, in its direct aid to the wounded, but in its advanced scientific sophistication, and in the extremely large number of donors he had registered.[13]

Bethune was not unfamiliar with Duran-Jorda's work. Early on he had informed himself about the situation in Barcelona where, fortunately, food shortages, and therefore the potential for malnutrition, were not as serious a problem. It would be necessary now to go to Duran-Jorda, to learn from him as a scientist, and to join forces with him as a militant.

Bethune left Cerrada's office and the next day he and Sorensen went to Barcelona and checked into the Hotel Continental. He spent the following two or three days with Duran-Jorda, examining his equipment and procedures, and absorbing his superior technique in blood preservation, before suggesting to him his proposal. Like Cerrada, Duran-Jorda was amenable to the plan. An agreement was reached: Barcelona would be the main collecting center for donated blood, which would then be sealed into sterilized bottles; this blood would be transported to Valencia, Madrid, and Cordoba, (the latter, southern, location was soon changed to nearby Jaen); Bethune and Sorensen would operate their original service out of Madrid, in conjunction with the bottles from Barcelona; Sise would be the principal driver from Barcelona to the various other fronts.[14]

Bethune cabled Spence in Toronto for permission to purchase a new, and much larger, truck and to send out a second driver to work with Sise: as it happened, no new driver was sent: Bethune found a willing recruit in Barcelona a week later. He then wrote to Sise in Madrid, requesting him to come to Barcelona. Bethune had already bought the equipment necessary to transform the new truck into a self-sufficient refrigerator car, and Sise was to outfit the new vehicle as soon as it was purchased.[15]

On 16 January, Bethune and Sorensen drove north from Barcelona, across the Pyrenees, then up to Paris to receive funds from the CASD; they then drove south again to the French seaport of Marseilles. Here they were able to obtain a two and a half ton Renault truck entirely adequate to their purposes. While in Marseilles, Bethune suggested that he and Sorensen make use of one of the city's many whorehouses. Later, coming out of his room, he said to Sorensen, "Now I'm refueled. Let's go." Earlier, in Madrid, Bethune had encountered Sorensen as he left Rothman in his bedroom: he had rubbed his hands together and said, "Here's a man who has just had a perfect fuck."[16] What's more, at about the same time, Greenspan had gone to Bethune's bedroom with some papers she needed him to examine. She knocked on the door and Bethune called for her to enter. Finding him naked in bed with Kajsa, she turned to leave, but Bethune disregarded her embarrassment and insisted on checking the papers without delay.[17] It is easily possible to misunderstand these incidents as expressing a simple extraverted exhibitionism. But we have seen that Bethune's exhibitionism, as far back as it can be traced it into his childhood was never simple; it always served

I Would Not Be Anywhere Else

the function of requiring that Others validate him *externally*, since he felt no permanent *internal* value: the Dragon's unlove had seen to that. Whether it was his professional competence, courage, or sexuality, invisible eyes were always upon him, measuring, judging, condemning. This profound unconscious need for valorization, which comes down in the end to the infant Bethune's consuming desire for his mother's love, had forced a deep division within him between love and sex. His lasting love for Frances Penney endured beyond and above any sexual component; or, in the case of Marian Scott or Elizabeth Wallace, entirely without it. But Bethune's sexuality, no matter whether his partner was merely one of many ultimately unfulfilling brief encounters, or a bourgeoning love affair, as it was with Kajsa Rothman, is an *inhibited* sexuality, as we have seen. When Bethune leaves a room and tells another man that he is "refueled," or has had "a perfect fuck," he is attempting to convince Others that this is true, *only in order to convince himself*. According to Sorensen, who appears to have been unusually perspicacious in this, "Bethune liked the conquest, but he was not very good in bed. He liked to impress people with his conquests, but had little fun out of sex."[18] Little fun, and less fulfillment.

Meanwhile, in Madrid, the work continued. Sise was distributing blood to the hospitals in the city and the nearby fronts, and assisting de la Loma. In a letter home, he described one of these transfusions:

> With a can of hot water I warmed up the bottle of nearly ice-cold blood while Loma lays out the little gleaming syringe-pump and examines the veins at the crook of the man's arm. The shells began falling closer, rattling the windows and making the instruments jump about in their glass cases. . . . The anesthetist grins cheerfully and sprinkles the ether. A doctor grunts. . . . Loma slipped in the needle and we started connecting the tubes, I holding the syringe, our arms intertwined in a complicated way. . . . The surgeons quickly sew up one wound in the abdomen and start on the leg. Loma begins to pump. Soon a doctor mumbles "350 cc is enough" and we're finished. We wash up, pack up, and as we turn to the door they call softly, over their shoulders, "Salud!"[19]

But not everything was going well. In a series of hand-written notes to himself, Sise had written: "Consolidation. Goyanes & Culebras. Beginning of xenophobia."[20] Evidently the two new Spanish doctors did not entirely appreciate the presence of the Canadians in the Blood Transfusion Institute. Within the larger situation of the war this was an unusual and peculiar sentiment. The Republican government was more than eager for whatever help they could obtain in an unequal war against fascism. The International

Brigades were considered heroic fighters who were risking, and frequently losing, their lives in the defense of Spanish democracy. Certainly the Spanish people, the proletariat and all the laboring classes, looked upon the foreigners who had come to their aid with immense affection. But the Spanish doctors, and especially Goyanes and Culebras, were in no sense proletarians; perhaps they imagined that their professional territory was being invaded by these outsiders and that they were entirely competent to run the blood transfusion service and the Institute without the Canadian interlopers.[21] In a sense this was true. But it was never a matter of competence, only of vision and diligence and the ability to force a situation through a complex bureaucracy towards a successful conclusion: the very qualities that Bethune had employed to bring the Institute into being. Furthermore, and perhaps even more importantly, Bethune was a Communist. He worked as a Communist; that is to say, with extreme dedication and commitment; he understood, as was common knowledge, that in battle it was the Communists who did most of the fighting, and in every sphere of activity were the most organized and efficient; he expected the Spanish doctors to work as Communists, to work as he himself did.[22] Goyanes was simply a doctor who happened to find himself living in the Republican zone. Indeed, at the end of the war, Goyanes was not shot by the Fascists, as he was likely to have been for aiding the Republican forces. Instead, he was interned in a concentration camp, escaped, and was subsequently exonerated by a military court. Without any apparent regret, he gave Dr. Elosegui, the head of Franco's fascist army transfusion service, "a detailed account of all the material and stock held by the Madrid center, and in the first paragraph of the report he included the material provided by Canadian aid." Culebras, on the other hand, while a member of the Communist Party of Spain, came into increasing conflict with Bethune and appears to have begun, toward the end of their time together, to virtually spy on Bethune and file possibly false or exaggerated reports on him to the Spanish authorities. What became of Culebras is more obscure.[23]

Possibly connected to the issue of xenophobia, Sise wrote in his notes, somewhat cryptically, that, "In Beth's absence – slow organization at Madrid – Kajsa language difficulty – recruitment of donors – Paulino – Radio." It is difficult to know precisely what these jottings mean. Why was organization slow? Bethune had worked unstintingly to establish and expand the Institute; he had only been absent from Madrid for a matter of days when this note was written. Did it imply that the Spanish and non-Spanish members of the Institute were having some difficulty integrating their activities? Did it imply that the number of blood donors had suddenly decreased, as the phrase "recruitment of donors" possibly suggests? And

I Would Not Be Anywhere Else

125

what, then is the connection between "slow organization," "recruitment of donors," and "Kajsa language difficulty," a phrase which Sise has underlined? Kajsa Rothman spoke Spanish; she was certainly capable of continuing the local radio broadcasts in search of new donors, although this seems never to have been one of her regular tasks. It is worth bearing in mind that Bethune's official translator, Henning Sorensen, was with him in Paris and Marseilles, and so the job of translation might well have fallen to her. But for whom, then, would she be translating? Everyone at the Institute spoke Spanish, except Sise. Was it a matter of translating between Sise and the Institute doctors, or perhaps between Sise, the Spanish doctors, and wounded patients of the International Brigades? It is doubtful that we will ever know what "Kajsa language difficulty" means, but the fact that Sise thought it important enough to underline is intriguing. The reference to "Paulino" is easier to interpret: Sergeant Paulino had newly been seconded to the Institute as the Assistant Secretary, and was responsible for the registration of blood donors, and the keeping of blood records, the daily reports, and the Institute diary. The final term, "Radio," might suggest that Paulino was also responsible for blood donor recruitment over the airwaves. In any event, while the details remain obscure, the general situation seems to have been one of increasing difficulties within the Institute exacerbated by xenophobic chauvinism and a certain degree of conflict or confusion between its members.[24]

Seven days after leaving for Paris and Marseilles, on 22 January, Bethune and Sorensen arrived back in Barcelona with the new Renault truck. Sise was waiting for them, and after he and Bethune visited Duran-Jorda to examine his truck, he spent the next ten days outfitting the Renault with bunk beds, batteries, a refrigerator, and a donkey engine – a heavy kerosene powered winch.[25] And it was in Barcelona that Sise introduced Bethune to Thomas Cuthbert Worsley, and possibly to Stephen Spender.

Worsley, a resolute antifascist, had arrived in Spain, on 6 January, with Spender, a noted poet and writer, and briefly a member of the Communist Party of Great Britain. Harry Pollitt, the leader of the CPGB, had asked them to find out what had happened to the crew of a Soviet ship, the *Comsomol*, which had been torpedoed by the Italians while it was bringing aid to the Republican government. Worsley and Spender had traveled south and crossed Franco's lines into fascist controlled territory: Cadiz and Gibraltar, where, it was discovered, the *Comsomol* crew had been interned. Their dangerous mission accomplished, they made their way back north to Barcelona where they arrived on 20 January and flew back to London two days later – the very day Bethune and Sorensen had arrived from Marseilles. Although Worsley could only have been acquainted with Sise for a day or two, and with Bethune for a few hours, it was somehow arranged that Worsley would no sooner arrive in London than he would return to Barcelona to join the Canadian Blood Transfusion Unit as an ambulance driver; an auxiliary driver to accompany Sise in the new Renault in bringing blood to the front lines.[26]

Worsley and Spender had had another, and more personal reason to come to Spain: they were both lovers of Tony Hyndman, a former Coldstream Guard and male prostitute; a man who was, in Worsley's words, "a real tart, a really high class tart." Hyndman had joined the International Brigades, but neither Worsley nor Spender had been able to contact him. At least part of Worsley's purpose in returning to join Bethune's unit, was that it would give him the opportunity to seek out Hyndman. Spender would return for the same purpose on 20 February,[27] and on at least one occasion, between 9 and 18 March, when he was in Madrid, he met and spent some time with Bethune.[28]

From Barcelona, Bethune intended to return to Madrid via Valencia. Sorensen was unable to accompany him: he had developed a serious case of bronchitis. Bethune prescribed medicine and told him to stay at the hotel and rest. He then drove the Ford wagon to Valencia and reported to Cerrada on Duran-Jorda's agreement to their proposal. Funding was worked out: the CASD would pay the salaries of the Canadians, and the Sanidad Militar would pay for the Spaniards. The CASD would further pay for the necessary equipment in Madrid, and make a contribution toward the costs of the blood distribution center in Valencia. Cerrada drew up and signed a contract that he was to have authorized by the Ministry of War.[29]

Bethune returned to Madrid, where he remained for a week, until about 2 February. Presumably, during these several days, blood was transported to the hospitals in the city and at the nearby fronts, and transfusions performed. Possibly there were arguments between Bethune and Goyanes and Culebras, although he seems always to have had quite friendly relations with de la Loma.[30] Bethune had forgotten to allocate funds for the Spaniards salaries while he had been away and had to apologize, at the same time pointing out that the new arrangement with Cerrada would guarantee their income.[31]

But it is possible also that at this time blood donations may have begun to fall off somewhat at the Institute. Celia Greenspan resigned her position, and with a letter of reference from Bethune,[32] she left Madrid and traveled to Murcia, a city close to the Mediterranean, several kilometers to the south of Valencia. There she visited her friends Jan Kurzke and Kate Mangan. Kurzke, who had been involved in anti-Nazi work, had fled Germany in 1933 for London where he met Mangan. With the outbreak of the war he had gone to Spain to join the German section of the International Brigades. Mangan lost contact with him and came to Spain in an effort to find him. She spent some months working at the press office in Valencia, where she joined the Communist Party of Spain. She eventually found Kurzke, wounded and seriously ill.[33] Mangan had met Hazen Sise several months ago at a London cocktail party, and had become reacquainted with him in Madrid where her husband Kurzke had been taken. Bethune had given him morphine and sent him to Murcia for an operation on his leg. Greenspan told Mangan and Kurzke that Bethune had temporarily given up collecting blood in Madrid since the people had become too malnourished to be healthy donors; she no longer had a functioning job.[34] Whether this was entirely accurate is open to question. Sise had said that there was never a time when donors did not flock to the Institute. It was true that Bethune was concerned about malnutrition, and the new arrangement with Duran-Jorda would have mitigated his concerns, but it is highly unlikely that he ever gave up blood collection in Madrid; at most there may have been a very temporary decline in new donors.

Bethune had no doubt that large-scale blood donations would eventually be re-established in Madrid, but what was important now was putting into practice the unified blood service that he had elaborated with Duran-Jorda and the Sanidad Militar; everything appeared to be ready. In recognition of this important new undertaking, the Spanish authorities had appointed him as director-in-chief and given him the honorary military rank of Comandante; Sise and Sorensen had been made Captains. It was in this context that the name of the Canadian medical unit was officially re-named as the *Instituto Hispano-Canadiense de Transfusion de Sangre* – no doubt as an acknowledgement of the important role that Duran-Jorda's Institute was also playing in this new venture.[35]

By the end of January Worsley returned from London to Barcelona to join Sise. On 31 January, Bethune made his way to Valencia, where Sise and Worsley were to meet him with the newly refurbished truck and several bottles of Duran-Jorda's blood. He had contacted Sorensen to join them, but his condition had worsened and he had been sent to a hospital.[36] While waiting for Sise and Worsley, Bethune met again with Cerrada, who informed him that shortly all medical facilities would be integrated under the control of the Sanidad Militar, but that, unfortunately, the Ministry of War had not yet approved the proposal for the unified blood transfusion service. He assured Bethune that if he returned on 6 February he would have final approval.[37] For Bethune, it was a moment of great triumph; of the concrete realization of a vastly important vision: he cabled the CASD to inform them of what had occurred:

We have succeeded in unifying all remaining Spanish transfusion units under us. We are serving 100 hospitals and casualty clearing stations in the front lines of Madrid and 100 kilometres from the front of the sector Del Centro. . . . We now have a staff of twenty-five, composed of a haematologist, bacteriologist, five Spanish doctors, three assistants, six nurses, four technicians, chauffers and servants. . . . We collected and gave ten gallons of blood during January. Expect to increase this to twenty-five gallons during this month. This is the first unified blood transfusion service in army and medical history. Plans are well under way to supply the entire Spanish anti-fascist army preserved blood. Your institute is now operating on a 1,000 kilometre front. I must leave for Paris immediately to buy fifty additional transfusion apparatuses. The Madrid Defence Junta has given us two new cars. We now have five cars operating here day and night in this sector. I have contracted with an English professional photographer to make a movie film of the work of the Institute for the Canadian public.[38]

As it happened, Bethune did not immediately go to Paris. On 6 February, Cerrada told him that he still did not have government confirmation.[39] But that no longer mattered to Bethune; signatures could wait. Rumors had been circulating about a massive new fascist assault in the south: they turned out to be true. Malaga was under attack; a bloodbath had begun; Bethune would go where he was needed.

14
Slaughter of the Innocents

General Queipo de Llano leaned into the microphone at the radio station in Seville: "The first sentence that we shall pronounce in Malaga is the death sentence."[1] He was true to his word.

The city of Malaga lay on the Mediterranean coastline not far from the southern tip of Gibraltar, hemmed in by the sea on one side and high mountains on the other. It was a city of one hundred thousand; swelled further by thousands of starving refugees. Three fascist columns had converged on the city: two led by Franco's officers, and the third composed of ten thousand Italian troops under General Mario Roatta. From the sea, it was bombed by Franco's cruisers, the *Canarias* and the *Baleares*; from the air by Italian aircraft and German Nazi Messerschmits. The assault on the civilian population was far worse than had been unleashed against Madrid: the bombing was more intense and concentrated; the target, civilian homes, were often flimsy and without cellars for shelter. The Nazi aircraft swooped down so low into the streets that, from ground level, the terrified townspeople could clearly observe the airborne machine-gunners engaged in their deadly work. In scattering crowds, the people ran – even though there was nowhere to run. The number of murdered is still unknown. On 8 February the fascists entered Malaga. During the first week alone they executed hundreds of men suspected of sympathizing with the legitimate government; in the weeks that followed 1600 more were lined up against the walls and shot.[2]

Paris was no longer possible. The newly required transfusion equipment would have to wait. Bethune called the members of his unit together. Sise and Worsley would return to Barcelona and fill the Renault's refrigerators with Duran-Jorda's blood ampoules. Bethune would wait for them in Valencia. The Republican forces at the front lines in Malaga would certainly require as much blood as Bethune could bring them; there was no other functioning transfusion service in the south. As important secondary issues, the very long journey to Malaga would provide a practical test of Bethune's blood preservation technique and of the quality of the truck's refrigeration system and other re-fittings, as well as allowing a general survey of the needs of the southern fronts.[3] It is probable that while he was waiting in Valencia,

Bethune met with Tina Modotti and Vittorio Vidali, both of whom had been summoned to the Socorro Rojo's Valencia headquarters to discuss the gravity of the situation unfolding in the south. In any event, it would appear to have been decided that Modotti and her friend Matilde Landa would go to Malaga on a humanitarian mission, and their paths crossed with Bethune's, as we shall see, at the crucial moment.[4]

The day before leaving for Malaga, Bethune, Sise, Worsley, and Claud Cockburn – who was coincidentally in Valencia – lay on the floor of their room in the Hotel Victoria examining a map and planning their route south and then west: Valencia, Murcia, Almeria, Malaga. Cockburn told them that when they arrived at Motril, a town halfway between Almeria and Malaga, they should not stop but drive through as quickly as possible as there was a considerable degree of political instability in the town. Pressed for details, he would say no more; much of what had happened, and was still happening, in the Malaga area remained mysterious and largely unreported. Still, Sise suspected that Cockburn, with his intimate political connections, knew more than he was permitted to reveal under conditions of war; a suspicion that was entirely valid: Cockburn had in fact recently been in Malaga and observed its repeated bombing.[5]

On 7 February, they left Valencia; Bethune in the Ford truck he had driven down from Madrid, Sise and Worsley in the Renault. South of Valencia they were met by a blinding sandstorm, but Bethune insisted on pushing through until they were forced to stop at Alicante, a city less than half the distance to Malaga.[6] Unfortunately, it was then discovered that the Renault's refrigeration machinery had failed: the dynamo that charged the refrigerator's batteries was damaged by repeated jolting on the rough roads and could neither be repaired nor replaced. From then on the truck's refrigerator would have to be manually plugged in to city circuits wherever they rested: with a rise of temperature, the blood would quickly spoil and be rendered useless. Happily, it was still early in February, the weather was very cold, and the town of Murcia was only eighty-five kilometers distant from Alicante. Murcia was home to an International Brigade hospital and was an intended stop on their itinerary.[7]

Bethune came to Murcia for two reasons; one professional, and the other somewhat more personal. Certainly he was carrying out his mandate to discover the medical and blood transfusion requirements of the hospitals along the southern fronts, and no doubt the International Brigade hospital was of particular importance in this regard. He spent the day of his arrival and the next day inquiring into the hospital's needs, and discussing the new unified blood transfusion system with the medical personnel.[8] But he had also promised Kate Mangan that he would look in on her husband Jan,

Slaughter of the Innocents   **131**

check on his recovery, and advise if further treatment was required.[9]

The problem of the broken refrigeration system remained: there was still some three hundred kilometers between Murcia and the undoubted hundreds, if not thousands, of wounded soldiers in Malaga. Clearly there was no going back. Bethune left his Ford truck in Murcia and joined Sise and Worsley in the Renault. They would need to stop in Cartagena to plug in the refrigerator, and again further south in Almeria, or even cool the blood in the fast-moving mountain streams if necessary. But one way or another they were determined that the blood would be taken to the wounded.

Bethune never arrived at Malaga. As the blood transfusion truck arrived in Almeria, 170 kilometers east of Malaga, they heard that the city had fallen to the fascists, but no one they spoke with knew precisely what had happened. Officials at the SRI in Almeria said that Malaga had fallen and that there had been attacks on fleeing civilians, but details were difficult to ascertain. Bethune intended to find out. There was only a single road connecting Almeria to Malaga, and as they continued along it, it began to rain. Sise later recalled that:

> then we ran into this pathetic procession of people, first little crowds, then thicker and thicker. The sun went down, it became dusk, and still this river of humanity came driving against us. . . . And Bethune, while we drove, was muttering and cursing to himself, and while the light still lasted he stopped the car, called me to get out the Leica camera, and take pictures of these refugees. We went on until nine or ten o'clock that night and in a little village people told us that the fascists were only a few kilometers ahead and that we shouldn't go any further. At this point Bethune had been so deeply moved . . . about this ragged procession of humanity, and the large numbers of children which we had begun to count, and we counted something like four or five thousand, and so he suddenly made the decision, in his characteristic way, that we would . . . forget about our stored blood for transfusions, and just try to save as many children as possible. We turned the truck around – the big truck – and began loading it with children, including two pregnant women in their last period – and we got nearly thirty jammed in and banged the doors closed. I drove it back with . . . Tom Worsley to Almeria, dropped the children off at one of the Socorro Rojo hospitals, went to the civic governor, reported to him this terrible crowd of people . . . on that road in terrible condition.[10]

Bethune, Sise, and Worsley were observing the head of a ragged column of perhaps a hundred thousand refugees fleeing the greatest atrocity in the

Spanish war. Not content to simply lay waste to Malaga, the fascists began to attack its people as they fled. Ten kilometers east of Malaga, two fascist aircraft dropped low out of the sky and began to machine-gun screaming women, infants, men with children on their shoulders. Two hours later, a fascist cruiser and a destroyer began shelling the desperate crowd from the sea. Bodies were smashed apart; others were buried under boulders blown out of the cliffs. For two days the refugees were shelled and strafed from both air and sea; at night, searchlights from the ships illuminated their targets and made them easy prey; behind them Italian troops rushed up the road in pursuit.[11]

At first, Sise and Worsley had been reluctant to drive forward to help the fugitives. But Bethune reminded them of the sign on the side of the Renault that read: *Servicio canadiense de transfusion de sangre al frente* – The Candian Blood Transfusion at the Front. "Service at the front," he said: "To the front we go."[12] For three days and three nights Bethune and his colleagues drove back and forth from Almeria to the roadway, not sleeping, scarcely eating, rescuing whomever they could. When Sise was driving back to Almeria, Bethune and Worsley walked among the refugees; when Worsley drove, Bethune walked again: just one more exhausted body in a column of the desperately tired and hungry.

On the dawn following the first night, one of André Malraux's contingent of Republican aircraft, which had been involved in a dogfight with three Italian aircraft over Malaga, crash landed on the beach eighty kilometers west of Almeria. As it happened, Bethune was nearby. He crawled down the embankment to see if he could help the downed airmen. Five of the crew were wounded. He tore electrical wires out of the plane and used them as tourniquets to stop the bleeding. By sheer force of personality, Bethune managed to harangue a group of *milicianos* from the road to come down and help him carry the crew back up, and somehow found a truck to get the injured men to a hospital in Almeria. Bethune gave them transfusions with the blood they had taken from Barcelona. Two lived; three died. On the second night, Bethune and Sise brought a truckload of children to a sanatorium on the outskirts of Almeria. Having walked for so long from Malaga, and in such fear, the children collapsed. When no one seemed to be doing anything about feeding them, Bethune became furious. He stormed into the kitchen, ordering the staff about and, with Sise, filled great, large saucepans with all the milk available, heated it up, and threw in all the bread he could find, cursing everyone in sight. Bowls and spoons appeared. Bethune fed the children, and Sise put them to bed. And then they went back to the road for more.[13]

Over the next few days, the last civilians fled Malaga; the Republican

Slaughter of the Innocents   **133**

forces had held out until they were overwhelmed and crushed; fascist tanks rushed up the coastal road to slaughter the last stragglers of the column of refugees that had stretched a hundred kilometers. Thousands died along the way in what the Spanish came to refer to as the *Caravana de la Muerte* – the march of death. At some point, Modotti and Landa joined in the evacuation: "Baked by the sun all day, Tina shivered as soon as it dropped into the sea, knowing that they could not build fires, which might draw more bombing." In Almeria, at the Socorro Rojo hospital, Modotti took charge of the children that Bethune and Sise and Worsley brought to her. Later, she told Vidali that, "War is hateful, but this massacre of women, children, and old people is the most horrible act." Of Bethune, she said, "He was marvelous, tireless. Instead of doing blood transfusions, he was concerned with saving children, and he saved hundreds of them."[14]

Bethune himself describes this horrendous event best. He wrote with an eloquence that only fury and rage can lend to words. His recollection, illustrated by twenty-six of Sise's photographs, was immediately published in Madrid in three languages: Spanish, French, and English. More than anything else Bethune wrote from Spain, it roused the conscience of the workers of the world. It has been said, with some justification, that "the Malaga tragedy was the climax of Bethune's career in Spain. Along that desolate, anonymous road, he lived his finest hours. . . . And he never performed so well as he did in those four days, walking with the Spanish people to Almeria."[15] The full text of Bethune's pamphlet follows:

The Crime on the Road: Malaga–Almeria
The evacuation en masse of the civilian population of Malaga started on Sunday Feb. 7. Twenty-five thousand German, Italian and Moorish troops entered the town on Monday morning the eighth. Tanks, submarines, warships, air planes combined to smash the defences of the city held by a small heroic band of Spanish troops without tanks, air planes or support. The so-called Nationalists entered, as they have entered every captured village and city in Spain, what was practically a deserted town.

Now imagine one hundred and fifty thousand men, women and children setting out for safety to the town situated over a hundred miles away. There is only one road they can take. There is no other way of escape. This road, bordered one side by the high Sierra Nevada mountains and on the other side by the sea, is cut into the side of the cliffs and climbs up and down from sea level to over 500 feet. The city they must reach is Almeria, and it is over two hundred kilometres away. A strong, healthy young man can walk on foot forty or fifty kilometres a day. The journey these women, children and old people must face will take five days and five nights at least. There will be no food to be found in the villages, no trains, no buses to transport them. They must walk and as they walked, staggered and stumbled with cut, bruised feet along that flint, white road the fascists bombed them from the air and fired at them from their ships at sea.

Now, what I want to tell you is what I saw myself on this forced march – the largest, most terrible evacuation of a city in modern times. We had arrived in Almeria at five o'clock on Wednesday the tenth with a refrigeration truckload of preserved blood from Barcelona. Our intention was to proceed to Malaga to give blood transfusions to wounded. In Almeria we heard for the first time that the town had fallen and were warned to go no farther as no one knew where the front line now was but everyone was sure that the town of Motril had also fallen. We thought it important to proceed and discover how the evacuation of the wounded was proceeding. We set out at six o'clock in the evening along the Malaga road and a few miles on we met the head of the piteous procession. Here were the strong with all their goods on donkeys, mules and horses. We passed them, and the farther we went the more pitiful the sights became. Thousands of children, we counted five thousand under ten years of age, and at least one thousand of them barefoot and many of them clad only in a single garment. They were slung over their mother's shoulders or clung to her hands. Here a father staggered along with two children of one and two years of age on his back in addition to carrying pots and pans or some treasured possession. The incessant stream of people became so dense we could barely force the car through them. At eighty-eight kilometres from Almeria they beseeched us to go no farther, that the fascists were just behind. By this time we had passed so many distressed women and children that we thought it best to turn back and start transporting the worst cases to safety.

It was difficult to choose which to take. Our car was besieged by a mob of frantic mothers and fathers who with tired outstretched arms held up to us their children, their eyes and faces swollen and congested by four days of sun and dust.

"Take this one." "See this child." "This one is wounded." Children with bloodstained rags wrapped around their arms and legs, children without shoes, their feet swollen to twice their size crying helplessly from pain, hunger and fatigue. Two hundred kilometres of misery. Imagine four days and four nights, hiding by day in the hills as the fascist barbarians pursued them by plane, walking by night packed in a solid stream men, women, children, mules, donkeys, goats, crying out the names of their separated relatives, lost in the mob. How could we choose between a child dying of dysentery or a mother silently watching us with great sunken eyes carrying against her open breast her child born on the road two days ago. She had

Slaughter of the Innocents

stopped walking for ten hours only. Here was a woman of sixty unable to stagger another step, her gigantic swollen legs with their open varicose ulcers bleeding into her cut linen sandals. Many old people simply gave up the struggle, lay down by the side of the road and waited for death.

We first decided to take only children and mothers. Then the separation between father and child, husband and wife became too cruel to bear. We finished by transporting families with the largest number of young children and the solitary children of which there were hundreds without parents. We carried thirty to forty people a trip for the next three days and nights back to Almeria to the hospital of the Socorro Rojo Internacional where they received medical attention, food and clothing. The tireless devotion of Hazen Sise and Thomas Worsley, drivers of the truck, saved many lives. In turn, they drove back and forth day and night sleeping out on the open road between shifts with no food except dry bread and oranges.

And now comes the final barbarism. Not content with bombing and shelling this procession of unarmed peasants on this long road, on the evening of the 12th when the little seaport of Almeria was completely filled with refugees, its population swollen to double its size, when forty thousand exhausted people had reached a haven of what they thought was safety, we were heavily bombed by German and Italian fascist air planes. The siren alarm sounded thirty seconds before the first bomb fell. These planes made no effort to hit the government battleship in the harbor or bomb the barracks. They deliberately dropped ten great bombs in the very centre of the town where on the main street were sleeping huddled together on the pavement so closely that a car could pass only with difficulty, the exhausted refugees. After the planes had passed I picked up in my arms three dead children from the pavement in front of the Provincial Committee for the Evacuation of Refugees where they had been standing in a great queue waiting for a cupful of preserved milk and a handful of dry bread, the only food some of them had for days. The street was a shambles of the dead and dying, lit only by the orange glare of burning buildings. In the darkness the moans of the wounded children, shrieks of agonized mothers, the curses of the men rose in a massed cry higher and higher to a pitch of intolerable intensity. One's body felt as heavy as the dead themselves, but empty and hollow, and in one's brain burned a bright flame of hate. That night were murdered fifty civilians and an additional fifty were wounded. There were two soldiers killed.

Now, what was the crime that these unarmed civilians had committed to be murdered in this bloody manner? Their only crime was that they had voted to elect a government of the people, committed to the most moderate alleviation of the crushing burden of centuries of the greed of capitalism.

The question has been raised: why did they not stay in Malaga and await the entrance of the fascists? They knew what would happen to them. They knew what would happen to their men and women as had happened so many times before in other captured towns. Every male between the age of 15 and 60 who could not prove that he had not by force been made to assist the government would immediately be shot. And it is this knowledge that has concentrated two-thirds of the entire population of Spain in one half the country that is still held by the republic.[16]

This was not just any atrocity – monstrous and unprecedented though it may have been – it was an atrocity against *children*. For Bethune, perhaps sitting in a hotel room in Almeria after the bombing of the innocents, scribbling down at white heat the outline of *Crime on the Road*, the children – the dead and the wounded – would without doubt have been foremost in his thoughts. The children of Malaga, and all those other children: all those children coughing up blood from their small diseased lungs, dying every day from tuberculosis; the children of Sacré Coeur, and of all the sad children's wards in every hospital from London to Detroit to Montreal; all the children living out their few and sickly years in the shadows of the slums; all the children condemned to misery and to early death by a voracious and blood-soaked capitalism that cared not at all whether they lived or died, who would deny them everything, even life itself; all the children everywhere dead because fascism wished it so and because the wealthy classes of Europe and North America preferred oppression and brutality to liberty and freedom. The dead children of Spain; the infant corpses of Spain: always the dead children, the wounded children, the hungry and the starving children, and his own aborted child, and his own lost and wounded and aborted childhood.

What he had seen on the road to Malaga transformed Bethune. He was no longer the same man he had once been; there was a new tension inside him, a new impatience; there was so much that needed now to be done. From Almeria, Bethune, Sise, and Worsley retraced their path to Murcia, where Bethune would pick up the Ford truck and again visit briefly with Jan Kurzke. "He returned," Kurzke observed, "a changed man . . . he had come back looking like a Biblical prophet, his face burned . . . by the southern sun making his disheveled white, wispy hair the more striking."[17] The change, of course, was not merely a matter of appearances: the lightness and gaiety, always so near the surface, had been transmuted into something not sadder, but perhaps *sterner*. From Murcia, Bethune drove to the International Brigade headquarters in Albacete, to report on the situation in Almeria – and there a nurse, Anne Taft, recalled him as "towering

Slaughter of the Innocents

with rage" – and then on to Valencia, while Sise and Worsley returned to Madrid.[18] In Valencia he once again visited Cerrada, and was once again told that the authorities had not yet signed their proposal.[19] From Valencia, Bethune flew to Paris, on 18 February, to receive funds from the CASD for employee salaries and other Institute expenses, to purchase transfusion equipment, to write the *Crime on the Road*, to assemble the foreign press, and to stand as the world's eyewitness to the carnage at Malaga.[20]

15

Every Minute is Beautiful

With Bethune in Paris, and Sorensen still recovering in Barcelona, Sise had returned with Worsley to Madrid. There were evident difficulties at the Institute. The Spanish doctors were doing what was necessary to keep the hospitals within the city and at the nearby front supplied with blood, but it was obvious that the doctors tended to resent Kajsa Rothman and her enhanced role at the Institute due to her being Bethune's lover and, in some sense, his representative.[1]

More importantly, Franco's armies had launched a major new offensive aimed at isolating Madrid through cutting the road between the capital and the seat of government at Valencia. The fighting was taking place in the Jarama River valley, directly south and east of Madrid, and would last, on and off until June. The fascist army, numbering forty thousand men, was met by two Republican battalions who fought fiercely and steadfastly until they were all dead. Fresh Republican reinforcements were accompanied by the XI and XII International Brigades – the Thaelmann, Dombrowski, and Garabaldi battalions. They were soon joined by the newly formed XV Brigade consisting of British, French, and Belgian volunteers, and by Americans and Canadians almost all of whom were in their first combat missions. It was an extraordinarily bloody campaign, often fought for control of a mere few kilometers. The losses were terrible; the Volunteers fell in their hundreds, but they held the front.[2]

Two days after arriving back in Madrid, Sise and Worsley, accompanied by Rothman, drove to the Jarama River front with blood for the field hospitals near the XV Brigade. At the Arganda Bridge, Rothman apparently asked a number of questions of the Republican soldier guarding the bridge, arousing his suspicions to the point where he was about to arrest her; only Sise's safe-conduct pass, which bore not only his own name and Worsley's, but also Kajsa Rothman's, convinced the guard not to detain her.[3] While at the front, Worsley had word of Tony Hyndman, who had suffered what may have been something of a nervous collapse and whose actions appeared to his comrades to have been little more than cowardice and desertion. Worsley found Hyndman and was "shattered" by his emotional condition.[4] A few days later Sise drove to Barcelona to work on the Renault accompanied by Worsley who, presumably, had contacted Stephen Spender in

Every Minute is Beautiful

England about their mutual friend. Spender left London immediately en route to Madrid.[5]

In Paris, Bethune made an important decision. For some weeks he had been extremely concerned about the situation of the Spanish children. Malnutrition was spreading quickly among them; he had seen its effects in the quality of blood donated by their parents at the Institute. Appeals had gone out across the world for shiploads of food and milk, and the working class had responded. But it was not enough, and as the war deepened and extended, much more would be required. And there were the orphans, more every day, thousands of them. And the imperiled: no matter how valiantly their fathers and mothers fought, every town and village bombarded and attacked by the fascists yielded its quota of dead children. The monstrous assault on the refugees from Malaga only underscored the depth of the problem and the necessity of a solution. For Bethune, two things became clear. Firstly, he had, against all odds, established the foundations of a wide-ranging and effective blood transfusion service; what needed to be done *could be done* if there was sufficient will to do it. Secondly, he understood the nature of propaganda; the working people who had responded to the call to finance the Blood Transfusion Institute would no doubt rally to the plight of children in danger of their lives. The children must not die. He could not permit it. Their silent sad eyes had looked up at him from the square at Almeria; their cries haunted him in his sleep; in dreams they were *his* children, he was their father.

Bethune sought out Ione Rhodes. A Belgian teacher, Ione, together with her American husband Peter Rhodes, later developed the International Office for Children in November 1937. But for almost a year Ione Rhodes had been engaged in collecting food and milk for Spanish children. She had been to Madrid and spoken with the central authorities in Valencia. She "understood that the Spanish Republic was seeking to realize a well elaborated plan for its children. They particularly wanted to have children's camps established outside the danger zones, where the children would be safe from the bombing . . . "[6] After some discussion with Rhodes he met with the Spanish Ambassador's wife, Gertrude Araquistain, who, with some enthusiasm, requested a written proposal, which Bethune provided.[7] He then sent a telegram to the Spanish government suggesting "that a Children's City should be erected with the assistance of international finances."[8] He sent another telegram to Sise at the Hotel Continental in Barcelona; it was simple, brief, but explosive: "Mobilize your architect friends in Barcelona to plan a whole new Children's Village to be put in the foothills of the Pyrenees. I'll be back in two days time – let's get this thing going."[9] Decades later, Sise recalled:

This was typical with Bethune; his idea was perfectly sound and imaginative. He had been worried for months about the evacuated children. They would be mostly evacuated from Madrid to Valencia, and it now looked as if war might come to that region and he was determined to get them further away, nearer to safety. He conceived this idea of new children's communities – whole villages – and his artistic imagination immediately got to work on it.[10]

On 25 February, Sise wrote Bethune a long letter. He acknowledged Bethune's "astonishing telegram about the Children's City," but his primary concern appears to have been to inform Bethune of the problems developing at the Institute, of Kajsa Rothman's activities, and of the mutual resentment between Rothman and the Spanish doctors. According to Sise:

> Kajsa was in fine form . . . she was of the greatest help to me – she has the whole situation at her fingertips and will be able to give you all the details as soon as you arrive back. . . . Kajsa and I arranged with Navarro that the Sanidad should order refrigerators to be paid for by you when you arrive . . . there isn't anyone amongst the crowd with the guts to smash through all the obstacles and get things done – no one except Kajsa and her position is difficult being a woman.

As always, propaganda for more blood donors was urgently required, but "actually the only stuff along this line was arranged by Kajsa – articles and photos in one of the illustrated papers." Importantly, a cable had come through from Tim Buck, the leader of the Communist Party of Canada, concerning the alleged capture and execution of General Kleber, the military commander of the International Brigades. If true, the claim would have seriously demoralized not only the Brigaders, but antifascist supporters everywhere. The claim was false:

> Kajsa did a good job. She got through to Valencia and had them make a public denial. But I wasn't satisfied it had got through to Toronto, so Kajsa and I went to Party headquarters and had them send a cable to Tim Buck from the Spanish Party.

Despite what Sise saw as her evident value, the Spanish doctors rarely made much use of her, much to her annoyance. On one occasion, after she had accompanied Sise on a blood delivery, the Spanish doctors needed her. "They asked Kajsa to go too and she went although it was her second trip that day – it was the first time they had asked her to do something and

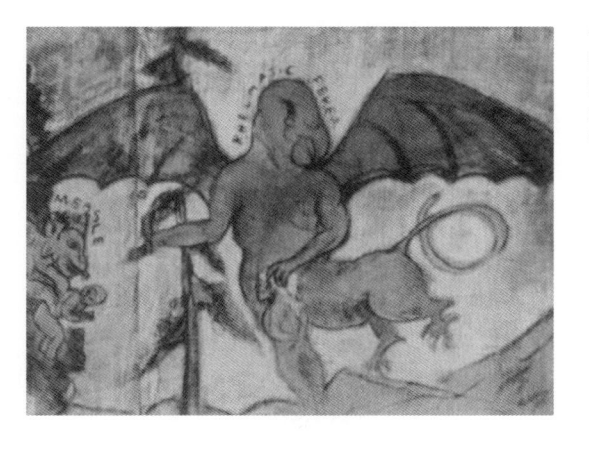

1 Mural Scene III. "Journey in Thick Woods – Childhood." Detail. Does this dragon represent Bethune's mother? Courtesy of Larry Hannant.

2 Professional photograph of Bethune taken in Paris (late February 1937). Courtesy of Library and Archives Canada.

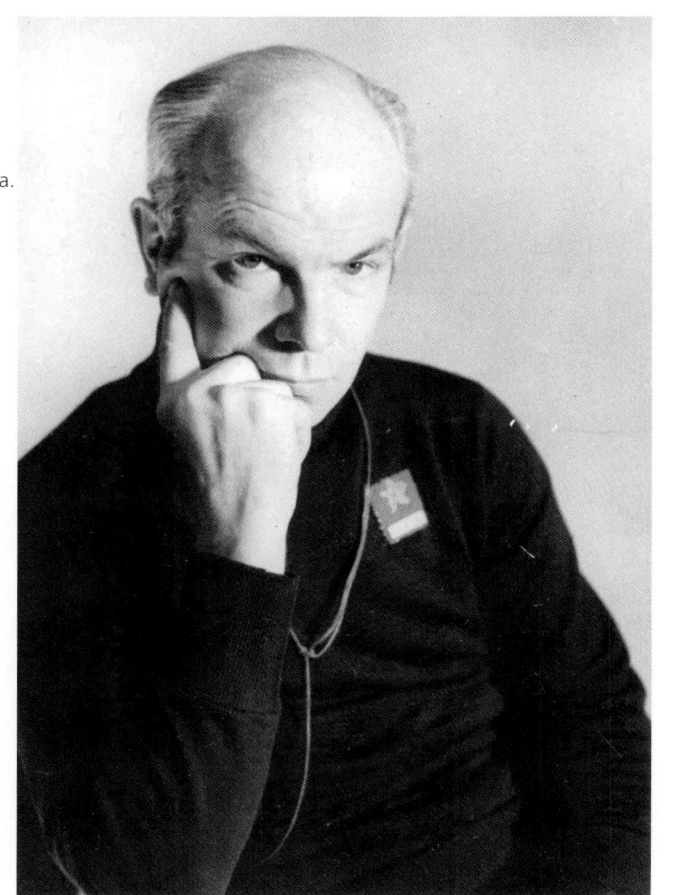

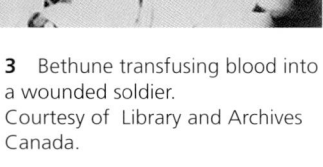

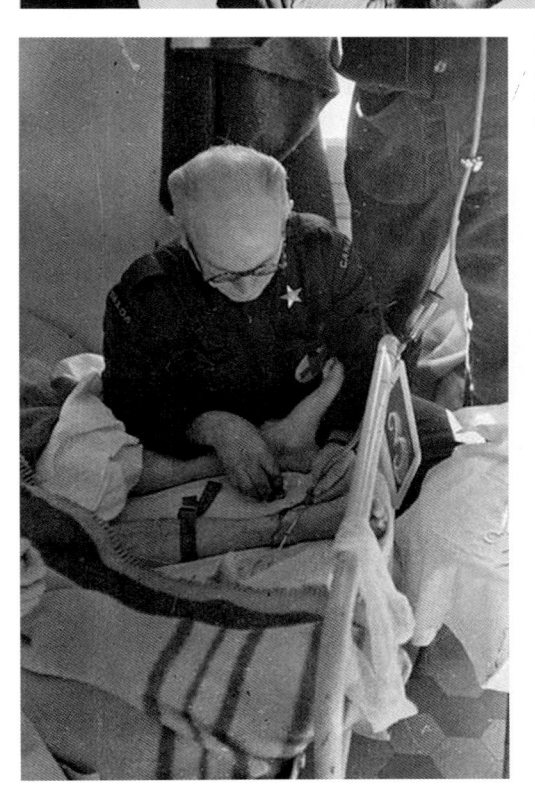

3 Bethune transfusing blood into a wounded soldier.
Courtesy of Library and Archives Canada.

4 Bethune transfusing blood into the foot of a patient.
Courtesy of Library and Archives Canada.

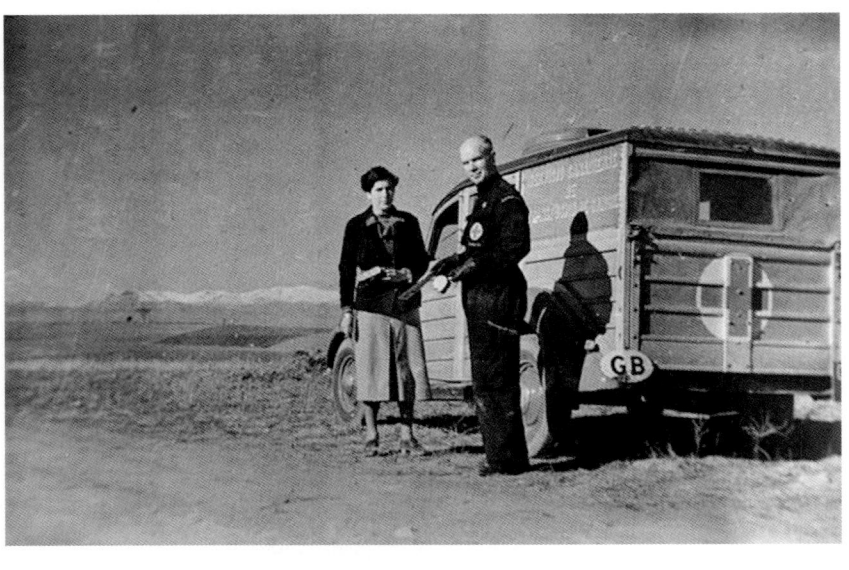

5 Bethune with ambulance and unknown woman, possibly a Spanish nurse.
Courtesy of Library and Archives Canada.

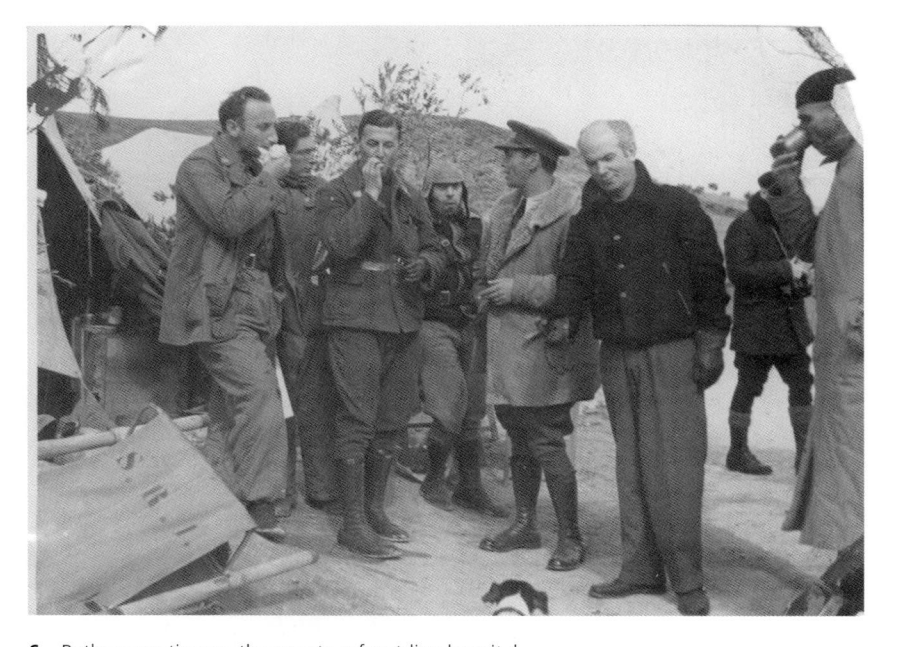

6 Bethune resting on the way to a front-line hospital.
Courtesy of Library and Archives Canada.

7 Bethune examining the remains of a downed Nazi aircraft. The British government consistently denied any evidence of German or Italian military presence in Spain.
Courtesy of Library and Archives Canada.

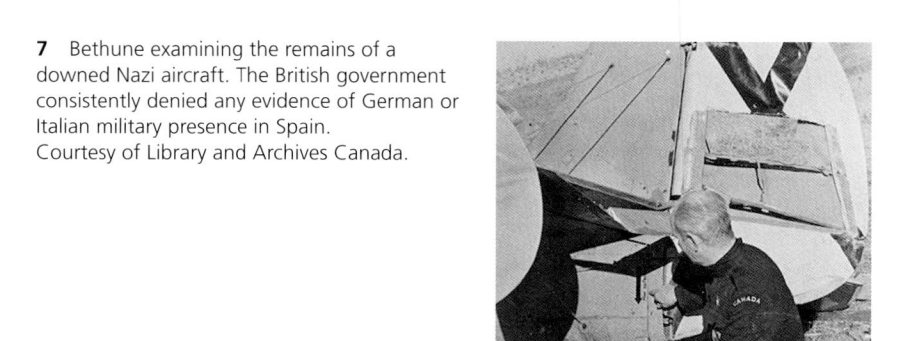

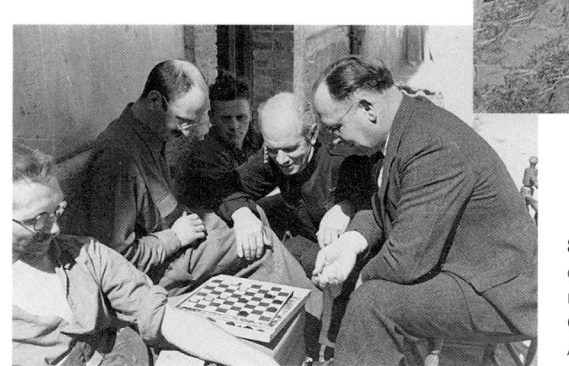

8 Bethune observing a game of checkers. Haldane is on the right.
Courtesy of Library and Archives Canada.

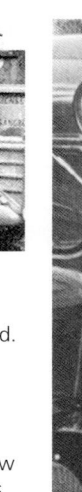

9 The Canadian Blood Transfusion team. From right to left: Sorensen, Bethune, Sise, and unknown Spaniard.
Courtesy of Library and Archives Canada.

10 Bethune standing beside the new Renault truck purchased in Marseilles (January 1937).
Courtesy of Library and Archives Canada.

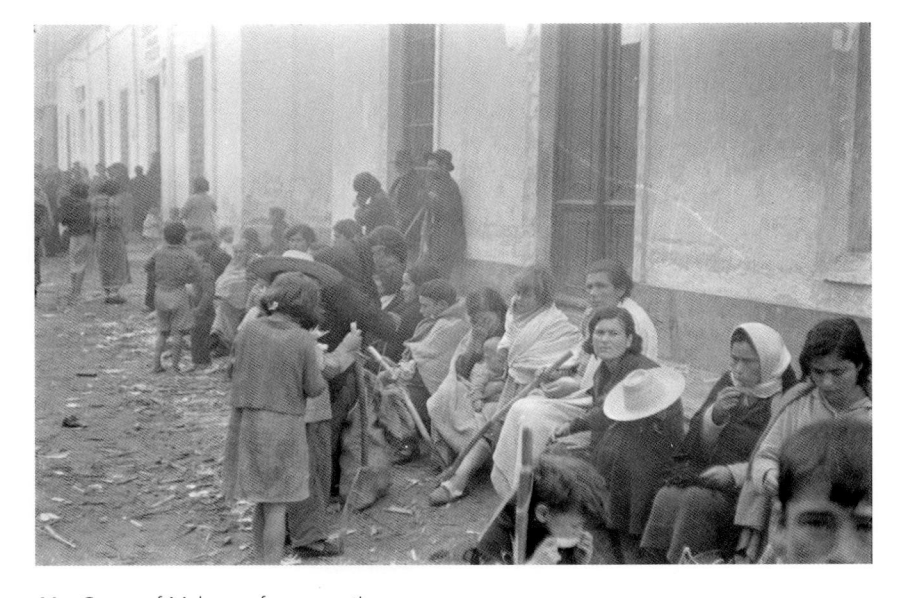

11 Group of Malaga refugees resting.
Courtesy of Library and Archives Canada.

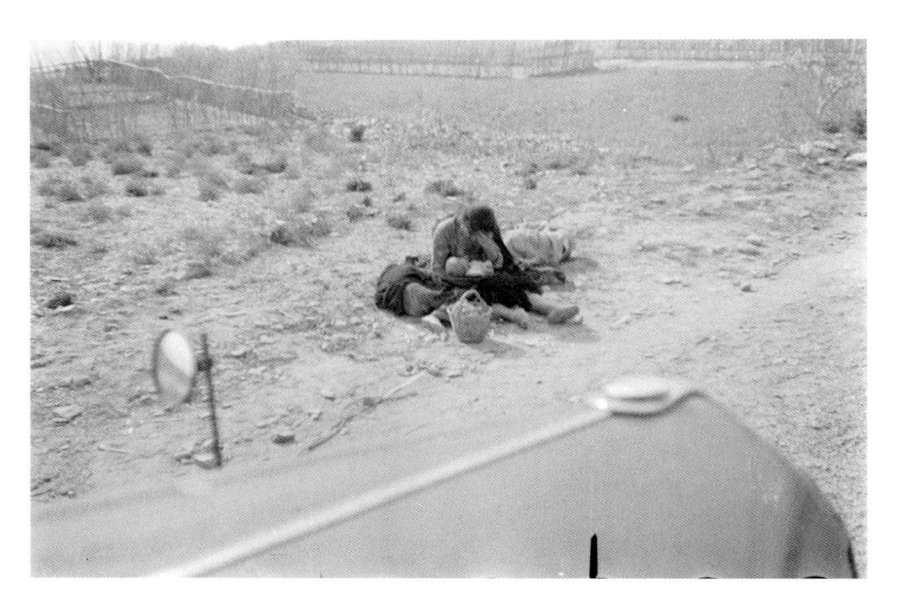

12 Refugee mother feeding baby.
Courtesy of Library and Archives Canada.

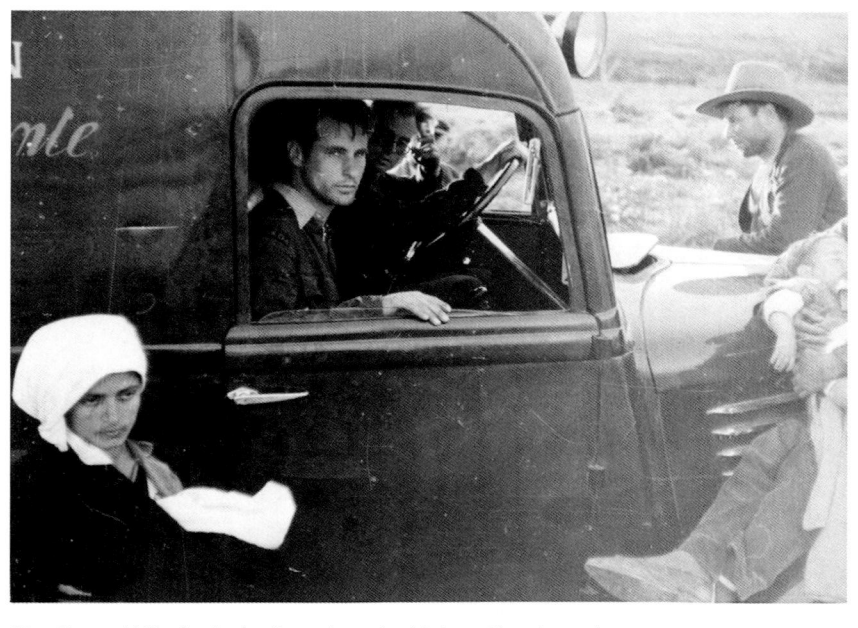

13 Sise and Worsley in the Renault on the Malaga-Almeria road.
Courtesy of Library and Archives Canada.

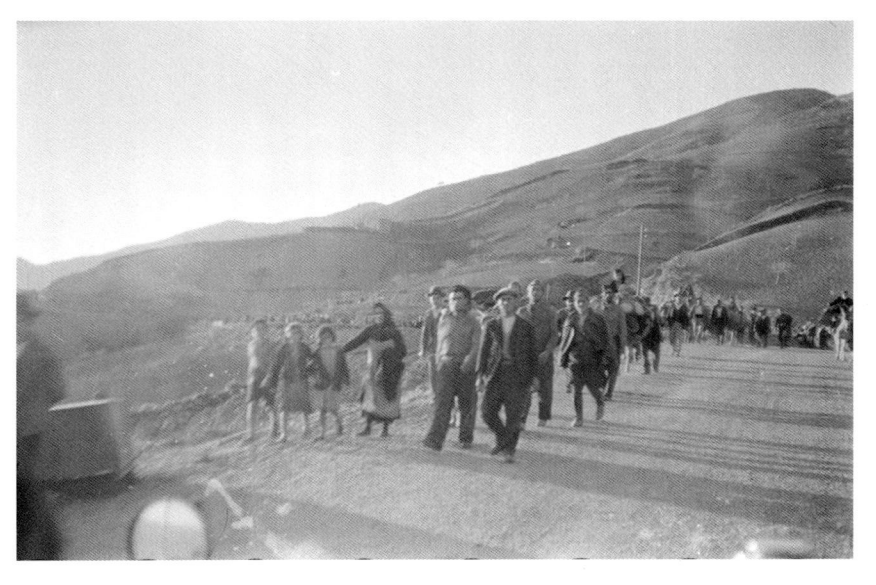

14 Malaga refugees walking the Caravana de la Muerte.
Courtesy of Library and Archives Canada.

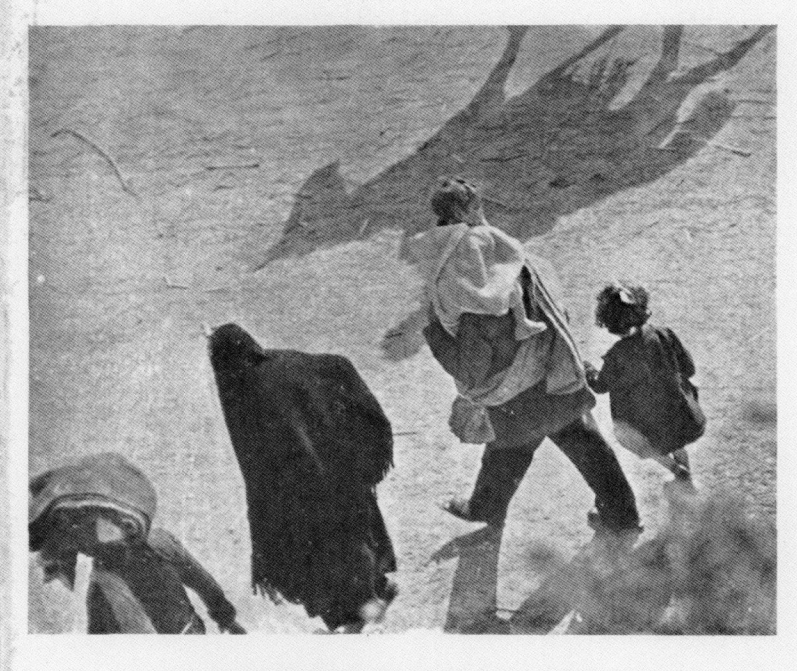

15 Front cover of Bethune's passionate indictment *The Crime on the Road: Malaga–Almeria*. The book was published simultaneously in English, Spanish, and French. Courtesy of Paul Preston.

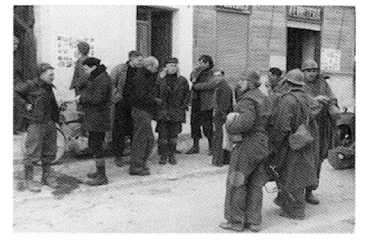

16 Bethune during filming of Heart of Spain (April or May 1937).
Courtesy of Library and Archives Canada.

17 Bethune at the front with Sorensen and May (April or May 1937). Courtesy of Library and Archives Canada.

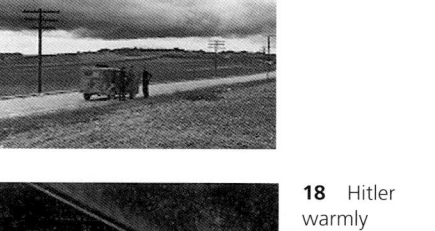

18 Hitler warmly greeting Franco (1938). Photograph by Ned Bayne. Courtesy of Paul Preston.

Every Minute is Beautiful

she was damned if she was going to refuse." When Sise had left for Barcelona with Worsley to repair the Renault, Sorensen had returned to Madrid on 20 February; Kajsa and Sorensen were alone together. "However," Sise continued, "things may be better now as Kajsa has the energy to get things done – with Henning there she can make herself seem to act under his orders so as not to hurt their pride."[11] Ultimately, Sise was mistaken. Certainly there were serious frictions between Rothman and Culebras and Goyanes, but an equal difficulty was to emerge between Rothman and Sorensen.

On the last day of February, Bethune returned from Paris to Barcelona. He was not alone; he had brought with him Allen May. Of all the men and women who intersected through Bethune's life in Spain, May is perhaps the most obscure. Virtually nothing is known of him, other than he came from the small village of Elfros, Saskatchewan, the son of the local hotel keeper, attended the University of Saskatchewan, and that he had been, most recently, a writer for *Liberty Magazine* and staff reporter for the prominent Toronto newspaper, the *Globe and Mail*. His political affiliation is unknown. After Spain, his name all but disappears. Either in December 1944 or January 1945, mysteriously "he was found one morning lying on the curb near his home, shot to death," possibly a suicide.[12]

The first reference to May is in a 25 February 1937 letter from the CASD to the Prime Minister of Canada, William Lyon Mackenzie King.[13] The Canadian government was preparing legislation to make it illegal for its citizens to fight on behalf of the legitimate government of Spain. It was not in the best interests of the ruling class of Canada, or of any of the capitalist powers, for the working class to learn how to fight for democracy, or for the exploited to learn that the terms "capitalism" and "democracy" did not in fact mean the same thing, but were far more frequently opposites; certainly the ruling class was quite consciously afraid that the working class, once trained in the use of weapons, and steeled in the practice of combat, would, returning from Spain, turn their weapons against their domestic masters. The CASD was immediately concerned that Bethune and his colleagues not be thrown in prison and forced to pay heavy fines on their return from the war, and that their Spanish status as "Commandante" or as "Captain" not be held against them nor as indicating any actual membership in the Republican army. The CASD sought, instead, that the Blood Transfusion Unit be considered exempt from the pending legislation as a "recognized Canadian humanitarian society." No doubt it goes without saying that the CASD's effort was ignored. It was, after all, in this same year that the Canadian Minister of Trade and Commerce, William Euler, was demanding that printing newspaper stories critical of Hitler be made a punishable crime, and that the Prime Minister himself was having a grand time touring Nazi Germany.

Still, it is in the CASD letter that we can read: "At the present moment our Committee has a Medical Mission operating in Spain. This Mission consists of Dr. Norman Bethune, Hazen Sise, Henning Sorensen and Allen May."[14] But May was most certainly not in Spain at the time this letter was written; he was unquestionably still in Paris. In a later letter of 9 March to Ben Spence, Bethune wrote, regarding May: "We met in Paris and between us sent over 100 posters to you and Norman Lee in Montreal. If you have not received them it must be the fault of the censors either in France or Spain, or the customs in Canada."[15] The 25 February CASD letter continues: "Further help may be required or replacements found desirable, indeed only last week we sent an additional man to re-inforce the staff already there . . . " This "additional man" could be no one but May himself, dispatched from Toronto with orders to meet Bethune in Paris and travel with him into Spain. But what was his intended function? There were serious problems developing at the Institute in Madrid, as we have seen. Indeed, there had been difficulties of one kind or another since Sorensen had made himself responsible for the police raid of 4 January. Had May been sent to look into these problems?[16] Such a possibility seems unlikely: no report from May to the CASD on these matters seems to exist; he stayed in Spain long after Bethune's departure; and A. A. MacLeod was sent to the Blood Transfusion Unit for precisely this purpose not long after. What's more, Bethune had written to the CASD on 27 January, stating that since he was working eighteen hours a day he could not be "war correspondent and doctor too."[17] Most probably May had been sent precisely to fill that role. On the other hand, May's trajectory in Spain would seem to indicate that he was something more than simply a newspaper reporter who wanted to serve the Republican struggle. Almost immediately he became the "official secretary of the unit," publicity agent, and liaison with the CASD.[18] Within weeks he had been appointed the Associate Director of the Blood Transfusion Institute's outpost at Jaen, responsible for blood extractions at this southern-most corner of the Republic, a city always in immediate peril of fascist occupation.[19] Whether he actually ever fulfilled this function is difficult to say; Sise maintains that they had "set up a number of centers,"[20] but whether Jaen was one of them, or how long it may have survived in operation is distinctly unclear. In any event, Bethune was full of praise for May, writing, "He has made himself universally beloved by his tact and courtesy to the Spanish people and by his organizational ability."[21] After Bethune eventually left Spain, it was May, and not Sise or Sorensen, who became head of the entire Institute at its headquarters in Madrid, and after

Every Minute is Beautiful

Sise and Sorensen followed Bethune back to Canada in the fall of 1937, Allen May was the sole remaining Canadian at the Institute and liaison officer between the CASD and the Sanidad Militar.[22] Near the very end of the war, when all was irretrievably lost – the precise date is uncertain – he escaped from undoubted fascist execution by swimming out to a British battleship where he was rescued.[23]

Sorensen had left Barcelona on 17 February and returned to Madrid three days later. Sise and Worsley left Madrid, arriving in Barcelona on 23 February, and the following day Sorensen left for Valencia. When Bethune arrived in Barcelona from Paris, he, Worsley, and May went directly to Valencia where they met Sorensen.[24] With Sise still in Barcelona, and temporarily out of the way, Sorensen took Bethune aside and gave him his appraisal of the situation in Madrid: there was jealousy and resentment at the Institute; the situation was deeply unhealthy; Sise and Kajsa had aligned themselves against the doctors; Kajsa was overstepping her position and lording it over everyone else; Kajsa's activities were suspicious; sensitive documents disappeared when she was alone, including Sorensen's safe-conduct pass.[25] Bethune listened. It was always the same, he thought. There were important things to be done, that needed doing immediately, and he was surrounded, as usual, by petty minds, enmired in jealously and endless backbiting. Fascism had to be defeated; orphaned children saved and fed; he was in the process of setting up a unified mobile blood transfusion system to serve the entire fighting front, from Madrid to Jaen, and he had to be confronted by gossip and ill tempers, and Sorensen's paranoid suspicions about Kajsa. Bethune thought about Kajsa. He had missed her and was eager to see her again; to take her to bed. Did he love her? Yes; but he had fewer illusions than he had before: there had been other women that he had loved, and they never stayed and never would.

But in Valencia, there was business to conduct. The plan to provide a fully unified blood service had yet to be approved by the Ministry of War.[26] Cerrada had always led Bethune to believe that it was merely a matter of time. Consequently, Bethune called together a gathering of foreign correspondents and told them that on the following day he would he would meet with Colonel Cerrada and return with a final agreement in hand. But the next day he was forced to tell the reporters to hold the story: the agreement had still not come through.[27] Things had changed rapidly since Bethune had been in Paris. The catastrophe at Malaga had very seriously called into question the strategy and policies of Largo Caballero's government, and the stunning incompetence of his primary military adviser, General Asensio. Both the military and the civilian population were insisting on a radical change in policy. The Communist Party of Spain had long criticized the practice of de-centralized armed resistance, so dependent on the quasi-independent militias, and called for the establishment of a unified Army of the Republic. Asensio was forced to resign: the Army of the Republic, the unified People's Army, was born. The objective necessity of a centralized, reorganized, and unified response to fascism meant not only that the days of the militias were coming to a close, but that *all* independent institutions, *all* independent activity, had to end or to be transformed: Malaga had changed everything.[28]

In Cerrada's office, it had been put to Bethune that it was no longer merely a matter of the *approval* of a unified blood service – that was certainly possible and entirely necessary – but that Duran-Jorda had objected to Bethune, or any non-Spaniard being in charge. Furthermore, the Blood Transfusion Unit in Madrid would henceforth be amalgamated into the Sanidad Militar and placed under a control board of consisting of two Spanish doctors – Goyanes and Culebras – and himself.[29] Although it was fully recognized that Bethune had conceived the blood service, and would retain his titular position as director, it was made clear to him that the service would necessarily become a mainly Spanish operation primarily staffed by Spaniards.[30] Bethune exploded. He was utterly opposed to any amalgamation of the Blood Transfusion Unit into the Sanidad Militar. He would refuse entirely to cooperate with any such scheme. It was left, as so often, for Sorensen to soften Bethune's language through careful translation, although his rage was perfectly obvious to the authorities.[31] Perhaps if Goyanes and Culebras had been as dedicated to his plans and projects as he himself had been, the transfer of control would not have appeared as problematic. But he had read Sise's letter; he knew of the difficulties and factions developing at the Institute in Madrid. He did not trust Goyanes and Culebras to control a project as complex as delivering blood to the entire war front. He was right not to do so: some months after Bethune left Spain, Sise noted in a letter to A. A. MacLeod, that Goyanes had "considerable ability, though it is usually hidden under a monumental but engaging laziness," and that he had been guilty of signing false employment certificates on behalf of Culebras's wife, and that Culebras himself was claiming that Sise and the other Canadians "were out to get him because of his hostility to Bethune in the past."[32] But perhaps most importantly – although he could not yet recognize it in himself – Bethune was still infected by the internal structure of the bourgeois artist: Spain had yet to burn it from him. Deep in his core he remained the man of *generosity*, the artist, who had laid his precious gift at the feet of the Spanish people. He was offended because they had not recognized his generosity and had, by appointing a control board, therefore rejected the individual *uniqueness* of his gift. No matter how

Every Minute is Beautiful   **145**

generous he might feel himself to be, he insisted on retaining control over whatever he gave away. The blood transfusion service was his creation, his to give or his to keep as he willed, but never to be stolen away from him. Barely listening to Sorensen's translation of the details of salaries and other shared responsibilities that would need to be worked out between the Blood Transfusion Unit, the CASD and the Spanish government, he sat in frozen and furious dignity until the interview was concluded and then stormed out.

As enraged as Bethune was at the Sanidad Militar, Sorensen was equally furious with Bethune, and rightly so. In Sorensen's eyes, Bethune had behaved abominably. They were guests in Spain; their function was to aid the Republican government, to follow its lead and its command. The blood transfusion service did not belong to Bethune, nor even to the Canadian contingent as a whole: it was an arm of the Spanish resistance. Bethune's behavior was an insult to Spain and reflected poorly not only on the blood transfusion unit, but on the CASD, on the Communist Party of Canada, and on the working people of Canada as a whole. Bethune had not behaved as a Communist, as an internationalist, ought to have behaved: it was totally incomprehensible for a member of the Communist Party to act in such an individualist manner.[33] If Sorensen told Bethune any of his perfectly reasonable concerns, we cannot know, although it is very doubtful. But within three weeks he would do precisely what he had done on 4 January: he would go above Bethune and voice his complaint directly to the Party.

In any event, it was, to a degree, irrelevant whether Sorensen spoke to Bethune or not. Bethune was nothing if not entirely sensitive to others; he could easily read Sorensen's contempt in his face, in the movements of his body. But Bethune was irritated; Sorensen was so often full of complaints. And where had Sorensen been when the thousands of starving and dying children had been dragging themselves along the bitter road from Malaga? What had *he* seen of horror and abomination? Who was he, after all, to criticize, he who had lain rather comfortably in hospital, or sat safely in Barcelona or Valencia, and who could not wait to "inform" him about the situation in Madrid, and to try to drive a wedge between him and Kajsa?

There was one more necessary meeting in Valencia. The project for a unified blood transfusion service throughout Spain would not be sanctioned by the Ministry of War without the agreement of Duran-Jorda, and of Dr Edward Barsky, the chief physician of the extensive American medical contingent of the Abraham Lincoln Battalion, and later commander of all International Brigade hospitals in Spain.[34] Duran-Jorda's assent had already been secured, even if he was opposed to the idea of Bethune's leadership; only Barsky's approval was pending. As so often with Bethune, his rage dissipated as rapidly as it had arrived; he was prepared now to be eloquent. The struggle for the independence of the Blood Transfusion Institute could wait; what was at issue was the completion of the final agreement for the unified blood service. Barsky was accompanied by his assistant, Dr. Albert Byrnne. The three sat down somewhere to discuss the issue, and Barsky seems to have approved the project. It was an important moment for Bethune, but it brought no joy. The serious conflict with the Sanidad Militar and the unspoken falling out with Sorensen ate at Bethune. He had to get away, to get clean of all these petty and idiotic entanglements. Bethune turned to Byrnne and said, as if speaking only to himself: "I must get back to the front. It is the only place that is real. . . . The front is reality. There is the most beautiful detachment there. Every minute is beautiful because it may be the last . . . "[35]

16

The Blood of the Dead

Bethune returned to Madrid two days later. There was little time to worry over the autonomy of the unified blood transfusion service, or the authority that Goyanes and Culebras would soon be exercising; Franco was on the march. Without delay, he began driving to the embattled Jarama front with blood for transfusion; within the first week of March he had placed no less than nine refrigerators at front line hospitals to keep their blood supplies fresh. Kajsa Rothman was his assistant; in the evenings they were lovers.[1]

While Bethune had been in Paris, Dr. Reginald Saxton, a member of the Communist Party of Great Britain, in Spain since September, had been sent by the International Brigades to establish a field hospital at Villarejo, a town on the main road from Madrid to Valencia, to service the Jarama wounded. Along with two medical colleagues, he drove slowly through the darkness in his truck, the headlights turned off to avoid attracting fascist fire; they arrived in Villarejo some time after midnight. Saxton commandeered the largest building, a mansion once owned by an Austrian aristocrat. They turned the bar room into their operating theater, gathering three tables on which to operate, and assembled benches moved from the meeting hall to create a makeshift ward of twenty-five beds. Within the first five days, seven hundred wounded were brought to the hospital, many in desperate condition. It was evident to Saxton that blood transfusion facilities were an absolutely necessary requirement, but it seemed to him there was nothing he could do about it. Then, "like a fairy-godmother," Bethune "appeared on his doorstep," ready to help. They discussed the matter, and Bethune promised to return with the needed supplies. On a second visit, snaking his way with Kajsa through the battle lines, Bethune delivered transfusion instruments, syringes and cannulas, and a quantity of citrated blood. Saxton, who was unqualified to engage in major surgery, learned quickly and soon became Villarejo's transfusion expert. Gratefully, he accepted "what Norman Bethune had to offer us and I gladly took everything he could give or advise."[2]

Initially supplied by Bethune's daily blood delivery service, Saxton was soon extracting and collecting his own blood supply not only from the local villagers, but from the increasing numbers of doctors and nurses arriving at the Villarejo field hospital.[3] He was much impressed by Bethune's work, and appears to have visited him more than once in March and April.[4] On 7 March, Saxton came to Madrid to examine Bethune's Institute, and wrote a brief report, *A Study of the Madrid Transfusion Service*, in which he listed the names of all the Spanish personnel, noted that there were some eight hundred civilians currently registered as donors, and that four hundred liters of blood were collected monthly. He further observed that because of the possibility of a toxic effect, no more than a single liter of citrated blood was to be administered, and if more was needed, direct person-to-person transfusion was the preferred method.[5]

Some months later, in September 1937, Saxton published an article in the prestigious British medical journal, *The Lancet*, entitled *The Madrid Blood Transfusion Institute*, in which he described Bethune's unit in extensive detail. But much had changed between March and September; Franco's forces were in the ascendancy and the war had become increasingly bloody. Toward the end of his article, Saxton wrote of the vast numbers of wounded and the mounting difficulty of finding a sufficient number of donors for blood transfusions.

> The only possibility of saving these lives appears to rest with the use of stored cadaver blood as described by S.S. Yudin. In my opinion it is the duty of the Sanidad Militar of the Spanish Republic to organize the large-scale supply of cadaver blood, which of course is readily available, to their front line hospitals in the same way as they now supply citrated blood.[6]

Saxton's article, although written in the usual colorless language of a technical report, is exceedingly interesting on a number of grounds. He was, in effect, proposing to combine the mobile blood transfusion system pioneered by Bethune with the use of stored cadaver blood initially developed by the Soviet researcher Sergei Yudin. This is, by any account, a rather stunning proposal, and it is unlikely that Saxton would have used *The Lancet* as the primary avenue to make such a recommendation to the Spanish government; presumably he had already spoken directly with the Sanidad Militar. But to propose that the Republic "organize the large-scale supply of cadaver blood" implies not only that Saxton thought such organization feasible, but that he reasonably believed that any technical problems with cadaveric transfusion – such as blood clotting or issues of preservation – had been effectively solved. Otherwise, for Saxton to make such a serious recommendation would have been absurd. And yet, what was the basis for this belief; how could he have arrived at sufficient certainty to approach the Sanidad Militar with such a wide-ranging proposal? Finally, why did Saxton

The Blood of the Dead

think that cadaveric transfusion was "the *only* possibility" for saving the lives of the wounded? The issue came down, in the last instance, to a reliable supply of blood. Bethune was convinced that antifascist sentiment among the people would help to resolve the problem of supply; indeed it was an important aspect of his contribution in Spain to recognize that blood transfusion was not simply an instrumental question of supply-and-demand, but a *political* question: that the ties between the civilians in the cities and the combatants at the front could be immeasurably strengthened by the very personal and intimate exchange of blood. But as the war went on, the savagery of the fascist offensive led, on the one hand, to a vastly increased demand for blood donations and, on the other, to a progressive deterioration in the quality of civilian blood due to widespread malnutrition. Cadaver transfusion seemed to Saxton, then, to be the only solution.

Even though there is no evidence to suggest that the Republican government embraced Saxton's proposal, he seems not to have been entirely deterred. According to Paul Preston, "Saxton explored the possibility of making transfusions from cadavers but eventually abandoned the experiment because of ethical considerations and technical obstacles."[7] It is apparent that Saxton did indeed engage in such transfusion, the extent of which we shall soon explore. But the more important question then immediately arises, crystallizing all the questions we have raised above: where did Saxton learn the technique of cadaveric transfusion?

Duran-Jorda had authored a pamphlet – undated, but probably written in mid-1937 – in which he indicated an early interest in Yudin's research "the more so since, even in the political press, the work done by Judine [Yudin] in the use of preserved blood from corpses had been given wide publicity." Although Yudin was without doubt the world authority on cadaveric transfusion and, as a Soviet scientist, held considerable weight among certain circles within the Spanish government, Duran-Jorda quickly dismissed the use of cadaveric blood which, he wrote, "is no longer considered practicable, because it has been demonstrated that the blood of those who die a violent death does not coagulate properly," and that the problem of cadaveric transfusion should be given up "as impossible of solution."[8] Where Duran-Jorda feared to tread, Bethune would soon apply his enormous energy and innovative talents.

The history of the civilian blood bank and the history of cadaveric blood transfusion form a perhaps surprising unity: both of these practices were first established in Russia in the immediate aftermath of the Soviet Revolution. During the early 1920s, Alexander Bogdanov began studying blood transfusion, and subsequently contacted his friend and former comrade, Soviet leader V. I. Lenin, for permission to set up a blood institute. Lenin consented, government funding was released, and in March 1926 the State Institute of Blood Transfusion was founded in Moscow with Bogdanov as Director. Such an institute was a historical novelty; no such specialized institution of this type existed in the Soviet Union or anywhere else in the world. Bogdanov died of a transfusion accident in 1928, but by 1930 the institute had expanded to Leningrad with Alexander Bogolomets as Director.[9]

Charles Drew, a pioneer in American blood transfusion, documented the primacy of the Soviet Union in the development of the blood bank.[10] While blood banking in the United States was not put into practice until 1937, when Fantus instituted the practice at Cook County Hospital in Chicago,[11] Bogdanov's institute established the world's first blood bank as early as 1932, creating "the first civilian blood centers as well as the basis of a centralized blood service for the entire country."[12] During the period from 1930 to 1935 the institutes in both Moscow and Leningrad were actively providing units of preserved blood to hospitals in their respective cities. In 1935, at the First International Congress of Blood Transfusion, in Rome, "delegates noted that none of the countries had an organized blood service like that of the Soviet Union."[13] Simultaneously, beginning in 1930, Sergei S. Yudin had introduced a new and innovative technique for which he became justly famous: the successful transfusion of stored cadaver blood into a living man.[14]

In a March 1936 article Yudin reported on 924 human transfusions with cadaver blood, noting that there were only seven fatalities in the living recipients: five resulting from a variety of technical errors, and two from "faulty blood typing": the blood type of the donor was incompatible with that of the recipient. In his view, "the therapeutic effect of cadaver blood does not differ from that of blood from living donors." Such blood, he wrote, could be preserved for more than three weeks in a refrigerator and, in a sodium citrate solution, for as long as four weeks and, unlike the rather limited amount of blood from living donors, "from 2.5 to 3 litres of blood can be easily obtained from a cadaver that is not damaged." He further indicated that blood from those who had died suddenly was preferable to that of those who had not. So successful were his experiments that "before long we not only had enough blood for our own clinic but we were able to supply it to a number of hospitals and even send it to distant points."[15]

A longer August 1937 article was essentially an expanded version of the earlier work with in-depth vignettes of a number of clinical cases. In this article Yudin repeated that blood extracted from those who had died a sudden death was preferable to blood taken from those who had died from a slow and lingering disease. He also noted that cadaveric blood did not

The Blood of the Dead

require the addition of anticoagulants such as sodium citrate since "once dissolved, it remains liquid" – essentially the blood has already clotted and then lysed – and that furthermore, anticoagulants, in significant amounts, could result in serious negative reactions in recipients. Importantly, both articles made the point that the technique of extracting cadaver blood was rather simple: the corpse being placed on a table, the head lowered relative to the feet, and the blood taken from an incision in the jugular vein.[16]

Was Bethune aware of these Soviet developments? As a physician who was also a member of the Communist Party, it seems quite likely that he would have followed Soviet medical advancements with some interest; moreover Yudin's brief 1936 article describing his experimentation was easily available (although the more detailed August 1937 article would not have been published until Bethune had left Spain) and, as Duran-Jorda noted, widely discussed in the left-wing political press. Furthermore, Bethune had traveled to Moscow and Leningrad in 1935 to attend Pavlov's International Physiological Congress. The details of his itinerary are not available, but it is known that he struck out on his own to visit several hospitals and clinics where there is some possibility that he became aware of the activities of Bogdanov's institute and of Yudin's research.[17] Certainly it is true that in Madrid, at the beginning of February 1937, Bethune stated: "I will use the latest Russian–American methods of blood transfusion . . . ," which seems to suggest a more than glancing familiarity with Soviet technique.[18]

It is evident that Bethune planned, relatively early in his service in Spain, to engage in associated fundamental research and to establish a laboratory to that end. It may be recalled that in speaking with the reporter Frederick Griffin, Bethune spoke of engaging in experimentation on the very nature of blood. It is clear that Bethune saw his blood service as more than a vehicle for the vitally necessary transportation of blood to the wounded at the front. Some few weeks later Bethune would begin to probe into whether the blood from human cadavers could revive the living. Indeed, according to Ted Allan, writing as early as 1942, Bethune "conducted the first experiments with cadaver blood in Spain in conjunction with J. B. S. Haldane and Hermann Muller."[19]

Shortly after Saxton first visited Bethune at Madrid, the Blood Transfusion Unit was joined by Hermann J. Muller, a renowned American geneticist who had been instrumental in discovering the effect of x-radiation on gene mutation and chromosomal change; discoveries which would eventually lead to his being awarded a Nobel Prize. An ardent communist, Muller had, in 1934, accepted an invitation to work with Nikolai Vavilov at the Institute of Genetics of the Academy of Sciences of the USSR, in

Leningrad and Moscow. In 1936 Muller wrote a lengthy letter to Stalin suggesting that, appropriately employed, genetic science could provide a path to human betterment within a socialist context. The letter was not well received: Stalin had become increasingly convinced that Trofim Lysenko's, utterly mistaken Lamarckian approach to evolution was superior to Muller's approach; it promised more rapid results in agricultural improvements, and human genetics had become tainted as inherently racist due to the Nazi and Anglo-American eugenics programs. A December 1936 public debate between Muller and Lysenko did nothing to improve matters. In early 1937 an ideological attack on formal genetics was launched at the highest levels of the Soviet state. It was evident to Muller that scientific genetic research was no longer possible; he requested a leave of absence. In order to avoid any unfounded suspicion that he might be planning to criticize Soviet biological policies while abroad, he decided to volunteer for the antifascist struggle in Spain. He discussed the matter with Vavilov who readily concurred. Muller appears to have known about Bethune's Institute through Julian Huxley, a good friend of J. B. S. Haldane, and it was with Bethune that he decided to work. N. F. Gorbunov, the Secretary of the Academy of Sciences, cordially agreed to the proposal. Muller spent his last days in Moscow preparing notes on blood transfusion, and took several books and articles on blood research with him. He left Moscow on 8 March and arrived in Madrid before the middle of the month.[20]

For eight weeks Muller worked in Bethune's laboratory developing a method for harvesting the blood of recently killed soldiers, in an effort to adapt Yudin's basic technique to battlefield conditions; his notes of 30 March 1937, entitled "Work on Cadaver Blood," explicitly refer to "putting it into use at the front." An undated page entitled "Equipment Needed for Getting Cadaver Blood," notes a long list of required materials, while a further three pages entitled "Technique of Obtaining Cadaver Blood," details a procedure initially "worked out by the Central Institute of Blood Transfusion [of the USSR] before 1932."[21]

Muller's project was carried out with the direct participation of Bethune, Dr. Grande Covian, a prominent Spanish physician, and, to some extent, Haldane, who had recently returned to Spain. He learned how to extract blood from cadavers, and was investigating the difference between such blood and that freshly donated by the living. Initial preparatory work involved the comparison between freshly-donated blood stored in a refrigerator and blood kept for two weeks at room temperature; freshly donated blood transported by truck for seven hours over rough roads was observed to differ not at all in terms of hemolysis – cell rupture – from a control sample in the laboratory.[22] Early in April he began to work with cadaver blood

The Blood of the Dead

itself. On 14 April he recorded in his notebook: "blood of a cadaver who died at 5 am with both legs blown off was obtained at 11 am from the right internal jugular vein. . . . It was mixed with the blood of Allen May. . . . In all cases the mixture clotted soon."[23] Bethune himself functioned as Muller's primary assistant, surgically inserting the glass cannulas into the veins.

After various experiments, Muller became increasingly confident that cadaver blood could be used effectively. He volunteered to have it transfused into himself. On 20 April he wrote in his notebook:

> I had earlier suggested to Bethune my being injected with this blood except for its too small quantity. Bethune answered that anything more would be too much to be safe, so I have decided on using it after it is four days old, unless the Wasserman group is bad or if sterility or other tests contraindicate. Questioning Grande as to his view of the safety of this experiment in view of his believing the blood to be weakly clotted, he says "well, we can try anyway and see." So on with the experiment. Later we found it full of small clots, so we discarded it.[24]

Further work involved comparing "records of manner of death of men where blood shows de-clotting and those where blood does not."[25] Much effort appears to have been spent on obtaining "blood from different organs,"[26] pumping, for example, the "liver for extra blood,"[27] and comparing the volume of cadaver blood that flowed from "the direction of the head," as opposed to that from the "direction of the heart."[28]

Muller received letters from Vavilov on 5 April and again on 8 May, concerning genetics, and congratulating him on his work in Madrid. And when Muller, along with Bethune and others, helped remove and save a number of scientific books from the biology museum of the University of Madrid following a fascist bombing attack, news of the incident was well received in Moscow. Shortly afterwards Muller concluded his experiments on cadaveric transfusion and left Spain, traveling to Paris, then to Texas to visit his son, and then returning to Soviet Union to pack his belongings. He left Moscow permanently in October for Edinburgh.[29]

Muller felt the "profoundest admiration, as well as a deep attachment" to Bethune, considering him a man of "heroic character" underlying an "unassuming exterior."[30] While there is no reason to doubt his assessment, it is evident that Muller's tenure at the Blood Transfusion Institute coincided with the final period of Bethune's work in Spain; Muller would leave the country less than a month before him.

Undated documents written by Hazen Sise – probably toward the end of April – indicate that Muller's experiments were much appreciated;

indeed it would appear that there was some definite expectation that Muller might continue at the Blood Transfusion Institute even after Bethune's departure. Sise was advocating that the Sanidad Militar, in the context of a general reorganization, relocate the Institute to a much more extensive building than they presently occupied, largely to accommodate a more sophisticated laboratory for Muller, Grande Covian, and their assistant Jean Picone. Sise pointed especially to the "unique advantages of cadaver blood as outlined by Judine [Yudin]," noting that "Prof. Muller of Moscow" was not only undertaking such research but would be attempting "to find and isolate an anti-coagulant in the plasma of cadaver blood which could be used in place of sodium citrate which sometimes has harmful reactions." Interestingly, in neither the detailed list of proposed room allocations, nor the equally detailed list of job responsibilities, was Bethune so much as mentioned; on the contrary – for reasons to which we must return later, and at length – Sise suggested one or more new doctors be sent out from Canada, and that Dr. Valentin de la Loma take on the role of director of the Institute.[31]

Muller's work would appear to have had a profound effect not only on Sise but, more importantly, on Reginald Saxton. Nor does it seem unlikely that since both Saxton and Muller worked closely and simultaneously with Bethune during this period that Saxton learned the technique of cadaver transfusion at Bethune's Institute in Madrid, and thus felt confident in advocating its widespread use to the Sanidad Militar.

As we have noted, Preston appears to hold that very little of value even-tuated from Saxton's apprenticeship in the transfusion of cadaver blood. The historian Victor Howard has agreed, maintaining that although Bethune's medical research was a legitimate "subordinate function of the unit," the work of Muller and others in "the research programs conducted at that time came to nothing . . . "[32]

But with the recent publication of the diary of James Neugass, an American ambulance driver with the International Brigades, we now know that Saxton applied what he had learned in Bethune's laboratory on a far greater scale than has hitherto been recognized. In this context, the diary entry for 14 January 1938 is revelatory. Neugass had driven into Cuevas, a small village slightly northeast of the city of Teruel, where the fascist offensive had been particularly brutal, with thousands of casualties. He wrote:

Entered Cuevas . . . with heart in my throat because town had obviously just been bombed. . . . Had the hospital been hit . . . ?

Four dead cavalrymen fully dressed and unspotted by blood lay on stretchers in the hospital courtyard. Saxton, blond tall young English

The Blood of the Dead

doctor, knelt beside one of them. He had rolled a sleeve up past the elbow of a gray arm.

"What do you think you're doing, Saxton?" I asked. . . .

He did not answer.

Angry, I leaned over the doctor's shoulder. The single vampire tooth of a big glass syringe was slowly drawing the blood out of the vein inside of the dead cavalryman's forearm. The vessel filled and Saxton stood up.

"New Soviet technique," he said, holding the syringe between his squinting eye and the late winter sun. Purple lights shadowed the glistening bar of ruby.

"Seldom we get the chance. Most of them are pretty well empty when they go out. Those four over there were in one of those clay dugouts in the wall of the main street. No timbers on the roof. Direct hit. Asphyxiated, all of them. Their comrades dug them out before they were cold and brought them up here. Thought we could help. Their bad luck" – Saxton pointed to the four gray young faces with clay-stuffed mouths – "was our good luck. We're running short on donors and the transfusion truck is too busy."

"You mean . . . that you're going to . . . "

"Well, first I'll have to type and then test it . . . why not? . . . have to hurry."

I touched the bright tube with my hard black fingertips. Was the glass warm with the sun or with human life?

Now I understand why we must win. Men die but the blood fights on in other veins and their purpose fills our hearts.[33]

Neugass's description of Saxton's work has the virtue of being undeniably moving, even poetic, while simultaneously providing an aura of true authenticity. But more importantly, what does it suggest about Saxton? There is no indication here of hesitancy or experimentation; on the contrary Saxton appears confident, assured, and knowledgeable, as if he had obviously done what he was doing many times before. He appears to be well-practiced in a well-established technique, typing and testing the blood of the cadavers before beginning transfusions into the living. In the light of Neugass' diary, it becomes necessary to reconsider the extent to which cadaver blood transfusions were carried out during the Spanish Civil War. For a brief few weeks in the spring of 1937, Bethune, Muller, and Saxton, came together in an at least partially successful attempt to apply Yudin's groundbreaking discoveries to conditions prevailing within an active war zone. And Saxton, having established his own mobile blood transfusion service, carried the method into practice.

There is scant mention of Bethune's laboratory, its purposes, functions, research program or participants in any of the standard biographies on Bethune: the nature and content of his medical research program has been almost entirely overlooked. His work on cadaver blood transfusion is a much undervalued aspect of his medical innovations in Spain, another facet of his total medical devotion to the Republican government and the international antifascist movement.

17

I Killed My Own Son

March was an intensely active month for Bethune, full of new and important accomplishments, but at the same time of increasing complexities and conflicts. To Sorensen's undoubted consternation, new faces were constantly appearing and disappearing at the Institute; not only Saxton and Muller, but Leonard Crome, Greg Moller, Geza Karpathi and Herbert Kline, Jean Watts and Ted Allan.

Dr. Leonard Crome came to Spain with the Scottish Ambulance Unit run by the indomitable Miss Fernanda Jacobsen, the same unit with which Kajsa Rothman had been associated, and from which she had later been expelled. Crome, and others in the unit, were repelled by Jacobsen's unprincipled position during the crucial Jarama campaign, that they were in Spain to help both sides: Republicans and fascists alike. Crome had become acquainted with Bethune, and he, along with other members of the Scottish Ambulance Unit – Maurice Linden, Roderick MacFarquhar, and George Burleigh – left Jacobsen and lived for a time, at Bethune's invitation, at the Blood Transfusion Unit where they were, reportedly, "royally entertained with political gossip and whiskey." Shortly afterwards Bethune drove Crome and the others to Saxton's International Brigade hospital at Villarejo on his near daily round of blood deliveries. Crome and Saxton became close friends, Crome rising to Chief Medical Officer of the Division Medical Services within the year.[1]

About this time, early in March, Greg Moller, an American who had been living in Scandinavia, was working as a war correspondent for the Danish newspaper *Politiken*, as well as aiding in the Republican government's evacuation of women and children from Madrid. He happened to encounter Bethune and Kajsa Rothman when they were delivering blood to Villarejo, and he and Bethune became close. Moller, who lived in the street next to the Blood Transfusion Unit, came over almost every day. He donated his blood regularly, and managed to bring a little of the food intended for the evacuees to help feed the blood donors. Often, Bethune took him on transfusion missions to the Jarama field hospitals or to the various battlefronts. On one occasion Bethune, Moller, and a reporter – Dennis Weaver of the *News Chronicle* – were "almost wiped out by a bomb that exploded nearby, while Norman was happily prowling around for souvenirs." A few years after the war Moller maintained that he had "smuggled letters out of Spain," presumably to Denmark, for Henning Sorensen; what might have been in these letters, or to whom they were addressed, he did not reveal.[2]

Moller knew very well that Bethune was in love with Rothman and was certain that she was, unknowingly, the cause of serious friction between Bethune and Sorensen. Certainly we have seen that Rothman had become a focus of Sorensen's paranoiac fear of spies infiltrating the Institute. Information in a Spanish intelligence document indicates that Sorensen was now reporting that, during Bethune's recent absence in Paris, Rothman had made allegedly suspicious "frequent trips to the front, morning, afternoon, and sometimes even at night," claiming that she was "gathering information with regard to the needs for transfusions at the front." As a result of these forays, and entirely on "Kajsa's initiative . . . there exists . . . a series of detailed maps, similar to military maps;" although it should have been obvious to both Sorensen and the Spanish authorities that such maps were a necessity for the rapid and expeditious delivery of blood. Moreover, according to Sorensen, when Bethune took photographs of hospitals, "the negatives disappeared when Kajsa was left alone." It would not be long before Sorensen was demanding that Bethune abandon Rothman and remove her from the Institute's premises.[3]

For some time, even before the events on the Malaga road, Bethune had been planning to make a film on the work of the Blood Transfusion Institute intended for Canadian and American audiences. He had convinced the CASD to purchase a camera and pay for the film. While in Paris, in discussions with Gertrude Araquistain and Ione Rhodes, he had met Ione's husband Peter. Bethune told him that he was looking for a photographer to help him make a film. Rhodes introduced him to Geza Karpathi, a handsome young Hungarian who had been educated at the Sorbonne in motion-picture photography. Bethune offered him $50 a week for his services, but Karpathi refused: he did not want a job, he wanted to help defeat fascism; he would accept only $25.[4]

Following Bethune and May from Paris, Karpathi came to Herbert Kline's hotel room in Madrid and suggested they collaborate on the film.[5] Kline was a writer who had traveled to Spain in December 1936 to report for the Communist magazine, *New Masses*. Together, they would ride with Bethune to the war zones and document the transfusion unit in action. The two filmmakers would live at the Institute, huddling over maps with Bethune, determining each day's shooting schedule. Kline would direct; Karpathi would be in charge of photography. The film they made together,

I Killed My Own Son 159

Heart of Spain, shot under often difficult battlefield conditions, would become a classic depiction of the resistance of the Spanish people to fascism and of the bond of blood that united them. Many years later, when Karpathi had changed his name to Charles Korvin and was working in Hollywood, both he and Kline were blacklisted as unfriendly witnesses before the House Committee on Un-American Activities: but they knew fascism, they had seen it first-hand; and they were not about to divulge the names of their comrades to its current American representatives.[6]

The filming of *Heart of Spain* appears to have begun early in March and lasted well into May. The finished film opens with a series of scenes depicting the nature of the fascist offensive and of the peoples' resistance: a fascist bombing raid over Madrid, the daily lives of the civilian population, an International Brigades cemetery, a notable speech by Commander Lister of the Fifth Regiment, and footage of the Army of the Republic moving into action. Only in the latter half of the film do we witness the functioning of the Blood Transfusion Institute: hundreds of civilian blood donors lining up on Principe de Vergara, and then Bethune himself explaining the process of blood transfusion, engaging in the extraction of blood from the donors, and transporting the blood, under fire, to Barsky's American hospital. Internal evidence suggests that the core of the film was shot in March and early April, during the period of the Jarama and Guadalajara campaigns; an article published in the *Daily Clarion* indicates that scenes portraying life in Madrid and the surrounding villages were still being filmed as late as the first week of May, and perhaps even later.[7]

Victory had eluded the fascists on the Jarama front; the road from Madrid to Valencia had not been severed; the attempt to form a wedge between the two cities, isolate them, encircle them, and destroy them, had failed. With the winding down of the Jarama campaign, the fascist armies moved north-east of Madrid toward Guadalajara, intending to penetrate Madrid's defenses from the north and capture the city. At the same time renewed attacks launched from the Jarama valley were intended as a secondary front; when the fascists rushed down from Guadalajara, they would be joined by troops moving up from Jarama, and Madrid would be overwhelmed. With the fall of Madrid, the majority of the Republic's best soldiers would be annihilated; the death of the Republic would inevitably follow, and the darkness and horror of Franco's fascism would swallow the entire country.[8]

This renewed attempt to capture Madrid was led by the Italian-Fascist general, Roatta Mancini, commanding four divisions: the Blackshirts, the Black Flames, the Black Arrow, and the Littorio, with the armored support of two hundred and fifty tanks and one hundred and eighty units of mobile artillery. The German-Nazi troops at Mancini's disposal included an infantry brigade and four companies of machine-gunners; seventy-two aircraft – half Italian, half from Franco's own forces – provided air support. The Guadalajara campaign began on 8 March and continued throughout the month. At first, the Italian divisions were successful, moving with lightning speed toward their target. The situation was critical. But within days the Republican forces and the International Brigades rallied and held their ground. Casualties mounted on both sides. On 18 March the Republican army went on the offensive; within the day, the whole Italian army was routed and in panicky flight; the towns and villages taken by the Italians were liberated by the Republicans.[9]

For the fascists, the Guadalajara campaign was a disaster. Sporadic fighting continued for several weeks, but the back of the fascist assault was decisively broken. Italian losses numbered three thousand dead, six thousand wounded, two thousand taken prisoner. In Madrid, hundreds of Italian prisoners were exhibited and photographed, mountains of ammunition, shells, grenades, trucks, and other war materiel was inventoried. The Republican government telegraphed the League of Nations stating that captured documents and the confessions of Italian prisoners of war proved without doubt "the presence of regular military units of the Italian Army in Spain." But the British government, as the leading power of the farcical Non-Intervention Committee, continued its outrageously hypocritical position, announcing publicly that "there was no official confirmation of the rumor of Italian troops on the Madrid front."[10]

Guadalajara was simultaneously the victory of democracy and the death of democracy. Guadalajara demonstrated that if the legitimate government of Spain had been permitted to purchase arms on the open market it would have unquestionably defeated Franco's fascism within a few short months. But Guadalajara also demonstrated, once and for all, that the Western Powers were determined to bury the Republic alive. And while the euphoria engendered by the defeat of the fascist armies in open country swept the Republic and buoyed for a time its hope of ultimate victory, Guadalajara was the last campaign, of any true significance, it was ever to win.

For his part, Bethune poured himself into the Guadalajara conflict, as he had at Jarama. He was everywhere at once in March, with Moller, and Saxton, and Muller, and Allan May, and Geza Karpathi, and so many others. There was the endless need for blood: extraction in Madrid, transport to the hospitals, transfusions to be given.

On the morning of 11 March, Bethune, Sorensen, Geza Karpathi, and Dr. Culebras drove from Madrid to Guadalajara in the Ford truck, carrying ten pint bottles of preserved donated blood and an extra refrigerator. The weather was cold; a piercing north wind blew down from the snow-capped mountains of the Guadarrama range. Bethune and the others were dressed in warm brown coats – a gift of the Madrid Syndicate of Tailors. The previous day, Mancini's Italian divisions had broken through the Republican lines, inflicting serious damage on both the army and the International Brigades, especially the Thaelmann Battalion. A Republican counter-attack on the fascist forces north-east of Guadalajara was now in progress. Driving at considerable speed, Bethune passed a convoy of open trucks carrying Republican troops and, up ahead, a string of tanks hurtling down the road.

Arriving at the five-hundred-bed Guadalajara hospital – only a week earlier bombed by fascist aircraft – Bethune noticed a long row of blood-stained stretchers leaning against a wall, waiting to be washed. The air in the operating room was heavy with ether. The chief surgeon looked up from his work at the operating table and nodded a quick sign of recognition. Bethune went over to the refrigerator standing in a corner and opened it: seven empty blood bottles, three full. It was agreed that he would leave six new bottles, and return the next day with more.

Bethune left the operating room and, with his colleagues, made his way down the corridor to Dr. Jolly's department. They were well acquainted from earlier days in Madrid. Jolly asked if they had brought him a refrigerator. They had. It was retrieved from the truck, plugged in, and the four remaining bottles of blood placed inside. Jolly's room was crammed with the wounded, bloodstained bandages were everywhere. There was a soldier with the International Brigades lying on a stretcher that no one could understand; he spoke neither English, French, Italian, nor German. He had been hit by a bomb and lost a hand and an eye on the battlefield. At the hospital it had been necessary to amputate his remaining hand. It was evident that he badly needed a blood transfusion. From his pallor and feeble pulse rate, Bethune estimated that he had lost at least two quarts of blood. He prepared the transfusion equipment, and then called to Sorensen for assistance. At sound of the name, the wounded soldier turned to Sorensen and began to speak: he was Swedish. Sorensen translated: the man had been in Spain only three days. He had been wounded on his first engagement. He felt now only regrets: he was of no more use to his comrades; he had done nothing for the cause. Bethune and Sorensen looked at each other in frank astonishment. Later, recalling the incident, Bethune wrote movingly: "Yet that is the spirit of the International Brigade; of ten thousand determined unconquerable men, with no thought of themselves, with no thought of sacrifice, but simply and with a pure heart ready to lay down their lives for their friends."[11]

They left the hospital and drove half an hour further up the road, toward the front, in search of more wounded. Unaware of the precise location of the battle line – the fighting having ebbed and flowed all day – they found themselves, without warning, in disputed territory between the Republican and fascist forces. As they approached the village of Trijueque, a shot rang out and struck their fender. Bethune attempted to turn back, but he flooded the engine and the truck stalled. Out of nowhere, two Republican soldiers leapt on to the running boards. Suddenly they were under fascist fire; a hail of bullets struck all about them. One of the soldiers was struck and fell to the ground. Bethune and the others jumped out of the truck. Bethune helped the remaining soldier drag his wounded comrade into a ditch. A second later, a bullet smashed through the windscreen directly over the steering wheel; a moment earlier and Bethune would have been dead, shot through the chest. Flattening themselves against the ground, Bethune and his colleagues crawled slowly through the fields, bullets whizzing closely over their heads. Worn out and filthy, Bethune and Culebras made their way back to the safety of a casualty clearing station near the Guadalajara hospital; Sorensen and Karpathi returned to Madrid separately. The next day, a retreating Republican soldier returned their truck.[12]

Bethune's commitment to the Republic was total; he was fearless, even reckless, in its defense. But he was becoming increasingly over-extended and exhausted. Working so hard and so long with only one lung was beginning to take its predictable effect. He needed more sleep. Often, in Madrid, he would grab a blanket, go into an empty room, and lie down for hours at a time. "Sometimes," as Sorensen observed, "fatigue would come over him . . . and he looked twenty years older."[13] And yet there was so much to be done. When blood supplies ran low at the field hospitals, Bethune would be called out at three or four in the morning to make emergency deliveries; a few hours later he would be making his regular daily rounds. And although he had said he preferred to be at the front, that it was "the only place that is real," it was at the front that the wounded lay, bleeding and dying, begging, in their pain, for their agony to end. As had been so obvious to so many in Detroit and in Montreal, his kindness and caring for the wounded was without parallel, and the language used to describe it is both significant and revelatory. According to Sise: "With the wounded, with anybody in distress, with children, Bethune became one of the most warm and solicitous people you can imagine."[14] According to Sorensen: "He was very tender with the wounded, very concerned. His whole personality changed when he was with the wounded . . . There was love, and they felt it. He communicated it to the wounded. He was so excited when they recovered."[15] He remembered a day when Bethune was required to give a transfusion to a young girl in Madrid. She was sixteen, and remarkably

I Killed My Own Son

163

lovely: a fascist artillery shell had blown off both her legs. She was moaning and crying, not only because of the agony of her wounds, but because, as she said in Spanish: "Who is going to marry me now?" Bethune held her, and quietly hushed her, and with loving gentleness he stroked her cheek over and over again, whispering to her that she was beautiful. Although she understood not a word of Bethune's English, her face slowly became calm, and she smiled up at him. The blood had kept her alive, but Bethune's touch had given her the will to live.[16] As Sorensen put it, most significantly: *"He was like a father to the wounded."*[17]

But when the wounded died it touched Bethune deeply, no doubt in a way that neither Sise nor Sorensen could understand. An eighteen-year-old Norwegian boy, whom Bethune described as "a mother's dream of a son," had volunteered with the International Brigades. He was wounded, he was transfused, and then he died. For Bethune, "It was like I had killed my own son."[18] Who was this boy who should not have died? He was not the first who failed to live. Not everyone into whom Bethune transfused blood thrived; an unavoidable proportion died. Perhaps the wound this boy carried was not so great. Perhaps it was nothing; a stray bullet to be easily excised, a loss of blood that was far from extreme. But there was something about this boy whose death was not at all predictable; perhaps he received the blood that Bethune put into his veins with a certain eagerness, his eyes opening with fervid gratitude and then, suddenly, he was dead in Bethune's arms.

It was not the first time that a death had torn at Bethune in this way; there is a history. There was the young priest at Sacré Coeur, and other patients who, inevitably, did not recover after their operations. And we can recall what Dr. Deshaies said: "I couldn't stay around when he lost a patient because he was so sorry . . . he would cry or be mad . . . at that time I preferred to be away from him." Bethune's grief could be overwhelming; not even he could comprehend it, but the words he uses provides us with the key. What does it mean to be *a mother's dream of a son?* Perhaps he was beautiful: young, strong, clean-limbed, and handsome; an open, honest face, unlined by compromise or cynicism. But what else could this mean to Bethune? This boy, this young Norwegian lad, this *mother's dream of a son*, is, suddenly, for Bethune the very symbol and crystallization of failure. The critical gaze of the mother – his own mother – is upon him; he is no dream for *her* but a curse; the son who has been rejected, cast out, who has been told that his sickness was God's retribution, that he was no longer her son. The fear of inadequacy, of mediocrity, bred by unlove, rises up within him again like a recurrent disease. And now there is this dead boy whom he mourns as though he were his own; the son he had always wanted but who had been denied to him: *it was like I had killed my own son*. Killed; another life aborted. Analysis is no longer necessary: we know our man: every lost boy is himself. This uncomplicated Norwegian lad is who Bethune himself wanted somehow to be. This beautiful boy is both the son he never had and the man he could never be – a man who could stand secure on the rock of his mother's love, who could sleep in peace within his mother's dream. As Sorensen said, with true perspicacity, there were times when Bethune "was like a lost child in search of his mother."[19]

If there had been occasions when Deshaies could not bear to be around Bethune, equally there were occasions when Bethune could not bear to be around himself. His grief and sense of failure went to the root. His solution: to drink, and in drinking, not to forget but to yield to the rage within him. He was aware of his anger, of his fury. He knew very well the division within him, although its true origin, submerged and unconscious, necessarily escaped him. He was proud of the work that he had accomplished, and was still accomplishing, in Spain, but increasingly it seemed to him that everywhere he turned new barriers and roadblocks confronted him. The Spanish doctors at the Blood Transfusion Unit appeared endlessly resentful and resistant to his projects and his authority. The problem was not new, but far from being resolved, it continued to escalate. On 9 March, Bethune had written to Ben Spence: "The Spanish doctors who work with us seem to be incapable of accepting responsibility or acting on their own initiative. Consequently, I am forced to attend to every detail myself."[20] And Culebras was openly flaunting him by attaching his many relatives to the Unit and encouraging them to draw double pay – both from the CASD and the Sanidad Militar. Furious, Bethune would lose his temper, cursing wildly and pounding his fist on the table.[21]

To make matters worse, the Sanidad Militar, having finally and irrevocably rejected Bethune's plan to have all the blood transfusion services in the Republic placed under his leadership, was nevertheless demanding that he provide funds not only for the Madrid unit, but also for the central Valencia transfusion service. Bethune refused to cooperate.[22] Twice Spanish authorities ordered him to report to Valencia to discuss the matter, and twice he ignored them. Only when they sent a third telegram, threatening him with arrest, did he comply. As so often, Sorensen was there to translate and to soften Bethune's fiery language. Cerrada insisted on knowing why Bethune had not sent the money for Valencia. Bethune replied that he had been occupied doing his job: transfusing the wounded at Jarama and Guadalajara. He also noted that Cerrada had not paid the salaries of the Spaniards at the Madrid unit, as *he* had promised. Cerrada, referring almost certainly to secret, and no doubt slanderous, reports sent by Culebras, accused him, according to Sorensen, of not behaving as a communist should. It was a low blow, and Bethune was hurt. His temper dropped, and Cerrada became more conciliatory. In the end, new promises and arrangements were negotiated.[23]

Every setback redoubled his smoldering anger, and then his fatigue and exhaustion. To Sise, it seemed as though Bethune was "living on the raw edge of his nerves" and "close to end of his tether as far as his physical strength and his nerves were concerned."[24] In Sorensen's view: "The strain of war began to tell. He would lose his temper. He drank too much. It affected his work. His hands were shaking when he had to do a blood transfusion."[25]

And then the final blow: Sorensen demanded that Bethune give up Kajsa Rothman. He insisted she was a spy; he insisted that the central problem between Bethune and the Spanish doctors, especially Culebras and Goyanes, stemmed from Rothman's presence in the Unit. And although none of this was true, Bethune could see no other way out. According to Greg Moller, Rothman's "loveliness almost broke up the Canadian Blood Transfusion outfit," and lost Bethune "his best friend," Sorensen. "Finally, he had to give her up to keep his staff together for the splendid work of which he was so justly proud."[26] For Bethune, the loss was devastating. He was in love with Rothman. Since the collapse of his second marriage to Frances Penney, there had been any number of women; with some of them the relationship, no matter how intense, had remained unconsummated; some had been brief affairs – a night or two of purely sexual enjoyment, or a few weeks of deeper intimacy. But there had been no one like Rothman. She not only fulfilled him sexually, but he was able to lose himself entirely with her, to overcome, to the degree that he was capable, the inhibitions that followed him into every liaison. She was generous and cheerful and capable as no other woman had been, of kindness, and devotion, and caring. Perhaps they both knew that a wartime romance would not last; quite possibly they did not, given the circumstances, think of the future: sudden death was always a possibility. And although we cannot know the precise details of the situation – who said what to whom; how Rothman received the news of the necessity of their separation – their break-up must have tragically fulfilled what had become a deep-seated belief for Bethune, the old formula repeating itself once again: *Whoever I love will not love me; whoever I love will leave me.* Inevitably, such a profound loss could only have exacerbated the cycle of drinking, rage, and irrationality allegedly increasingly evident throughout the final weeks of Bethune's tenure in Spain.

As for Kajsa Rothman, it may be that, with whatever regrets, she knew it was time for her to go. She had worked well with Sise and was devoted to the Blood Transfusion Unit, but it cannot have escaped her that Culebras and Goyanes distrusted and resented her, and that Sorensen's nagging suspicions were utterly paranoid. In any event, she seems to have rebounded from the affair with Bethune rather quickly. We do not know the exact date on which Bethune and Rothman said goodbye to each other, but an article in the *Daily Clarion* of 12 March, filed from Madrid, indicates that she was still working with Bethune's unit at that time.[27] The final break must have occurred only days later, since she appears to have been employed with the Republican press office very shortly thereafter. By late April she was acting as a guide and interpreter for a number of notable journalists including Virginia Cowles, Herbert Matthews, Philip Jordan, Willie Forrest, and Josephine Herbst.[28] In the fall of 1937 she was recruited by an organization called the Swedish Relief for Spain to work with refugee children and raise money for an orphanage in which to house them. She returned to Sweden in December 1937 to tour the country, talking about the situation in Spain and raising money for the orphanage. Later, she wrote the text for a book of drawings these refugee children had made about the war. She appears to have traveled frequently between Sweden and Spain until, with the Republic's collapse, she fled to France and finally to Mexico where she died in 1969.[29] It should be noted that there were certain parallel and mutual interests between Bethune and Rothman: both were much concerned about the increasing numbers of orphaned Spanish children – and about children's art – and both went to great effort to raise money for their support. It is interesting to speculate what influence Bethune may have had on Rothman in this regard.

And yet, we are now confronted with a serious problem. We have been told by both Sise and Sorensen that Bethune was "living on the raw edge of his nerves," exhausted and "close to the end of his tether," that fatigue would so overwhelm him that he would "look twenty years older," that "his hands were shaking" to the point where he could scarcely transfuse blood, and that he was given to rages and outrageous drunken behavior. *But is this true?* We have already observed that Bethune was making daily rounds to the hospitals in Madrid, and that throughout the Jarama-Guadalajara campaign he was delivering blood and providing transfusions at the front line field hospitals. He was training Saxton in the practice of blood extraction and transfusion; he had hosted Crome at the Blood Transfusion Unit and driven him to Villarejo; he had regularly taken Moller and a number of journalists to the front; he had worked extensively with Muller on experiments with cadaver blood; and he had been engaged in the planning and filming of *Heart of Spain*. While it was no doubt the case that such a heavy work load would have been tiring, the mere fact that he could accomplish so much in such a short period of time does not at all give evidence that he was "at the end of his tether;" quite the contrary. It is similarly significant that neither Saxton, nor Crome, nor Moller, nor Muller, nor Karpathi, nor many others who were acquainted with him make any mention of overwhelming fatigue, or, for that matter, of fits of rage or drunkenness. And yet it is not possible to simply discount the testimony of Sise and Sorensen. We know the effect, for example, that Kajsa Rothman's departure must have had on Bethune. It is more a question of exaggeration, perhaps even quite excessive exaggeration: the fits of rage and drunkenness may well have been less frequent and less severe than Sise and Sorensen indicate, the exhaustion and fatigue less onerous and grave. But why then these knowing, these deliberate, exaggerations? The answer is both simple and astonishing: they provided a *post facto* excuse, a plausible cover, for a conspiracy to remove Bethune from Spain.

18

The Conspiracy

Despite the significant role he would come to play in the conspiracy, surprisingly little is known concerning Ted Allan's activities in Spain. He seems not so much to inhabit the Blood Transfusion Institute, as to merely haunt it as a transitory ghost; he appears less a comrade or colleague of Bethune, than a tangential visitor pulled into a quarrel about which he knew little.

Allan had intended to go to Spain as a reporter for *The Clarion*, the daily newspaper of the Communist Party of Canada; Fred Rose, the head of the Party in Quebec, had made the necessary preparations. But Leslie Morris, the paper's editor, had already arranged for Jean Watts, a wealthy young woman who was prepared to pay her own expenses, to fill the position.[1] Allan, undeniably irritated, was not to be deterred. One version of events was that he decided to join the International Brigades and "fight in the trenches," traveling from Montreal to New York to take ship to France and from there to Spain. And yet he is said, while in New York, to have "called in at the office of the Federated Press, a wire service for the trade union movement, and convinced it to accredit him as a Spanish correspondent."[2] To make matters more complex, Pat Stephens, a Canadian volunteer who served in the Lincoln Battalion, recalled that he met Ted Allan on board the S.S. *Paris* sailing out of New York on 21 January 1937, and that Allan had told him he was indeed going to Spain as a reporter for *The Clarion*.[3] Also on board was John Lenthier, a young actor who became friendly with Allan, and Jean Watts, the actual *Clarion* reporter, whom Allan accused of having an affair with Lenthier.[4]

Six months later, in July 1937, *The Clarion* reported that Allan had "enlisted as a soldier,"[5] and Allan himself much later claimed that he had been in "a fighting unit,"[6] but he could not have been with the Brigades for very long and almost certainly he never engaged in combat. When his ship arrived in France at the port of Le Havre, Allan, like so many other volunteers, undoubtedly would have made his way to Paris and then traveled south, crossing the Pyrenees mountains into Spain. Hugh Garner recalled meeting Allan at the fortress of Figueras, a few kilometers south of the Spanish border some time in February.[7] From there, Allan continued on

The Conspiracy

to Albacete, the headquarters of the International Brigade. Perhaps Allan received a few days of arms training. He may possibly have been at Albacete when Nazi aircraft bombed the barracks in mid-February. But that was certainly the last Allan saw of the Brigades. Events then become unclear.

Allan was already an accredited correspondent for the Federated Press when he left New York, and it would appear that after a few days at Albacete he obtained a transfer to work as a press correspondent in Madrid.[8] Years later, Allan claimed that he left Albacete as a chance result of having dinner with Peter Kerrigan and several other commanding officers. Once Kerrigan discovered that Allan was from Montreal, he inquired whether he knew Bethune. Allan said they were good friends and that Bethune had previously asked him to come and work with him in Spain. Kerrigan then informed him that there were serious morale problems at the Blood Transfusion Unit, that Bethune was drinking heavily and arguing with the Spanish doctors, and that Allan should go at once to Madrid, investigate the situation, and report his findings directly to Luigi Longo (known in Spain as "Gallo"), the chief Political Officer of the entire International Brigades.[9]

It is difficult to determine how much, if any, of this story is true. Bethune had scarcely known Allan in Montreal, and there is no evidence that he ever asked him to join him in Spain; it is unlikely that he would. What's more, if Kerrigan asked Allan to make investigations and report to Gallo, Allan, in all of his various and contradictory reminiscences of his Spanish adventures, never so much as mentions Gallo again, let alone recalls submitting a report. What is certain is that Allan went to Madrid in February, working as a press correspondent, and at some point inserted himself in the activities of the Blood Transfusion Unit.

Meanwhile, Jean Watts, after disembarking ship, parted ways with Allan and made contact with Loto Katz at the *Agence Espagne* press office in Paris, who put her on an airplane bound for Valencia, most probably on 13 February. Unable to arrange further transportation, she was forced to stay in Valencia "in a ghastly place with no windows for about a week," until the Scottish Ambulance Service was able to take her on to Madrid.[10] According to the diary of Hazen Sise, she arrived at the Blood Transfusion Institute on 21 February.[11] Bethune himself was not there: he had gone to Paris on 17 February in the aftermath of the Malaga atrocity, and would not finally return to Madrid until 3 March. Sise and Tom Worsley were in Madrid on 16 February, but left again for Barcelona on 21 February. Sorensen returned to Madrid from Barcelona on 20 February, but left again for Valencia four days later.[12] In short, the only Canadian member of the blood transfusion team present with Watts from the day of her arrival at the

Institute, until the return of all its members on 3 March, was Sorensen. What did he tell her during their four days together?

Decades later, Watts told an interviewer that she "really didn't like Bethune at all," while conceding, significantly, that she saw little of him. Her duties at the Institute consisted primarily of writing articles for *The Clarion*, and helping out with the making of *Heart of Spain*, traveling about the countryside with the blood delivery truck and keeping a record of filming locations. Ted Allan, she maintained, was in Madrid entirely "as a civilian."[13]

Allan, however, claimed in an interview that he first went to the Blood Transfusion Institute "about February 11, 12, or 13," and that he and Watts greeted each other "fulsomely." When he asked where Bethune was, she allegedly said, "Oh that son of a bitch," and told him "that he was vicious, he drank, he was violent, and the Spanish hated him."[14] Undated research materials that Allan collected – or invented – for his autobiography contain a number of typed pages in a diary format. The page for 12 February 1937 states "I got here on the 9th. Made my first notes on the 10th. Beth lovely but isn't he drinking too much? He's very impatient with the Spanish staff. Says they're mostly incompetents and suspects some of them are fascist sympathizers. . . . Jim [Jean Watts was known to almost everyone as 'Jim,'] had a long talk. Says Beth's an egomaniac and she hates him." The diary page for 14 February states "Showed Beth my dispatch about Albacete bombardment. He said it was very good."[15]

Again, it is exceedingly difficult to take Allan at his word. Bethune simply was not in Madrid on the dates of the alleged "diary" pages, nor is it possible for Watts to have formed any opinion concerning Bethune on the dates in question since she had not yet arrived in Madrid and had not yet met him. It remains true that, in the interval, she could have absorbed Sorensen's increasingly hostile attitude toward Bethune, but there is a good deal of emotional distance between the dislike Watts admitted and the hatred ascribed to her by Allan. It is perhaps possible that Allan may have visited the Blood Transfusion Unit once or twice in February: he published a short article on the blood service during that month, although, significantly, the article possesses not a single direct quotation from Bethune himself, indicating strongly that Allan did not interview him – which he surely would have done had he been available – and that the article as a whole could easily have been cribbed from existing press reports.[16]

If we are to believe Greg Moller, Ted Allan rarely made an appearance at Bethune's headquarters until a month later, in mid-March. Moller, it will be recalled, lived close to Bethune, saw him "almost every day," and rode with him to the frontlines following the fascist defeat at Guadalajara, and yet, he said: "I don't know Mr. Ted Allan."[17] Moreover, the war-time diary of British International Brigader David Crook supports a position that Allan probably did not encounter Bethune until late into February, or in early March, and that for some time thereafter he was at best an infrequent visitor. In the first week of March, Crook met Jim Watts and "fell very hard at first sight." On 14 March, Crook notes that Allan is a journalist, and that Herbert Kline "is working here with Ted Allan who is doing some stuff for the *New Masses*. Allan has been to the front and described the attitude of the men."[18] Crook never mentions Allan again, despite the fact that Crook was living with Watts "the last twelve nights – and most of the days" at the Blood Transfusion Institute and "through Beth's goodwill," during the last two weeks of March.[19]

Crook's diary possesses yet another value: in the space of a few pages it provides some real insight not only into Watts, but into Bethune's character and habits at the time. According to Crook, Jim Watts, who was an enigmatic figure, and almost certainly bisexual, was "neither timid nor frigid but has some physical or psychological inhibition which makes intercourse painful – probably with anyone." Even so, they spent much of their time "in bed, in a gluttonous sort of way" – whatever that might mean. As to Bethune, Crook did not observe the exhaustion and fatigue maintained by Sise, but noted that, on the contrary, he displayed "drive and energy and is apparently highly qualified technically." Like Watts, however, Crook found Bethune to be "a colossal egotist, though a party member, which makes his relations with his coworkers, and with most human beings, very bad." A few days before he left Madrid, Crook got drunk at the Institute, later writing in his diary: "unfortunately Beth came in and saw me – people in glass houses," indicating that if he had not seen Bethune drinking, he had at least been told of it.[20]

And yet, where was Ted Allan? What was he doing? Without doubt, many of Allan's tales are entirely fictitious. His claim that when he met Bethune in Madrid, "he greeted me like a brother, or perhaps a son, hugging me and saying 'God, I need you,'" and that "right then and there he appointed me political commissar," has been dismissed as a total fabrication by both Sise and Sorensen.[21] In his alleged "heavy role of the political commissar," Allan "began to insist" that Bethune "go home, and that he conduct a propaganda tour of the USA and Canada."[22] He also claims that during a meeting held by himself, May, and Sise, in which they were allegedly discussing this matter, Bethune came out from behind a curtain where he had been hiding and said: "So that's what you're planning to do with me":[23] a highly dramatic event which Sise, in the multitude of interviews he later gave, not once recalled. None of these stories are true, as we shall see. But even if we recognize Allan's further confessionary *mea culpa*: "I was mainly responsible for his going home" as an equally false, and an all too typical exaggeration, it is nevertheless the case that he certainly became a major player in the conspiracy to remove Bethune from Spain.[24]

We have already recorded the claims that Bethune was excessively fatigued, that he was at "the end of his tether," that his hands were shaking to the point where he was incapable of transfusing blood, that he looked twenty years older, and was "living on the raw edge of his nerves." And it must be asked again whether it is possible for someone in such condition to have done what we know he was doing: transporting blood to the front lines, training Saxton, working with Muller on research into cadaveric transfusion, engaging in the shooting of *Heart of Spain* where, in point of fact, we can actually *see* him performing blood transfusions with hands that are perfectly steady? Was he drinking more than usual? Quite probably, and we know why: the forced loss of Kajsa Rothman. Was he angry with the Spanish doctors in the unit? Again, certainly; and again, we know why. But were these really mad, insane rages? Ted Allan would have it that one night "Bethune, infuriated by the doctor with whom he'd had all the problems, gulped four straight whiskies, got drunk, and smashed his fist through the front-door window."[25] Sorensen too has his stories of rage: one legitimate, the other not. In the first, he recalls that Bethune, probably after an argument with Culebras, threw a chair against a wall and broke it. In the second, Bethune had returned late at night from delivering blood, and after knocking repeatedly on the door of the Blood Transfusion Unit, and finding that no one was going to get out of bed to answer it, he smashed a pane in the door with his gloved hand and let himself in; hardly an act of rage at all, and one is left wondering what else he was supposed to do?[26]

And yet, so many who were with him did not remark on Bethune's anger and bouts of drinking; neither Moller, nor Saxton, nor Crome. According to Muller, who was with Bethune precisely in that period when Bethune's rage and fury were said to be at a peak – March and April 1937 – he not only "felt the profoundest admiration, as well as deep attachment" toward Bethune, but he specifically refers to "the heroic character that underlay Dr. Bethune's unassuming exterior."[27] Anne Taft, who was Dr. Barsky's chief surgical assistant, knew Bethune well. She first met him when he delivered the first blood refrigerator to Barsky's hospital at El Romeral, and throughout the later period when *Heart of Spain* was filmed. Her impression was that he: "was interested in everything. He was the most vital human being. In a quite pleasant way, you could feel his personality. He was a compassionate, vibrant, vital person."[28] It is also worth noting that at precisely this time, transfusions given by Bethune and his unit had increased from about three

The Conspiracy

a day in early January, to upwards of 100 a day in March,[29] and that quite recent Spanish estimates suggest that Bethune was responsible for eighty per cent of all transfusions delivered during the war.[30]

Why then did the conspiracy to remove Bethune choose the middle of March to take action? Why at this time when Bethune was evidently so active in so many fields and with such apparent efficacy? And since the chief conspirator was most certainly not Ted Allan, who was?

Despite a complexity that we will necessarily do our best to unravel, the true heart and origin of the conspiracy comes down, in the final analysis, to a single factor: Sorensen's purity. He thought that Bethune was not communist enough, that he was insufficiently egalitarian, that he was egotistical and autocratic, that he spent money – money collected from hard-pressed Canadian workers – frivolously and individualistically, especially when he was away from Madrid, in Paris or elsewhere. Sorensen had been saving up these grievances, savoring them, almost cherishing them, to use when the time was ripe. When Bethune returned from Paris with Allen May, he brought Sorensen a gift: a set of Beatrix Potter books, and a portrait of himself signed "To Comrade Henning:" a photograph which Sorensen destroyed "in a fit of anger." May once complained to Sorensen that, in Paris, Bethune "certainly did not act like a revolutionary," and that he "would tell a lie if he was cornered." Sorensen "lost a lot of respect for Bethune when he heard this."[31] There was, of course, the on-going and overriding issue of Bethune's individualist refusal to cooperate with the absorption of the Blood Transfusion Institute into the Sanidad Militar, and, in Sorensen's mind, the worst sin of all – that Bethune spent time in bed with Kajsa Rothman, the primary focus of Sorensen's obsessive and almost pathological fear of fascist spies.

The truth was that Bethune was indeed guilty of most of these shortcomings and moral failures, but for reasons that Sorensen could never have understood. Sorensen wanted some sort of communist saint – as he himself later recognized – not a whole man, and especially not a whole man such as Bethune whose failings were so intimately and inextricably enjoined with his outstanding virtues.[32] Ted Allan too sought an angel in Bethune and was disappointed to find only a man. For his own deeply neurotic reasons, Allan needed a father to replace the father who had not loved him; quite possibly this was the source of Allan's endless fictionalizations and exaggerations. If he came to both love and hate Bethune, we should not be surprised. As he later wrote, Bethune "did not act as a hero is supposed to act, and he did not act as *my* hero was supposed to act."[33] In any event, given their mutually interlocking fantasies, Allan became the perfect ally for Sorensen.

When Bethune had delivered blood to Dr. Jolly's hospital in Guadalajara, he had returned to Madrid and dashed off a long article for the *Daily Clarion* detailing his experiences, and in which he had written: "This is great! Isn't it grand to be needed, to be wanted!" Ironically, on 18 March – not a week later – Sorensen, together with Ted Allan, wrote a letter to the Communist Party of Canada condemning Bethune and demanding his replacement. A brief note in the chronology written by Sorensen reads: *Pinto. Wrote the Party in Canada.*[34] Sise had been away from Madrid, in Perpignan and Barcelona, tending to truck repairs, until the 18th, and so could not have been part of this letter writing.[35] But a secret report, composed on 3 April by an intelligence officer of the Communist Party of Spain, refers to "Henning Sorensen, Dane, and Ted, Canadian" having sent a letter of complaint to the CPC, via a member of the Provincial Committee of the Party in Madrid.[36] The reference to "Pinto" is obscure; it may be the name of this Committee member, but Pinto was also the name of a pivotal village in the Jarama sector where fighting continued to break out.

It should be noted that the complaint was sent to the CPC, not the CASD who, it would seem, were not informed of the matter. There is nothing mysterious in this: Bethune was a Party member and his recall was entirely a Party matter. It was important to the Party, both in Spain and in Canada, that Bethune's work, and therefore his reputation, be kept intact, and for that reason neither Bethune nor the CASD were to be enlightened concerning the complaint that Sorensen and Allan had lodged. What was now imperative was to discover a method to remove Bethune from Spain with his honor intact.

It is evident that Sorensen and Allan could not have requested the CPC to recall Bethune without leveling specific charges against him. No document exists that details these charges, but the Spanish secret report of 3 April, and another undated secret report most probably written in July, contain a variety of charges and suspicions, many of which almost certainly originated with Sorensen, while the origin of others remains unknown.[37] These charges range from the likely to the absurd. Jewels which were said to have been present when Bethune and his team arrived at 36 Principe de Vergara, had allegedly disappeared, and it was said that Bethune took them to Paris and sold them, keeping the proceeds for himself, and that he also squandered money raised by the Canadian proletariat. It was alleged that he was frequently drunk and "was never in a condition to lead a mission as delicate as blood transfusion." It was heavily implied that Kajsa Rothman may have been a spy, and that on her own initiative she made a series of "very detailed maps similar to military maps." Even Bethune himself was not free from the false taint of espionage: it was said that he frequently went

The Conspiracy

to the front whenever there were troop movements, but not to make transfusions; and that he, "without concealing it, took detailed note of the state of bridges, road crossings, distances between certain points, the time it takes to travel them, etc., writing it all down carefully."[38] Whatever charges Sorensen and Ted Allan provided to the CPC, the Party certainly could not have evaluated them from such a distance; they would have had to rely on the capabilities of their comrades in the Spanish party. Presumably the Communist Party of Spain was in regular contact with the Canadian party, following Sorensen's complaint, since it is highly unlikely that the Spanish party would have acted alone, or taken any steps regarding Bethune without clearing them first through the CPC. Negotiations, no matter how brief, must have been entered into between the two parties, and an agreement concluded on how to proceed. However it came about, a decision was reached: the July report, written after Bethune left Spain, states explicitly, if somewhat mysteriously, that Bethune was expelled by the Blood Transfusion Unit and returned to Canada *"in a clever way."*[39]

This reference to a "clever way," not only alerts us to the reality of the conspiracy, but speaks to the importance of Bethune's work in Spain; other foreigners would simply have been removed from the country without anyone bothering to concoct a cover story. But it was necessary, from the Spanish government's point of view, that the moral and political support of the Canadian working class should continue. It was true that the Canadian volunteers that would make up the Mackenzie–Papineau Brigade had begun to arrive in substantial numbers, but Bethune and his blood transfusion unit were internationally famous and justifiably so; it was important that Bethune's name and person not be tarnished. The Communist Party of Canada, for very similar reasons could not but have agreed.

According to Sorensen's chronology, he and Ted Allan left for Valencia the very day after making their complaint to the CPC.[40] Perhaps significantly, it is the *only* mention of Ted Allan in the chronologies of either Sorensen or Sise. Why they went to Valencia is not recorded, but the likely explanation is that they needed to present themselves in person to either the central authorities of the Communist Party of Spain, or the Sanidad Militar, or both, to explain their complaint to the CPC. In any event, while in Valencia, Sorensen, through the intervention of Dr. Juan Planelles, the medical officer for the Fifth Regiment, became formally attached to the Sanidad Militar. What he did for them remains obscure since he seems never to have ceased working for the Blood Transfusion Unit in Madrid.[41]

Over the next several days, the details of the "clever" plan must have been worked out. The Spanish party contacted Vittorio Vidali, the one Spanish official that Bethune would be likely to have fully trusted and whom he would have regarded with incontrovertible esteem. Vidali was, after all, not only the head of the Socorro Rojo, but had been the political officer and organizer of the celebrated Fifth Regiment that had been primarily responsible from preventing Franco's entry into Madrid. He had met with Bethune prior to his intended journey to Malaga and had received sterling reports of Bethune from Tina Modotti. Moreover, Vidali had encountered Bethune very recently during the crushing defeat of the fascist forces at Guadalajara, on one of the many days and nights that Bethune was tending to the wounded.[42] It fell to Vidali to persuade Bethune to leave Spain. It would be a delicate thing. There could be no mention of the complaints and charges against him, of his alleged personal failings, nor even of his conflicts with the Sanidad Militar. Instead, Vidali would concentrate on the enormous propaganda value of Bethune's work to the people of North America.

Precisely when Vidali met with Bethune it is impossible to determine, but it must have occurred sometime in the last week of March. Vidali called Bethune to his office. He was fully aware that Bethune was engaged in making a propaganda film about the Blood Transfusion Unit, and he put it to him that he should complete the film and return with it to America.[43] Vidali suggested to Bethune that since the transfusion unit was well established and operating efficiently, he could now best help the Republic by taking on a lecture tour of Canada and the USA, "bringing the plight of Spain directly to the people," and advocating for the end of the non-intervention pact that was starving Spanish democracy of the weapons necessary to defeat Franco.[44]

It was a convincing proposal, not least because it came from Vidali, but for some days Bethune resisted.[45] To leave Spain while the Republic was in peril, and men fought and died, and there was so much left to do, could not have sat well with him.

But it was the fate of the blood transfusion unit that was uppermost in his mind. Goyanes and Culebras were nothing more than "bourgeois loafers," and one of them, he thought, was probably a fascist sympathizer.[46] Still, even if he could no longer lead the unit in Madrid, or the unified blood transfusion service across the whole of the Republican zone, it had come into being, it existed, and at his hands. As Sise later remembered: "We had the main centre in Madrid. We had another extraction centre in Valencia, and another in Jaen in the south;"[47] and, "I suppose we had a total of two or three dozen people scattered across Loyalist Spain."[48] But Bethune remained deeply unsure whether the blood transfusion work would continue effectively if it was absorbed into the Army of the Republic, and not sink into a tangle of bureaucratic regulation. He had come to feel that

The Conspiracy

Cerrada had been less than open with him, and their last encounter had not gone well. Certainly it led to a further alienation from Sorensen who, furiously, told Bethune he was leaving.[49] And then things took an even more sinister turn. After Bethune returned to Madrid the next day, Sorensen met with the military police, apparently at their behest; the interrogation led to the secret report of 3 April, and reflected Sorensen's unfounded accusations that both Rothman and Bethune were guilty of theft and espionage.[50]

Although Sorensen had apparently broken with Bethune, it was to some degree an empty threat. Sorensen followed him on 4 April and wrote, cryptically: "I arrived Madrid – things had happened."[51] Indeed they had. At the same time, he informed Bethune that on 8 April all foreign services in Spain would lose their autonomy; the blood transfusion service would cease to exist as an independent entity and become an integral part of the Army of the Republic. It was out of Bethune's hands. Two days later there was a conference at the Institute; Vidali's suggestion was thoroughly discussed. Bethune's initial resistance was overcome, and he "admitted this proposal was correct."[52] Sorensen wrote: "We persuaded Beth to leave. He wrote a letter of resignation to the Party."[53] It is unlikely that Bethune resigned his directorship of the Blood Transfusion Unit on 6 April, as Sorensen implies; a letter to the CASD of 19 April suggests that the resignation more likely occurred some two weeks later. Nor did Bethune leave Spain immediately; as events turned out, he remained until the middle of May.

In the meantime, Bethune wrote two letters in which he attempted to come to terms with the reorganization of the blood transfusion service, and its implications for the Canadian Blood Transfusion Institute and its personnel. The first, a cable to the CASD dated 12 April, clarified the political situation. Bethune reported that the Republic had decreed that all foreign organizations were to be placed under the control of the Ministry of War, that the Sanidad Militar had taken control of the Canadian unit, and that the position of the Canadian personnel had become purely nominal. He drew the inevitable conclusion: "Our work as Canadians here is finished." He therefore requested that the CASD authorize him to "first withdraw Canadian personnel, second hand over to government cars, refrigerators, and equipment, third agree to provide two hundred dollars monthly six months for maintenance institute, fourth return Canada with such Canadians as desire with film for antifascist propaganda." Perhaps suspecting Sorensen's hidden hand behind much that had happened, Bethune concluded: "Only future cables signed Beth Bethune are from me."[54]

The second letter was written a week later, on 19 April, and addressed to the director of the Sanidad Militar. In it, Bethune reversed his former position. After considering the political and military situation in the country as a whole, he now maintained that he was "firmly of the opinion that all services of the Republican Army should be controlled by the Spanish people," and that since the "Instituto Hispano-Canadiense de Transfusion de Sangre" as conceived by him in January was "now operating as an efficient well-organized institute," it had become clear to him that his "function as chief of the organization here in Spain has come to a natural end." He then delegated his "authority as Chief representative of the Canadian Committee to Aid Spanish Democracy to the following members: Allen May, Ted Allan, Hazen Sise and Henning Sorensen." The order of names is interesting, and quite possibly was intended as a snub against Sorensen, who appears last. As a further insult, he designated Ted Allan as "political commissar," a role he never played, and a function the Institute never accepted; indeed it appears likely the members of the Institute were never even made aware of the designation. Finally, Bethune offered his resignation "as chief of the organization," stating that if his resignation was accepted – as he knew it would be – he would "at once proceed to Canada to carry out propaganda work in connection with the Institute and in support of the Popular Front," and adding that "in view of the urgency of the situation and the necessity of showing our propaganda film as quickly as possible, I would like my resignation to take effect immediately."[55]

There it was, in print. There was no turning back. His resignation was now irrevocable. The conspiracy to remove Bethune from Spain had been successfully consummated. Bethune's departure from Spain was simply a matter of time.

19

They Are In Me, They Have Changed Me

Fascism has always meant mass murder; since its policies can, by their very nature, have little appeal for the people, massacre becomes a necessity, and organized terror a weapon to defuse civilian resistance, and to coerce a reluctant submission.

Guernica was a small town in the Basque country in northern Spain just south of the western border with France. The capital of the region, Bilbao, lay a few kilometers to the west. On 26 April 1937, German Nazi airplanes, accompanied by a few of Mussolini's aircraft, bombarded and completely destroyed the town on Franco's explicit orders. Bombers dropped heavy explosives and incendiary projectiles, while fighter planes flew low to strafe the townspeople with machineguns. Showers of grenades dropped from the sky. Guernica was engulfed in flames and systematically destroyed; there were craters in the middle of town twenty-five feet deep. Innocent farmhouses for kilometers about were deliberately blown up; a tiny nearby village was machine-gunned for fully fifteen minutes without respite. Guernica was never a military objective. The attack was intended to demoralize the Basque people preparatory to a full-scale fascist invasion. The barbarous tactic they employed was the terror-bombing of innocent civilians in an undefended town.[1]

Franco denied bombing Guernica, madly accusing communist saboteurs of having destroyed it, or alternatively claiming, even more absurdly, that the people of the town had dynamited it themselves. These fascist lies were happily trumpeted by Father Joseph Thorning, an American Catholic propagandist devoted to Franco, and by pro-fascist elements in the British military, press, and government. The Franco regime continued to deny all responsibility for Guernica well into the 1970s.[2]

News of the massacre reached the world through the journalist George Steer, whose magnificent reporting appeared in *The Times* of London, and in the *New York Times*, on 28 April 1937,[3] the same day that Sorensen, Sise, and Allen May returned from Valencia to Madrid with the Sanidad Militar's written acceptance of Bethune's resignation.[4]

Bethune's reaction to these events is nowhere recorded, but it is possible to speculate on their effects. First Malaga, now Guernica: what images did these similar atrocities evoke in Bethune's mind, what emotions? The refugees straggling down the road to Bilbao; the children, the little lost children weeping softly in the night for mothers and fathers they would never see again; these pitiable, orphaned children that, somehow, he knew, needed him. He must have been torn. The strength of Vidali's proposal was all the more evident: the world must know the true nature of the fascist attack on Spain; the people must grasp the despicable game the Western powers – and Britain above all – were playing: the pretence that there were no Germans, no Nazi arms behind Franco; the utter fraud of the non-intervention pact. Bethune was needed in Canada and America to expose the lies and to tell the truth. At the same time, there were the unhappy children now crowding into Bilbao: they needed him too. And if Sorensen and Sise and Ted Allan and Allen May wanted to take the Blood Transfusion Institute away from him, let them have it. Let them deal with that snake, Culebras, there were other and better things to do.

For his part, Bethune appears to have spent his last few weeks in Spain continuing to do what he considered necessary. Much of his time was still occupied with Muller in the laboratory, and in the filming of *Heart of Spain*, both in Madrid and in the surrounding countryside. He carried on with the transfusion service, collecting blood and driving it to the various hospitals on his regular delivery route.

At some point during this latter period, Bethune, Sorensen, and Sise became acquainted with the American novelist Ernest Hemingway, and saw a good deal of him.[5] He was staying at the Hotel Florida, a short distance from the Blood Transfusion Institute, and part of the hotel was serving as one of the many temporary hospitals to which Bethune habitually drove his cargo of blood. According to the journalist Virginia Cowles, Hemingway's suite at the Florida was frequented by "a strange assortment of characters" including Kajsa Rothman with whom Bethune had so recently and reluctantly broken, and who was now acting as in interpreter for Cowles and a guide for Hemingway.[6] Sorensen avoided Hemingway on the grounds that he "appeared too detached" and "did not create the impression that he felt for the people of Spain's fight against fascism."[7] Sise held an entirely opposite view, maintaining that Hemingway was "definitely a partisan of the Spanish republic," a man whom he "liked enormously, . . . a wonderful person to be with and to talk to . . . and there was much sitting around and drinking . . . and damn good conversation."[8] Bethune left no record of his response to Hemingway. It is possible that he would have been as attracted to the conversation as much as to the whiskey – both of which seems to have flowed abundantly in Hemingway's rooms – but there was, quite obviously, much on his mind in those days. In Sorensen's memory, neither he nor Bethune "took to Hemingway particularly,"[9] and whether this alleged indifference accurately corresponded to Bethune's true feelings, or was simply a reflection of Sorensen's own antipathy, it is not possible to say.

Martha Gellhorn, the writer, journalist, and Hemingway's lover, arrived in Madrid at the very end of March. She came often to visit at the Blood Transfusion Institute, although never with Hemingway,[10] and found Bethune likeable. In April, she went with him several times to help deliver blood to the front line hospitals in the Jarama battle zone.[11] On one such occasion she drove with Bethune and Haldane to the town of Morata, near the Jarama river, on a road that had been shelled by the fascists that very morning; gunfire continued throughout the day. They were driving fast; Bethune was "afraid the hospitals would run out of blood for transfusions to the wounded." They arrived at the first hospital and made their delivery. They drove quickly to the next hospital, a dim room in an unused farmhouse. They moved on to three other hospitals receiving "orders for the bottles that were to be taken up the line the next day." By then it was dark, "a smooth, black night, with high stars." They drove back to Madrid in quiet without talking.[12] The next day, Bethune carried on with his work.

Meanwhile, ever since Bethune had cabled the CASD on 12 April and suggested that the Canadian personnel be withdrawn from the Institute, the CASD had been, quite understandably, extremely concerned. Rumors of discord had apparently been leaking back to them through other channels, but they were unable to gauge their accuracy. Eventually, they decided to ask A. A. MacLeod, a leading member not only of the CASD, but also of the Communist Party of Canada, to look into the matter.[13] MacLeod was already scheduled to go to Paris on other business. He would be leaving shortly, following on the heels of ranking Party member, William Kashtan, who was en route to Spain primarily to organize the nascent Mackenzie–Papineau Battalion of the International Brigades.[14]

Bethune had already sent the CASD a number of cables informing them of the on-going process of reorganizing all foreign organizations under the control of the Ministry of War, and the repercussions this was bound to have on the Institute. He had concluded his 12 April cable to the CASD, written a week before his official resignation to the Sanidad Militar, by saying, somewhat enigmatically: "Many schemes more urgent now than Blood Transfusion. Will inform you later."[15] At the end of April he was suggesting, in light of the events at Guernica, a proposal that was close to his always wounded heart: that the CASD consider the possibility of transferring some of their funds to the relief of the orphaned children at Bilbao, and of putting him in charge of such a project.[16]

However, on 5 May, Bethune cabled the CASD to reassure them that all was essentially well with the blood transfusion service. "Relationship with Sanidad Militar clarified and satisfactory," he wrote, adding that the name "Hispano-Canadiense being retained for Madrid sector," and that the "Bethune unit operating smoothly and efficiently." As to *Heart of Spain*, "All here agree Bethune return Canada with wonderful film now finished for propaganda work."[17] Indeed, with the exception of the addition of voice-over narration, sound, editing, and the usual matters of post-production work, the film footage itself had been completed and required only the government censor's authorization before it was ready to leave the country. Bethune's cable concluded with a highly significant sentence laying out the functions of the various Canadian members of the unit: interestingly, he appointed Allen May to replace him as "directing secretary," while Sise would be in charge of transport, and Sorensen would liaise with the Sanidad Militar – there was no mention whatever of Ted Allan, or his fictional role as political commissar – all this during what Bethune referred to as his impending "absence," indicating that he fully intended to return to Madrid after touring North America with the film.

Some days later, Bethune and, according to Sise, a large group of unnamed others left Madrid for Valencia to have *Heart of Spain* censored. Since the government was at war, it was of course necessary to ensure that the film footage contained nothing that might, quite by accident, have been of benefit to the enemy. In Valencia they were informed that the film could only be censored in Barcelona. The group then divided into two: Bethune and his "party" – which probably included Sorensen, with his excellent translation skills – went on to Barcelona, while Sise and "the rest of the party" remained in Valencia. Why it would have been necessary for the entire Blood Transfusion Unit – Bethune, Sise, Sorensen, May, possibly Jean Watts, and probably Herbert Kline and Geza Karpathi, given their direct participation in the making of the film – to have accompanied the film from Madrid, Sise does not inform us; but as the initial group was large enough to divide into two "parties" there must have been a minimum of six persons involved.

In any event, as Sise and his group made their way about Valencia, passing the days until Bethune's return, they realized they were being constantly shadowed by a mysterious Spaniard. This unknown stranger left a series of calling cards at their hotel requesting a meeting. Sise and his colleagues, justifiably suspicious, ignored the requests. Eventually, the

Spaniard came directly to their hotel room, demanded entrance, and showed them his papers: he was the Chief of Military Intelligence for Valencia. Although Sise later described him physically as "a great big burly guy," he did not suggest why a man holding such a high position of authority would have been tailing them through the streets. Sise and his group were taken to the Chief's office where a "six-shooter" was openly displayed on his desk. The Chief had a single question: Where was Bethune? Sise replied that he was in Barcelona to arrange the censorship of *Heart of Spain*.[18]

It is exceedingly interesting that the highest levels of Military Intelligence should have taken such an interest in Bethune. But why? Perhaps the answer is obvious. Despite his prominent role as director of the *Hispano-Canadiense de Transfusion de Sangre*, Bethune's security file must, by then, have become quite thick. It will be recalled that as early as his second day in Spain he had been accused of being a spy. Sorensen's complaint "of suspicious foreigners" at the Blood Transfusion Institute on 3 January led to Bethune's arrest, and Sorensen's endless insinuations that Bethune's lover, Kajsa Rothman, was a spy could only have added to the file. Finally, Sorensen and Ted Allan's denunciation of 18 March, which culminated in the secret police report of 3 April, completed an entirely false picture of Bethune as a potentially dangerous renegade, politically ambiguous, possibly a double-agent, possibly a spy, possibly a fascist sympathizer. How much of any of this was believed by Military Intelligence is open to question, but certainly they could not be faulted for doing their job. Spies and double-agents were not uncommon within the Republican zone, and only a very few days before the Chief of Military Intelligence had begun to follow Sise and his party through the streets of Valencia, Anarchist and Trotskyist elements had attempted to take control of Barcelona by force of arms, much to Franco's delight.[19] In the political atmosphere of May 1937, there was more than enough suspicion to go around.

The Chief of Military Intelligence, however, seems not to have fully accepted Sorensen's suspicions, nor to have aligned himself with the author of the 3 April secret report. According to Sise, once it was explained what Bethune was doing in Barcelona, the Chief became "chummier and chummier," going so far, in the end, as to ask whether Sise and the others would like to see, "for their amusement," the files that had been kept on each member of the Institute.[20] Most regrettably, Sise has chosen not to reveal anything that he saw within those most intriguing files.

Heart of Spain received the required censorship papers and was taken across the border to Paris in a British diplomatic pouch, oddly enough, to be picked up by Bethune at a later date.[21] Shortly after Bethune returned from Barcelona to Madrid, the CASD seems to have warmed to his earlier suggestion: they telegraphed him with the recommendation that he "explore fully possibilities child relief work Bilbao refugees," and that he not leave for Canada with *Heart of Spain* until he met with MacLeod in Paris for consultations.[22] What did Bethune imagine, at this point? Was he under the impression that the North American tour would only last a month or two and that he would then be recalled? That he would be appointed director of a project to bring relief and succor to the lost children of Spain? Did he believe that the construction of children's villages, which he had already advocated in the wake of Malaga, would soon be achieved? The conspiracy that had been hatched against him – the "clever way" – spoke only of the necessity of taking the film on a propaganda tour; there was no indication, as far as Bethune was concerned, that he would not, within a few short weeks, be returning to the Republic.

In any event, Bethune appears to have followed to the letter the CASD's requests. He readily agreed to meet with MacLeod and to stay in Madrid until further notification.[23] MacLeod sailed for Paris on 13 May, the same day Kashtan arrived in Madrid from Albacete, where the International Brigades headquarters had officially granted permission for the formation of the Mackenzie–Papineau Batallion.[24] The CASD cabled Bethune to come to Paris to meet MacLeod; he was to bring *Heart of Spain* with him so he could leave for Canada directly from Paris. He was further requested to take Sorensen with him to discuss whether the Blood Transfusion Unit should continue, and in what form. The cable, written by Ben Spence, concluded by offering Bethune sincere congratulations for the "magnificent and successful culmination of the blood transfusion project," and assuring him that a warm welcome awaited him in Canada.[25]

On 16 May, Bethune left Madrid, never to return. He was accompanied to Paris by William Kashtan and Ted Allan; Sorensen declined to follow Spence's request and stayed in Madrid.[26] According to Sorensen, when he said goodbye to him Bethune "looked relaxed and happy for the first time in a long while. I think he was mighty glad to get out of there."[27] As to Sise, in a later interview he maintained that no farewell party was thrown for Bethune, and that he could not, in fact, "remember the occasion of his going actually."[28] Sorensen's reminiscence should be taken at face value. Bethune was not "mighty glad" to leave Spain, as we shall very shortly see. And perhaps the reason that Sise could not recall Bethune's departure is that he may well not have been in Madrid: he was spending a good deal of time in Valencia. It is certainly the case, however, that Sise, in outlining a formal proposal to the Sanidad Militar for the relocation of the Blood Transfusion Unit and its associated laboratories to a more extensive facility, wrote that the remaining Canadian members of the Unit "should not be judged by

Bethune."[29] It is hardly possible, in this context, to imagine that Bethune's departure from Madrid was a particularly cheerful affair.

Once in Paris, Bethune had to wait until 26 May to meet with MacLeod.[30] Kashtan had, by this time, gone back to Canada, and Ted Allan was to return to Spain on the 28th.[31] MacLeod had attended an international solidarity meeting with André Malraux, and the Spanish cabinet minister Leone, in Paris. He reported to the CASD that he would be going to Geneva the next day, the 27th, with a delegation to the League of Nations. The delegation had already conferred with the Basque Committee, and they had proposed that Bethune and MacLeod proceed to Bilbao immediately to investigate the situation regarding refugee children's homes. Spence and the CASD, while sensitive in principle to the issue of orphaned and displaced children, wanted Bethune back in Canada to begin the publicity tour.[32]

But Bethune and MacLeod continued to confer privately. It became apparent that Bethune was eager to visit Bilbao, to examine the situation on the ground, before returning to Canada, and that he had convinced MacLeod to change entirely the focus of the Institute's personnel: the blood transfusion service would be placed completely into Spanish hands, while Sorensen, Sise, and May would coordinate the maintenance and care of five hundred displaced children in a number of Basque villas.[33]

On 29 May, Sise was in Valencia, sun tanning on the beach, playing chess, and having lunch with Claud Cockburn, Jean Watts, and Allen May. Ted Allan arrived from Madrid very late in the day with a cable from Bethune indicating that he had indeed talked MacLeod around to withdrawing the blood service and announcing his intention to go to Bilbao. Sise was much alarmed. The next day he sent a cable to Spence personally, and had Allen May cable the CASD strongly advising that Bethune not be allowed to operate any further projects in Spain, and asserting the on-going need for the CASD to continue funding the Blood Transfusion Institute. Not content with simply offering his advice to the CASD, Sise was determined to ensure that Bethune would never again set foot on Spanish soil. He went to the Military Police and had them telegraph their consulate in Paris to prevent Bethune's visit to Bilbao. According to his diary, Sise had "a long chat" with the police – in the person of his "chum," with the six-shooter? – "saw and corrected Beth's dossier, and discovered they would have put out an order for his expulsion if he hadn't left."[34]

It must be said that, under the circumstances, it would hardly have been unusual for the Republican government to demand that Bethune leave the country: he had officially resigned his position as director of the blood transfusion service on 19 April, the resignation had been formally accepted, and therefore he no longer had any authority to continue to function within the country. The potential order for expulsion should not be regarded as a sign of the Republic's disavowal or repudiation of Bethune. Less than a week earlier, Tomas Piero, the Spanish Consul General in Montreal, had concluded a speech by saying, "I cannot finish without remembering Doctor Bethune, the friend of Spain, the friend of humanity, the man who has all the virtues of a peoples' son."[35] Malraux too had recently been in Toronto, and had spoken of Bethune and his associates "performing heroic deeds and saving countless Spanish lives."[36]

The CASD found themselves in somewhat of a quandary. While they were entirely in sympathy with the Bilbao project, they were not, in Spence's words, "prepared to throw over the Blood Transfusion Service," unless the Spanish government requested that they do so, and were of the opinion that the children's project "be additional not alternative to blood transfusion activities." More to the point, they needed Bethune back in Canada without delay, otherwise the scheduling of his propaganda tour would soon run into difficulties.[37]

Bethune and MacLeod capitulated. MacLeod informed Spence that Bethune would require a week in New York in order to deal with post-production work on *Heart of Spain*. Spence agreed, and on 2 June 1937, Bethune boarded ship to cross the Atlantic with Herbert Kline and Geza Karpathi.[38]

Shortly before leaving Spain, probably not long after his resignation had been accepted, and the fascists had laid waste to Guernica, Bethune wrote an article at the request of a Canadian communist periodical, *New Frontier*, and which they published in their May edition. It is by no means a simple document. Viewed from one perspective, it is a startlingly brilliant exercise in the application of Marxist dialectical methodology to the process of the artistic impulse. From another point of view, it again seems to reveal the deep contradiction in Bethune between his sincere antifascist solidarity with the Spanish working class, and his sense of individualist "generosity:" of standing above the very people he has served through his self-personification as an artist. At the same time the article indicates a recognition that he has been profoundly changed by his experiences in Spain; changed fundamentally but in ways which yet eluded him; he has lived his experience, but he comprehends it without understanding it. What's more, his internal contradictions, unsettled by the realization that he has in some way changed, leads to what amounts to a barely disguised attempt at self-clarification. Finally, this important document is an "apology" not so much in the sense of asking forgiveness, but in the more philosophical meaning of an "apologia": it is a justification, in this case, for a principled inaction.

Given the length of the text, it has been slightly abbreviated: omissions are indicated by ellipses.

An Apology for Not Writing Letters

This is an attempt at an explanation why I, who think of you so often, with love and affection, have not written – or so briefly – since my arrival in Spain.

I had thought to say simply (that is, shortly) – I have been too busy; I am a man of action; I have no time to write. Yet as I look at these words, I see they are false. They simply aren't true. In fact, I have had plenty of time to write to you, that is if I had cared to write, but, in truth, I did not care. Now why is this? Why have I not written to those of you who, I know, without illusion, would like to hear from me? Why is it I can not put down one word after another on paper and make a letter out of them?

I will try to be truthful. It is difficult to be truthful, isn't it?

First of all, I don't feel like writing. I don't feel the necessity of communication. I don't feel strongly the necessity of a re-construction of experience – my actions and the actions of others – into the form of art which a letter should take. As an artist, unless that re-construction take a satisfactory form which is truthful, simple and moving, I will not, nay, I can not, write at all. I feel that unless I can re-construct those remembrances of action into reality for you, I will not attempt it. To me, a letter is an important thing – words are important things. At present, I don't feel any necessity to communicate these experiences. They are in me, they have changed me, but I don't want to talk about them. I don't want to talk about them yet.

Besides, I am afraid to write to you. I am afraid of the banality of words, of the vocal, the verbal, of the literary re-construction. I am afraid they won't be true.

Only by a shared physical experience – tactile, visual or auditory – may an approximately similar emotion be felt by two people without the aid of art. Only through art can the truth of a non-shared experience be transmitted. To share with you what I have seen, what I have experienced in the past six months, is impossible without art. Without art, experience becomes, on the one hand, the denuded, bare bones of fact – a static, still-life – the how-many-ness of things; or, on the other hand, the swollen, exaggerated shapes of fantastically-coloured romanticism. And I will do neither. I refuse to write either way. Both are false – the first by its poverty, the second by its excess.

So I despair of my ability to transpose the reality of experience into the reality of the written word. Art should be the legitimate and recognizable child of experience. I am afraid of a changeling. I am afraid it would have none of the unmistakable, inherited characteristics of its original, true, parental reality.

I can not write you, my friends, because this art of letters is a second, a repeated form of action. And one form of action at a time is enough. I can not do both – but successively, with an interval of a year, or ten years, perhaps I can do both. I don't know. I don't think it matters very much.

I think that art has no excuse, no reason for existence except through the re-creation – by a dialectical process – of a new form of reality, for the old experience – transmitted through a man's sensorium – changed and illuminated by his conscious and unconscious mind. Exact reproduction is useless – that way lies death. The process of change from the old to the new is not a flat circular movement – a turn and return on itself, but helical and ascending.

The process of creative art is the negation of negation. First there is the change, that is, the negation, of the original, the positive reality; then the second change (or negation), which is a re-affirmation, a re-birth, through art, of the original experience, to the new positive, the new form of reality.

Let us take an example from painting – a moving object such as a tree swaying in the wind, a child at play, a bird in flight – any form of action, seen and perceived. This is the positive, the thesis. Reduced from the dynamic positive in time and space to a static form, by representation, (in this case, by paint on canvas) it becomes the negation of action, the denial of action. This is the antithesis. Then by a miracle of creative art, this static thing (of necessity static, owing, to the medium employed) is vivified, transformed into movement again, into life again, but into a new life, becomes positive again, becomes the negation of the negation, the synthesis – the union of life and death, of action and non-action, the emergence of the new from the old, but retaining the old within the new.

Now the same thing applies to the literary art, the plastic arts, music, the dance or what not – any art form. And unless that fresh emergent form, with its core of the old, is a new thing, a dynamic thing, a quick and living thing, it is not art. It arouses no response except intellectual appreciation, the facile response to familiar, recognizable objects, or admiration for technical skill.

And because I can't write you, my friends, as I should like to write you, because my words are poor, anaemic and hobbling things, I have not written. Yes, I could write, but am ashamed to write – like this:

"We were heavily shelled today. It was very uncomfortable. Fifty people were killed in the streets. The weather is lovely now although the winter has been hard. I am well. I think of you often. Yes, it is true I love you. Good bye."

I put them down and look at these words with horror and disgust. I wish I could describe to you how much I dislike these words. "Uncomfortable" – good god! what a word to describe the paralyzing fear that seizes one when a shell bursts with a great roar and crash nearby; "killed," for those poor huddled bodies of rags and blood, lying in such strange shapes, face down on the cobble-stones, or with sightless eyes upturned to a cruel and indifferent sky; "lovely" when the sun falls on our numbed faces like a benediction; "well" when to be alive is well enough; "think" for that cry rising from our hearts day by day for remembered ones; "love" for this ache of separation.

So you see, it's no good.

Forgive me if I talk more about art. It must seem to you that I know either a great deal about it or nothing at all. I really know very little about it. I think it is very mysterious, very strange. But it seems to me to be a natural product of the subconscious mind of man, of all men, in some degree. Arising into the realm of deliberate thought, its life is imperiled. . . . A theory of art is an attempt of the rational mind to impose its discipline and its order on the seeming chaos and seeming disorder of the emotional subconscious. . . . By its subjection to the conscious mind, to the deliberate directional thought of the artist and his theory, it lives for a while and then languishes and dies. It cannot survive its separation from the great breeding ground of the unconscious. The mind (that alien in the attic) by its dictatorship, destroys the very thing it has discovered. . . .

A great artist lets himself go. He is natural. He "swims easily in the stream of his own temperament." He listens to himself. He respects himself. He has a deeper fund of strength to draw from than that arising from rational and logical knowledge. Yet how beautifully the dialectical process comes in again – modified by thought, his primitive unconsciousness, conditioned by experience, reacts to reality and produces new forms of that reality. These particular forms of art arise, satisfy for their time, decay and die. But, by their appearance, they modify and influence succeeding art forms. They also modify and influence the very reality which produced them. Art itself never dies. Art itself is a great ever-blooming tree, timeless, indestructible and immortal. The particular art forms of a generation are the flowers of that immortal tree. They are the expressions of their particular time but they are the products also of all the preceding time.

The artist needs, among other things, leisure, immense quietness, privacy and aloneness. The environment in which he has his being, are those dark, sunless, yet strangely illuminated depths of the world's subconscious – the warm, pulsating yet quiet depths of the other-world.

He comes up into the light of every-day, like a great leviathan of the deep, breaking the smooth surface of accepted things, gay, serious, sportive and destructive. In the bright banal glare of day, he enjoys the purification of violence, the catharsis of action. His appetite for life is enormous. He enters eagerly into the life of man, of all men. He becomes all men in himself. He views the world with an all-embracing eye which looks upwards, outwards, inwards and downwards – understanding, critical, tender and severe. Then he plunges back once more, back into the depths of that other-world – strange, mysterious, secret and alone. And there, in those depths, he gives birth to the children of his being – new forms, new colours, new sounds, new movements, reminiscent of the known, yet not the known; alike and yet unlike; strange yet familiar; calm, profound and sure.

The function of the artist is to disturb. His duty is to arouse the sleeper, to shake the complacent pillars of the world. He reminds the world of its dark ancestry, shows the world its present, and points the way to its new birth. He is at once the product and the preceptor of his time. After his passage we are troubled and made unsure of our too-easily accepted realities. He makes uneasy the static, the set and the still. In a world terrified of change, he preaches revolution – the principle of life. He is an agitator, a disturber of the peace – quick, impatient, positive, restless and disquieting. He is the creative spirit of life working in the soul of man.

But enough. Perhaps the true reason I can not write is that I am too tired – another 150 miles on the road today, and what roads!

Our first job is to defeat fascism – the enemy of the creative artist. After that we can write about it. . . . [39]

A strange article, and a fascinating self-revelation: Bethune tells us that he can write about art, but he can't write about Spain; at least he can't write about Spain in a way that would make us feel, concretely, and in our blood, its savage reality. And yet, an article he had written for the *Daily Clarion* only a month previously, *With the Canadian Blood Transfusion Unit at Guadalajara*, is a small masterpiece of emotionally-charged reporting, and his speeches over the radio station EAQ were equally brilliant. What had changed? We do not need to speculate: he tells us himself: *They are in me, they have changed me, but I don't want to talk about them. I don't want to talk about them yet.* There are things he cannot talk about, they have changed him too profoundly, they have broken the back of his abstract generosity, they have made him more humble, more forthright, less self-divided, more determined, more devoted; he has less need to prove himself to others – the interior gaze of the all-critical Dragon eye has begun to close; he is more steeled for combat. And he is more wounded.

It is not simply, or not only, the quiet dignity of the Spanish people; not only their undiluted courage in the face of the murderous onslaught of fascism, of their determination to fight, to survive or to die; not only their warmth, their true and human generosity in yielding up their blood that others might live. It was not simply these fiercely determined people among whom he had lived. There were the *others*, the ones that tore at him: the Swedish soldier, only three days in Spain, now half-blinded with bloody stumps where hands used to be, apologizing because he was of no more use to his comrades; the hopeless, lonely, sad children staggering up the road from Malaga, and those other children, equally bereft, crawling out of the rubble in Guernica; the eighteen-year-old Norwegian boy, a mother's dream of a son, dying in his arms – the boy of whom Bethune had said: It was as though I had killed my own son. How could he write about *them*? They were in him; they had changed him. But he could not speak of them. Not yet.

But Spain was finished for Bethune, though he could not then have known it. What had he accomplished in Spain? He had brought hope to little children. He had brought blood to the wounded twisting in agony on the front lines. He had built with his own hands and his own determination the world's first unified mobile blood transfusion service. What more could be asked of any man?

PART FOUR

In Defense of the Republic

20
A Tumultuous Welcome

Bethune disembarked from the *Queen Mary* in the harbor of New York on 6 June 1937. He was greeted by Ben Spence and taken by taxi to a hotel; the press was waiting. In their hotel room, a reporter sent down from the *Ottawa Journal* questioned him on the purpose of his return from Spain. Bethune was ready. He had arrived, he said, "to report to those who sent me – the Canadian workers." In a single sentence he had exposed the class nature of the antifascist struggle. After describing the work of the blood transfusion unit, he struck out at the "non-intervention farce" in which Great Britain, Canada, and the United States, allowed the fascist powers to intervene in Spain while denying aid to the Republic. As to the civil war itself, Bethune said: "It is the third stage of the world war. The first was Manchuria and the second Ethiopia. Fascism has won both. But Fascism won't win this one if the properly-elected government of Spain can get free access to arms and ammunition." "Madrid," he said, as he had said so often before, "would never fall." Would he, the reporter enquired, be returning to Spain? This was the inevitable question to which there could be no easy answer. Although he knew nothing of the official report that had been lodged against him, he was well aware of the frictions and divisions that had opened up within the blood transfusion service, not least because of his relations with the Sanidad Militar. Would the Party permit his return? There was nothing for Bethune to do but give an official reply which, in any event, expressed his true intentions: Yes, he said, he would be returning shortly.[1]

To a reporter from the Montreal *Gazette*, stationed in New York, he repeated the same themes, but took them still further. The war in Spain was the pivotal war of democracy against fascism. "Franco," he said, "is nothing. The German General Staff is directing the war and there are 100,000 Italians fighting. Why, oh why, can't the democratic nations see this? That's what the Spanish people cannot understand." Grimly, he spoke of the slaughter at Guernica and at Malaga. "They are getting away with murder. Simply murder." But whatever happened, the Spanish people would never yield. They would never surrender to Franco and his Nazi overlords: "No, not until the last man, woman and child has been killed." And if the Spanish people were butchered, if Spain was lost to fascism, the fault would lie as much with England, the United States, and Canada as with the fascists themselves. Those who were refusing Spain the weapons they needed at the most crucial moment, were as guilty as those who used weapons against her. If Spain were defeated, he said: "war will surely spread all over the world."[2] He was not wrong.

The next afternoon, Bethune was sitting at Longchamp's bar with the Hungarian cinematographer Geza Karpathi. He knew that Irene Kon, his old friend from Montreal, was often in New York working at the American head office of the Young and Rubicon advertising agency, with whom she was employed. On the off chance that she might be in the city that day, he decided to telephone her. According to Kon, she was in a meeting when the phone rang. She was astonished: it was Bethune in an exuberant mood. "I'm at Longchamp's," he said, "hurry up, come on down." She left and arrived at the bar to find him with Karpathi and "a very pretty blonde girl" with whom "Beth was carrying on a very long conversation." He introduced Irene to Karpathi, pointing out that he spoke no English, and asking her to "be nice to him." Bethune returned to the blonde woman leaving Irene and Geza staring pointlessly at each other. A moment or two later, Bethune turned to Irene and enquired about a hat of hers that he remembered fondly, a straw hat with a ribbon, and wanted to know what had happened to it. "It's at the hotel," Irene said. Bethune insisted that the four of them should go there immediately. In Irene's room she put the hat on. Bethune admired it and said, simply: "That's nice." Later, Irene traded stories about Montreal for Bethune's personal report on Spain.[3] Although he remained in New York for another week, working on *Heart of Spain*, helping to edit the raw footage and the audio track, Bethune and Irene never saw each other again. The happy encounter of a single day, a brief reminiscence of what must have seemed a former life, forever past, was soon overtaken by events neither could have foreseen.

During the week that Bethune spent in New York, he was occupied primarily with working on *Heart of Spain*. Progress was slow and expensive: the film would not finally be ready for viewing until August, far later than anticipated, and by that time the cost of production had risen to between five and six thousand dollars, much more than had been initially budgeted.[4]

Did Spence speak to him about his behavior in Spain? Probably not; the subject did not, properly speaking, fall under the purview of the CASD; it was more a matter of Communist Party discipline and would be better deferred until Bethune met with Party leaders in Toronto. Certainly Spence would have wanted to broach the issue of the lecture tour; many details remained to be resolved. MacLeod had suggested that, apart from major

A Tumultous Welcome

cities, no other meetings should be arranged until Bethune arrived in North America. As it happened, whatever Spence might have discussed with Bethune was cut short: he was obliged to return to Toronto on 11 June to deal with the Canadian Legation in Paris which had denied MacLeod a visa to re-enter Spain.[5]

Meanwhile, on the west coast, the Communist Party in British Columbia was preparing for Bethune. The 4 June issue of the Party's provincial newspaper, *People's Advocate*, carried a long article entitled "Canadian Makes Medical History," not only chronicling the story of the blood transfusion unit, but tying Bethune's service directly to the International Brigades where, "in the trenches, Canadians are fighting and giving their lives that the tragedy of Spain may not be repeated in Canada." Whatever misgivings the Party leadership may have had about Bethune, they were to remain private. Publicly, and indeed entirely accurately, the newspaper asserted that "Canada has every reason to be proud of the significant achievement of Dr. Bethune." In the same issue another article, "Canadian Ambulance Campaign Opens," revealed that there were "plans to equip an ambulance which will be given to the Canadian Blood Transfusion Unit, headed by Dr. Norman Bethune." In order to raise funds for this new venture, to assist existing committees, and to organize new committees in "conducting Spanish defense work," and, no doubt, with an eye to Bethune's eventual appearance on the national speaking tour, the Provincial Executive of the Party sent Arthur Evans to conduct a circuit of the province. Evans was a popular speaker and a veteran communist who had helped to lead the workers out of the government internment camps and had played a major role in the historic On-To-Ottawa trek. In the space of less than two months, and starting on 6 June, the very day Bethune landed in New York, Evans visited no less than fifty-three communities across British Columbia from the biggest cities and towns to the smallest villages and hamlets. More than once police contingents tore down posters advertising the meetings, closed the meeting halls, paraded in menacing armed units through the streets, or threatened to jail Evans unless he left town. But the meetings continued, the money was raised, and the Party was ready to host its wandering boy, its prodigal son, its national hero.[6]

A week after arriving in New York Bethune took the train to Buffalo, New York. He was driven across the border and entered Canada en route to Toronto. Who accompanied him we do not know; almost certainly a representative of the CASD and most probably a member of the Communist Party. Of the many things they must have discussed, we can be sure that it was made very clear to Bethune that he must not publicly reveal his Party affiliation. His speaking tour was to stand as a vital expression of Popular

Front policy: it was necessary to speak not only to Party militants, but to convince the broader circles of progressives and democratic-minded people across the country of the legitimacy of the Republican government of Spain, the necessity of supporting its struggle against fascism, the inherent justice of her demand that the policy of non-intervention be abandoned, and that material aid and armaments be provided to her. The Party was deeply concerned that the CASD appear to be precisely what it was: an umbrella organization whose purpose was to unite antifascists of any political affiliation or of none. It was the Party's belief that if Bethune spoke openly as a communist it would not only limit the size of his audiences, but provide government agents and far-right elements an opening to attack the CASD and the Party and, by implication, the democratic nature of the Spanish Republic itself. How did Bethune feel about this restriction? He was aware that the Party had reason to be critical of his individualism, of his aggressive and uncomradely refusal to subordinate himself and his unit to the Sanidad Militar during the period of amalgamation, and he was anxious to make amends. But more than that, he not only understood, as a Party militant, the need for a Popular Front in Canada, he lent it his full and enthusiastic support. And yet, at the same time, he loathed hypocrisy and he chafed under the restriction it would put himself personally. He was immensely proud of his Party affiliation, and was eager to recruit others to the Party's ranks and to the ideology he had come to embrace with such unshakeable conviction; it was a contradiction that would, more soon that late, come to a head. In any event the secret police were to report only a few days later, on 18 June, that, "according to Ken Clark, secretary of the League Against War and Fascism, and secretary of the Committee to Aid Spain" in British Columbia, Bethune "naturally will not come out in the open" about his Party membership.[7]

Bethune entered Toronto on the evening of 14 June. A wildly cheering crowd of as many as twenty-five hundred men and women greeted him at Union Station. Surrounded by a milling throng shouting out his name and bearing banners in defense of Spanish democracy, he was escorted by Ben Spence to an open touring car where he hailed the crowd with the clenched-fist antifascist salute. Bethune was driven to the grounds of Queen's Park, a large grassy area in front of the Ontario legislature, followed by a tumultuous parade over a kilometer long, including two marching bands. A massive gathering of five thousand had come to hear him speak. The meeting was chaired by George Watson, president of the Toronto Trades and Labour Council; Stewart Smith eulogized the Canadian Blood Transfusion Unit; Louis Palermo, an Italian antifascist leader called for the day when fascism in both Spain and Italy would be destroyed; and Ben

A Tumultous Welcome

Spence asked for donations to continue Bethune's work in Spain. When Bethune took the microphone he saluted the crowd with the antifascist raised fist. The crowd cheered wildly and raised their fists in return. "Friends and comrades," he began, "salutations from the antifascists of Spain to the antifascists of Canada."[8] He continued: "The people of Spain are a grand people. Their fight is the fight of the workers of the world – the fight against fascism which is the world war that is on now!" A victory of the Republican government, he said, would be the beginning of the defeat of fascism throughout the world. Their triumph would be the direct result of the common front they had formed, and that if democracy were to be preserved in Canada and the United States, it would require a similar common front. "The Communists can't prevent fascism," he said, "nor can the CCF or the Socialists. No one party can fight this thing and defeat it. Only a common front of all you people can save democracy."[9]

The following morning Bethune was interviewed in his hotel room by a reporter for the *Toronto Star*. The reporter asked him bluntly: "Doctor, are you a Communist?" Bethune answered him the way he knew he must: "Most emphatically I am not. Let's get this thing straight. You can call me a Socialist if you like. I am a Socialist in the same way that millions of sane people are Socialists. I want to see people getting a square deal, and I hate fascism." He then asked the reporter if he knew what the fascists had done in Spain, and without waiting for a reply, answered his own question:

> They shot every trade-unionist they could lay hands on. They shot every man who had ever been on strike. They shot every mild Socialist. They shot schoolteachers who had at any time spoken favorably of democracy. Then after a while they went further than that. They rounded up everyone they could find who had worked for the democratic government of Spain – the legally elected government of their own country! And if these people could not prove positively that they had worked unwilling for that government . . . well, they shot them too.

What of non-intervention; what of Britain? "My own theory," Bethune said, is that:

> England is an imperialist, capitalist country possessed of enormous vested interests in various parts of the world, and these are loosely held together by a cement of sentimentality. . . . The British government is playing a deep game . . . and the British will do nothing as long as their commercial interests are not threatened.[10]

Later that day, Bethune spoke at the Carlton United Church hall both during the afternoon and then at an evening session to a much smaller group, of perhaps one hundred, called by the CASD. Tim Buck, Sam Carr, and other prominent Party leaders were in attendance. During the afternoon session he discussed the operation of the blood transfusion unit, but during the evening he expanded his remarks in a number of directions. Reiterating his disgust with England, he described the recent coronation of George VI as the "biggest build-up and advertising stunt for the next war." "Political democracies," he observed, were "a shell and a sham." The British Empire was maintained by nothing more than imperialist capitalists who sought to exploit and control its wealth; the Empire itself consisting of "blocks of gold scattered around the world." Bethune also took the opportunity to urge the CASD to more fully consider the plan which had so occupied him since the massacre at Malaga – the resettlement of children who had become the victims of war. He called for a national campaign to raise a million dollars to establish homes for Spanish orphans in Spain itself, opposing the suggestion that they be evacuated for fear that they would "lose that beautiful revolutionary spirit." The CASD, in committee, agreed to care for five hundred children; to launch a nation-wide campaign for that purpose; and to continue funding the blood transfusion effort.[11]

From Toronto, Bethune took the evening train to Montreal, the city where he had lived and worked for so many years; after Gravenhurst, his true home town. Here the reactionaries of the Catholic hierarchy had prepared themselves for his arrival. The Vatican was quite demonstrably on the side of Franco and Mussolini; they had spread a never-ending abundance of lies and misrepresentations about the legitimate Spanish government: bloodthirsty atheists, communists, and Jews were held to be slaughtering priests. From the Archbishop of Quebec to the local parish priest, from every pulpit the faithful were deliberately fed a hateful form of clerical fascism. Conrad Chaumont, the vicar-general of the Montreal diocese, was given the task of suppressing Bethune's testimony; he went to every newspaper and radio station requesting them, in the name of the Church, not to provide any publicity for his public speeches. For the most part, he was summarily rebuffed.[12]

Emerging from Windsor Station, Bethune was met by a thousand enthusiastic supporters. Eager young men surrounded him and carried him shoulder high while reporters mobbed him and camera bulbs flashed. Wellwishers called out his name in English and in French: "We're with you, Bethune!" "Vive le docteur Bethune!" In a long cavalcade of cars, bedecked with bunting and banners, their horns honking loudly, Bethune was driven through the downtown streets, then east into the francophone working class

A Tumultous Welcome

district, and finally looping back toward his hotel. On the sidewalks the people cheered; from the factory windows the night-shift workers waved. After a full day in his hotel, interviewing with the inevitable reporters, and spending what time he could with friends, Bethune was taken to the Mount Royal Arena; it was packed to a full capacity of eight thousand, while hundreds more listened in the streets at specially installed loudspeakers. On Bethune's entry to the arena a bugle sounded; the crowd stood, roared, threw their hands in the air in the clenched-fist salute. Bethune responded in kind. Suddenly they were one: speaker and audience united in a single passion. From the stage, two minutes of silence were observed in memory of the Canadian volunteers who had died on Spanish soil. Bethune began. He outlined the history of the Spanish conflict, praised the volunteers of the Mackenzie–Papineau Battalion, described the function of the Madrid blood transfusion unit, and condemned Britain's role in the non-intervention pact. "Canada," he said, "cannot avoid the moral responsibility for the death of five hundred thousand people. Every man, woman, and child sitting in this room has blood on his hands because he did not appeal to his politicians and insist on refusing to let Downing Street dictate Canada's foreign policy." Finally, Bethune paused. He looked out across row after row of eager faces. They were listening to him; they were with him completely. It was time to ask them for their help in the project that now mattered to him most. In simple and clear words, shorn of all verbal flourishes, he talked of the massacre on the road from Malaga, of the orphaned and starving children, and he appealed for aid to build a children's city in Spain. He told them that by his estimate each orphaned and needy child could be supported by one hundred dollars a year. The response was immediate: according to the press, "one, two, five and 10-dollar bills literally showered the platform, along with cheques, and in less than ten minutes nearly $2000 was collected for the project."[13]

It was a glorious evening: the adulation, the crowd hanging on his every word, and, especially, the mass raising of the antifascist salute. How could Bethune have felt? Could he have expected the wonderful and massive welcome he had received in both Toronto and Montreal? No doubt he was exhilarated and grateful, but as he spoke, especially about the blood transfusion work, he must also have experienced a certain regret, not for his accomplishments, but for the unconscionable behavior that had caused so many difficulties for his unit and led to what, in effect, was his official removal from Spain.

There was no doubt that Bethune's public appearances were inspiring. He was a master of public relations, an accomplished speaker who had the rare ability to make members of an audience feel as though he were speaking directly to each one of them. A fourteen-year-old boy, Dovid Kunigis, had been in the Mount Royal Arena and was "very much moved" by Bethune's description of the blood transfusion unit. The next day, he took a collection can into the café across the street from his father's bakery and asked permission of the owner to make an appeal for the Republican cause. The owner had him stand up on a chair and asked everyone to pay attention "to what Kunigis' son" had to say about Spain. Dovid made an ardent and eloquent speech and afterward went to each table, where the regulars were playing pinochle or gin rummy, and collected money in his can. "This," Dovid recalled, "was in the depression time, when a nickel or dime was the norm, a quarter was very good, but after my impassioned appeal . . . there were many who folded up one dollar bills, and even two men at one table who folded up two dollar bills in the can." This response was far from unique: wherever Bethune went men and women, and even small children, were moved by what he had to say, many giving a substantial donation from what little they had.[14]

Publicly, in Montreal, Bethune was an enormous success, but his private life was more bitter. This man who had no home, who was never at home wherever he was, had come home again, if only briefly. Who he saw in the few days he spent in Montreal we do not know: his contacts with friends and former lovers have gone largely unrecorded, but what little has been left to us bears the unmistakable signs of sadness. According to Thelma and Robert Ayres, art critics who knew Fritz Brandtner, "there was friction between Bethune and the Brandtners on his return" from Spain, the nature of which they do not disclose.[15] Whether it was political, or financial – the Brandtners were still operating the children's art center at the Beaver Hall Square apartment – or had some other origin is unknown, but it would appear that whatever had drawn them together had somehow come apart. He appears to have spent a little time with Frances Coleman and Marian Scott but few letters or reminiscences of these early days in Montreal appear to have survived.[16] Years later, Marian Scott said:

> I didn't see him so much after he had come back from Spain. He was moving about the country and I felt that he was a rather official figure and I had hoped that he was happier and was less lonely. He seemed always surrounded by people. It was only later that I realized this had been quite an unhappy and stormy period of his life. But I saw very little of him during this time.[17]

Georges Deshaies, the young surgeon at Sacré Coeur, "couldn't see him at that time because he was very busy."[18] But we know that Bethune visited

A Tumultous Welcome

the Sacré Coeur. Those of his former patients who were still recuperating in the hospital were delighted to see him, and he was warmly received by many of his former colleagues, but as for the nuns, entirely under the heavy thumb of the Catholic hierarchy, and thoroughly infused with its pro-fascist propaganda: "when the poor sisters saw him in the corridor, they ran away. They were afraid of [him]. The Mother Superior was afraid that she would meet the devil if she met him."[19] Later, when Bethune told the story to a friend, Dr. Roger Gariépy, he tried to make light of the incident, but it was clear to him that Bethune was most deeply hurt.[20]

These days in Montreal did not last long; he was soon again in Toronto, available to the headquarters of both the CASD and the Communist Party. The main issue for these interconnected organizations was finalizing the locations for Bethune's speaking tour, ensuring that the necessary funds were in place, and that adequate travel and lodging arrangements had been made. Bethune was to speak in a wide scattering of communities across Canada, and he was also booked into a number of cities in the United States. The CASD was connected to the American Committee in Aid of Spanish Democracy, which, not trivially, was sharing the expenses associated with *Heart of Spain*. What's more, the Communist Parties of Canada and the United States were intimately close both ideologically and organizationally. There was a joint and common need to raise public awareness on behalf of both national efforts, which were, in any event, one. And Bethune was, as we have noted, a superb public speaker and there was no one – certainly at this time – from the Abraham Lincoln Battalion who could have done the work, nor possibly any other figure so internationally renowned as Bethune who was so famously connected to the cause of the Spanish Republic.

But Bethune had not left Spain behind. If anything, the response of the enormous crowds in Toronto and Montreal had convinced him that he needed to go back where the wounded and the children needed him. Toward the end of June, he went to the central office of the Communist Party, and adamantly insisted on returning to Madrid. Joseph Salsberg, a member of the national executive, was the only high-ranking official present in the office. He watched Bethune "striding back and forth across the party's meeting room," with a strength that appeared "to derive from a seemingly limitless courage and energy." Bethune grabbed a pencil and quickly drew lines across a map of Spain indicating the advance of Franco's troops. "Joe," he said, "if I don't make it now, I'll never be able to get in." In his view, the Party and the CASD was perfectly capable of raising money, and *Heart of Spain* would show the people the barbaric nature of the fascist aggression, and the work of the Blood Transfusion Service just as adequately as his own words could do. Salsberg argued that Bethune's services were absolutely essential on the North American tour. The working class had shown their commitment to the antifascist struggle, and Bethune's presence at the upcoming rallies would ensure a broadening of their support and the raising of the necessary funds. In the end, Salsberg indicated that failure to follow Party orders was unacceptable; he would be disgraced within the Party. Bethune relented; the Party was his life.[21]

During the week or ten days Bethune was in Toronto, before finally embarking on the extended speaking tour, he stayed at the home of the artist Paraskeva Clark. She recalled that before he went to Spain Bethune was always elegantly dressed and indulged himself in luxury, and even later, just before heading west on the tour, he found a perfume in the family bathroom and sprayed it on himself.[22] There is no doubt that Bethune enjoyed fine things, and had an unusual sensitivity and interest in beautiful objects and in clothing. But at the same time this idiosyncrasy should not be overly exaggerated. Whether it was advocating for socialized medicine, or establishing a children's art school, or engaged directly with medical work in Spain, all this was far more important to Bethune than luxury. When he could afford fine things he enjoyed them; when he could not, he didn't care. On a Montreal street, in the dead of winter, before he went to Spain, he took off his overcoat and gave it to a cold and hungry unemployed worker.[23]

When he stayed with Paraskeva and her husband Philip, he had no money, and the CASD had little to give him. As Clark remembers, in her broken and impassioned language, "my husband was just as much taken with him as myself," and they "could do for him just anything we could. . . . We rented a car for him, we just wanted to take him; we wanted to do things for him. . . . He was worth it, you know. You could, you could, you felt that you were in the presence sort of a great wonderful person."[24] One day, Bethune approached Philip and told him he wanted to make love to Paraskeva. Philip replied that the choice was hers to make. She made the choice, and on the occasional night, both in June and again at the end of the year, they were lovers.[25] Most of the time he was a quiet houseguest, never raising his voice, never imposing, but at one point he and Paraskeva argued. Clark had consistently donated money to the CASD, even, to some extent, working with the organization. She had heard that Bethune had been drinking heavily in Madrid. She confronted him, berating him on the grounds that the money for his liquor had came from working-class men and women, and that they would "give their salary for a whole week" so he could drink. But things had changed; much of the time Bethune was out all day returning only to have dinner and to sleep; there was no drinking. And yet one day, Paraskeva and her husband were out late and returned to find Bethune brooding by a lamp, "returned from some-

A Tumultous Welcome

where," and he had drunk a whole bottle of rye. It had had no effect on him other than to make him unusually quiet. Bethune did not tell her why he had been drinking, but it must have been important and unpleasant.[26] It is quite possible that this had been the day that he had argued with Salsberg, and Spain had been denied him.

We know nothing more of these last days of June. Bethune seems to have recommitted himself fully to the Party and recovered his equanimity. He traveled to Kitchener to visit his sister Janet and his nieces. A few days later he wrote a quick letter to Frances inviting her to join his sister in Muskoka where she had taken a cottage. Bethune remained concerned about the pointless, apolitical, and apathetic life she was leading with Coleman. The letter had been written from the tiny community of South Porcupine, Ontario. Not a month after arriving at the New York harbor, Bethune had packed his bags and was prepared to tell the people of Canada – foremost among them the workers and the farmers – that fascism must not only be defeated in Spain, but right where they lived, in their very homeland.[27]

21

Sharply Raising the Question of Class Struggle

During the weeks and months of Bethune's speaking tour, the RCMP secret intelligence division kept detailed reports on every meeting he attended. Indeed, the police documents and newspaper articles of the period demonstrate that the speeches Bethune delivered across the country were among his most profound; they provide the richest source of his thought during this critical time, and add immeasurably to our knowledge of his evolving political position. It is evident that Bethune's experience in Spain had led to a true maturation of his understanding of socialism in both theory and practice. But it was not Spain alone that was responsible for the deepening of his revolutionary awareness: despite his long and grueling itinerary, he had a good deal of time on the series of endless railway cars and hotel rooms to absorb the daily left-wing press and any number of socialist texts; and his allegiance to Party ideology was strengthened by this intensified reading. His 1937 speeches were therefore not simply inspiring or merely radical, they were specifically revolutionary and Communist speeches: they analyzed imperialism, the Spanish war, and the growth of fascism in Canada and around the world, on the basis of class struggle.

Following Toronto and Montreal, the tour shifted to Northern Ontario. The first stop was at Kirkland Lake, on 6 July. Before addressing an audience of six hundred at the Strand Theatre, Bethune found the time to help the local Mine Mill and Smelter Workers Union prepare a report on silicosis, a condition which, he advised them, predisposed miners to tuberculosis; concrete evidence of his continuing commitment to working-class health.[1] Bethune was a revolutionary whose class consciousness had led him to Spain; but it was as a doctor that he served the Republic, and as a doctor that he served the working class wherever they needed him.

In Timmins, on 7 July, at the Arena, Bethune maintained, as the CASD and the Party required, that he was not a communist, but quite definitely an antifascist. Taking up the issue of the insidious growth of reaction at home, he held that Ontario premier Mitchell Hepburn "was a perfect type of fascist dictator," and condemned Prime Minister Mackenzie King for his

Sharply Raising the Question of Class Struggle

207

recent trip to Nazi Germany and for his evident friendship with Hitler. Antifascism required a struggle on multiple fronts – political, diplomatic, and through force of arms: the fight in Spain was not an isolated struggle of little concern to Canadian workers, but dialectically connected to the struggle at home. At the end of his speech he assured the crowd that he would be returning to Spain in September.[2] On 8 July he appeared in Rouyn[3] and on 9 July he spoke in North Bay at the District Medical Association.[4]

When Bethune had written to Frances from South Porcupine, he had told her that: "Although this public speaking is not to my liking, I will go through with it."[5] He was entirely sincere. He knew the Party needed him to speak, to raise awareness, and to encourage the necessary financial donations. What's more, it was now happily obvious that the CASD had put their backing behind his concept of providing homes for the Spanish orphans in the safety of children's villages, and the speaking tour would raise funds for their maintenance. But when he had completed his duty in North America he intended to return to active struggle in Spain. After meeting with the Party leadership in Toronto, he knew that his work in the blood transfusion unit was finished – nor would he be permitted any role in the children's villages – just as he knew that it would be impossible to publicly reveal such a truth: he would present himself at every public gathering as the director of the blood transfusion service recalled to Canada on merely temporary leave. But he had another plan in mind.

On 11 July, he spoke before seven hundred at the Grand Theatre in Sudbury. The International Nickel Corporation, which virtually controlled the city, scheduled an unexpected company picnic in a fruitless effort to lure the miners away from Bethune and sabotage the meeting.[6] That same day, Bethune cabled his former comrades in Madrid: "On Trans-Canada tour. Can I expect from all comrades Madrid same support as I am giving unit? Wire me committee Winnipeg." Hazen Sise and Ted Allan responded by immediately cabling MacLeod, who was then in Paris, that they were puzzled. They requested his advice on a reply they proposed to send to Ben Spence, in Toronto, for forwarding to Bethune: "Have heard glowing reports of your meetings. Of course we wholeheartedly and enthusiastically support the work you are doing in Canada. Please elucidate your cable. Institute working full blast. Transfusion team at front during these victories past week. Battle still raging. Salud. May, Sorensen, Sise, Allan." MacLeod recommended deleting the "elucidating sentence." On 16 July, Sise wrote Sorensen in Valencia: "About Beth's mysterious query from the wilds of Sudbury Ont – I was very suspicious and with the agreement of Allen and Ted sent the text to MacLeod in Paris together with a suggested reply on the lines you and Allen discussed on the phone and asked his opinion." Spence forwarded the amended reply to Bethune. The "mysterious query" of 11 July was soon clarified: on 22 July, from Regina, Bethune cabled that he would be returning to Spain with *Heart of Spain* and would be joining the International Brigade at its head-quarters in Albacete.[7] Since he knew that the film was not yet completed, it is evident that Bethune fully intended to complete the speaking tour before seeking to return to Spain in a new role as physician to the Mackenzie–Papineau Battalion; a position that would, in any case, require the consent of the Party. Such consent was not forthcoming. A. E. Smith, a member of the Central Committee of the Party, presently in Madrid, advised Sise to contact the Central Committee of the Communist Party of Spain and have them telegraph Tim Buck that Bethune's intentions were not acceptable.[8] Precisely how and when Bethune received this undoubt-edly disheartening news is unknown, but it would seem that this may well have occurred very quickly and, in any event, no more than several days before the end of the month.

Meanwhile, Bethune continued touring unaware of the flurry of cables and discussions regarding his new project. From Sudbury he traveled to nearby Espanola, and from there to Sault Ste. Marie where he spoke before a capacity crowd at the Technical School Auditorium, saying: "Do you think yourself a superior person to the man who served you at table today or the man at work on the streets? If so then it is wrong, for you and I are not supe-rior in any way to the man who lives by the work of his hands." At the Rotary Club, that same day, he again attacked premier Hepburn for using "the military and police forces against the workers' sacred right to strike," saying: "fascism is raising its head in Ontario."[9] On 14 July he wrote to his friend Louis Kon as he crossed Lake Superior: "Please convey to the Montreal Branch of the Friends of the Soviet Union my sincere thanks for their welcome on my return home. I am sorry I could not fit in my arrangements to meet you all, but I hope to see you on my return of my Trans-Canada tour."[10] From 15–18 July he spoke to audiences of several hundred in Fort William,[11] Port Arthur,[12] and Fort Frances.[13]

On 19 July he crossed from Ontario to Manitoba. On arriving at the Winnipeg railway depot in the morning, he was greeted by the deafening cheers of a massive throng of two thousand enthusiastic supporters. Just as in Montreal, eager hands lifted him high and he raised his fist in the antifas-cist salute. In the afternoon, he spoke to the Ukrainian Labour Farmer Temple Association 16th National Convention. He thanked the Association for the work they had accomplished on behalf of Spain and called for the unity of all progressive elements across the country. That evening he

Sharply Raising the Question of Class Struggle

addressed an overflowing mass meeting at the Walker Theatre. At his appearance on the platform, the audience rose in a thunderous ovation. Again calling for unity, he said, "We are all workers – white collared, doctors, lawyers, professors, bank clerks, and common labourers are all members of the working class and should all unite." Working-class unity, he said, "was the only weapon they had to fight capitalism." He spoke of his advocacy of socialized medicine and how that had led to his transfusion work in Spain. He bitterly denounced the pro-fascist attitude of Great Britain and the entire non-intervention farce. Finally, he called upon the audience not only to unify but to organize: "Say less and do more; don't say it but do it; and do it right now and today! Today!"[14]

The next evening, 20 July, a banquet was held in Bethune's honor at the St. Charles Hotel; it was a much smaller event attended by – in the words of a secret police document – "approximately one hundred persons prominent in the radical movement." It was, nevertheless, open to reporters. Bethune spoke of how, two years previously, he had visited London, England, and seen "women and children starving in the slums." But when he had gone to Moscow he had found the healthiest women and children he had ever seen. "I didn't care then," he said, "what the system was called, but I knew that what we wanted was the thing those Russians had got." Praising communism and decrying fascism, he told the audience that: "The men who are fighting in the government forces in Spain are fighting for you . . . It is a better thing to fight for democracy than to fight for your king and country." He eulogized the International Brigades, stating that Canadians in the Brigade had stayed in the trenches for ninety days without a break, a longer period than any brigade in the Great War of 1914–1918. And then he spoke openly of the possibility of revolution. "Canada's time of agony has not come yet, but it will come. Do not despair if the bourgeois class will not cooperate with you. When the clash comes, they will melt like snow. We bourgeois must humble ourselves before the workers, not go down to them but go up to them and ask them if we may help them in their work." At some point in the evening, perhaps in response to a question, he said: "I have the honor to be a Communist."[15]

This public revelation of his Party status was, of course, a breach of Party discipline. The very next day, in Brandon, Manitoba, he told another audience he was a "red, and proud to be one."[16] Why would he do this? His speeches were becoming increasingly class-conscious, his pride in his Party fundamental, and to hide his own partisanship must have seemed to him increasingly futile, false, and hypocritical. But it is also possible that breaking Party discipline was a conscious tactic to force the issue of his much wished for return to Spain and his anticipated enlistment in the

Mackenzie–Papineau Battalion. In any event, there is no extant record of the Party's response to the matter.

The Brandon meeting found Bethune again taking a thoroughly revolutionary stance. After his usual discussion of the blood transfusion unit, he suggested that unless the people organized a common front they would find themselves suffering a similar fate to that of Spain. He maintained that Mackenzie King had gone over to see Hitler to find out how to handle the communists and that it was necessary for the people to take action to prevent what might well be coming: the rounding up of "all those who kick" into jails and concentration camps.[17]

At Regina, Saskatchewan, on 22 July – the same day he cabled his former comrades in Madrid – he spoke to the medical staff of the Regina General Hospital at a noon luncheon, and in the evening addressed an audience of two thousand from an open-air platform in Wascana Park. He praised his Madrid colleagues and the International Brigades and denounced the British government. He said of Anthony Eden, the British foreign affairs minister, that at sessions of the League of Nations dealing with Spain, "he yawns and goes to sleep." As to the Spanish conflict: "This is the most important war the world has known." It would decide the fate of Europe, and of Canada, during the next five years. "If fascism," he said, "wins in Spain, it will encourage the fascists in other countries to such an extent that Europe – and then Canada and the United States – will be plunged into new dark ages of terror."[18]

From Regina he was driven north across the prairie to Saskatoon where he spoke to seven hundred, possibly half of whom were unemployed workers. He suggested that the Canadian people should assume responsibility for five hundred orphaned and refugee children in a Spanish village to be built and called "Canada." He maintained that the workers of Canada and all other countries could ensure peace by declaring they would not fight against other workers in other countries, but only against fascism wherever it arose. Most significantly he told the crowd, in the words of a police agent, "that there are only two classes in the world today, sharply raising the question of the class struggle."[19]

In Edmonton, Alberta, on 25 July, Bethune was received by fifteen hundred cheering people crammed to capacity at the Empire Theatre. He went beyond his now familiar themes, holding nothing back, indicting England's "capitalist government and diplomats, led by Anthony Eden, who are pro-Nazi and admire the Nazi form of government"; that fascism had begun in earnest in Canada, that it could only be defeated by a united front, and that "any progressive person who resists a united front is a traitor." Finally, to widespread applause, he said: "Today every progressive person is called a Red. These people on the platform are called Red and I am proud of it." He left on the midnight train to Calgary, and from there traveled west and south to California.[20]

22

You See Now Why I Must Go

On the very day when Bethune was opening his westward tour in Timmins, Ontario, the Japanese militarists, aligned with Hitler and Mussolini, attacked China with the intention of colonizing the entire country. The *Daily Clarion* printed an interview with Mao Zedong carrying the significant title: *Spain's Fight is Oppressed China's Fight*.[1] In the days that followed, the immediacy of the Chinese struggle gained such political prominence that articles on Spain were soon moved from the front pages to the interior of the newspaper, while banner headlines followed the relentless Japanese invasion.[2] Nor was this the concern solely of the Communist press. On 20 July, for example, the Winnipeg *Free Press* carried front-page stories on both China and Spain.[3] For many months, indeed until the ultimate collapse of the Negrín government and the bloody victory of Franco, the antifascist struggles in Spain and in China became politically linked and united. The global war that Bethune and the Communist Party had long predicted had truly begun.

On Wednesday, 28 July, Bethune arrived in San Francisco, California.[4] Had he by now been informed, through Party channels, that his plan to join the International Brigades had been denied? Almost certainly. And it seems equally likely that it was in California that he developed a new project: he would seek Party approval to travel to China on a new medical mission. It was in California, precisely at this time, that attention to China was at its height in the USA. The Communist Party in the United States, as well as significant sectors of socialists, trade unionists, and the burgeoning Chinese immigrant communities were determined to defend China against Japan's open aggression. On the day of Bethune's arrival in California, the Japanese army had smashed its way into Beijing, with Chinese troops and civilians in full retreat. Bethune's Party contacts in California would already have been organizing within their membership and mobilizing against this new front in the worldwide fascist assault. The invasion of yet another nation, and the militant atmosphere in California, would not have gone unnoticed by Bethune. Moreover, it was precisely at this time that reports were arriving of an appeal made jointly by Mao Zedong and the American leftist Agnes Smedley urging the Communist Parties of Canada and the USA to send medical supplies and doctors to Mao's headquarters;[5] together these were the deciding factors in the development of Bethune's determination to go to China.

Since Bethune left no diary, it is impossible to be certain of the exact date of Bethune's decision. But it is not the case, as some have maintained, that Bethune went to China because he had no choice, that he had burned his bridges to the medical community, that no hospital would take him, and that he had nowhere else to go. It should be recalled that he was a Fellow of the Royal College of Surgeons, a prestigious title in the medical world. He was a noted expert in the treatment of tuberculosis and one of a handful of recognized innovators in thoracic surgery. He was a member of the executive council of the American Association of Thoracic Surgeons. He had friends and amiable colleagues throughout North America; even if Sacré Coeur and the Royal Victoria Hospital would not have accepted him, he could quite readily have gone into practice in Toronto or New York, or any other North American city. Bethune's decision to go to China, almost certainly formulated in California, was not made by a man without choices, abandoned and lost. It was made by a man who hated and despised fascism, and who had the courage and tenacity to put his beliefs into action. Without question he was often sad, often lonely, wounded by his past, hollowed out by the absence of someone to share his life with, haunted by the ghosts of children he never had. But China was another matter. Bethune was a man who had been hardened by Spain, toughened by what he had seen and done. He was fully a Communist militant, as his speeches of the summer of 1937 so obviously attest: his decision was political and made on principle. As he would later write his friend, Marian Scott, from on board ship as it chugged its way out of Vancouver harbor and on to the Pacific: "You see Pony, why I *must* go to China. I feel so happy and gay now. Happier than since I left Spain."[6]

In a mass meeting in San Francisco, Bethune provided the audience with much the same themes that had occupied him previously, emphasizing the situation in Spain, but also making an allusion, for the first time, to Japanese troops. The following evening, 29 July, he spoke at a dinner, held at the St. Francis Yacht Club, under the auspices of the Medical Bureau to Aid Spanish Democracy.[7] The dinner was chaired by Dr. Leo Eloesser, a thoracic surgeon that Bethune had known for some years, and who himself was soon to depart for Spain. Intriguingly, some decades later, Eloesser would recall to an interviewer: "During a short trip back from China, he stayed with me in San Francisco for some days." Since Bethune never returned from China, the accuracy of this reminiscence was called into question. Eloesser replied: "I feel quite sure about Bethune's interruption of his work in China and his visit to the US to collect funds, for I remember his inflammatory speeches, not always too well aimed to grease the palms of staid medical audiences, who might, a priori, have been disposed to help him."[8] Eloesser's confusion is interesting: Bethune could well have stayed at Eloesser's house, and a yacht club gathering might well perceive his remarks as "inflammatory," and he was certainly visiting the US to "collect funds," but for Spain, not for China. And yet it is *China* that surfaces so strongly in Eloesser's memory: was this because it was China that was then at the forefront of Bethune's mind; was it not therefore China that Bethune discussed with Eloesser when they were alone together?

From San Francisco, Bethune traveled south to Los Angeles. Who he met there and to what ends we do not know. An itinerary published in the *Daily Clarion* notes, rather vaguely, that he attended "important gatherings";[9] a brief mention in the Los Angeles *Times* records that there was a "banquet in his honor," on 30 July, at an unidentified street address near MacArthur Park.[10]

Returning from Los Angeles to Canada on 1 August, Bethune spoke at the Orpheum Theatre in Vancouver, packed to the last seat, and with hundreds turned away for lack of space. He spoke again of Spain and of the blood transfusion service; his intentions concerning China he kept to himself. *Heart of Spain*, completed at last, received its long-awaited premiere, illustrating with stark realism the tragedy of the Spanish people. Defending the Republican government against unwarranted accusations, Bethune declared: "There have been atrocities on both sides, but the greatest atrocity is the clique of moneyed men who have banded together to kill the workers in Spain in order to regain their lost power." Toward the end of the meeting he said: "When fascism is defeated in Spain, it will vanish from the earth." The audience rose from their seats, cheering and applauding in a spontaneous demonstration of unity, and repeatedly thrusting their fists in the air.[11]

Interestingly, in the course of the meeting, a member of the Party stood and asked if Bethune was a Communist. Without hesitation, Bethune replied, "I have the honor to be accepted as a member of the Communist Party." Directly after the meeting, several members of the Party convened, including one who was evidently a secret police infiltrator. In a memo to his superiors in the police force he not only notes what the questioner asked, but *what he would have asked* – namely where and when Bethune joined the Party – had he not been immediately pulled back down into his seat. The Party member "received a severe lecture for 'bringing out the face of the Party' at a most inopportune time;" his question was called the "act of a provocateur;" and he was stripped of "voice and vote in his unit for three

You See Now Why I Must Go   **215**

months." Although the police spy's report is vague on the issue, it appears that Bethune himself was at least mildly rebuked. Taking some offence, Bethune responded that "he realized the propaganda value of his surgical work to the Party," but that he was more interested in blood transfusion operations than in "political manoeuvers." The reprimanded Party member is said to have immediately left Vancouver to join the Mackenzie–Papineau Battalion; an honorable response Bethune himself would have now been forbidden.[12]

After Vancouver, Bethune took a ferry to Vancouver Island and the capital of the province, Victoria, for a public meeting of nine hundred at the Chamber of Commerce, chaired by Party executive, Nigel Morgan.[13] On 3 and 4 August, Bethune spoke in Cumberland and Nanaimo, on Vancouver Island, to substantial audiences, raising money and screening *Heart of Spain*.[14] From there he crossed briefly into Washington State, speaking to the Medical Association in Seattle where, apparently overcome with exasperation at the political ignorance and self-satisfaction of the assembled physicians, he abandoned his usual impassioned but friendly manner and flew into a rage.[15] The next day found him in an equally truculent mood. A house party was held at the home of Dolly Stevens for the British Columbia Executive of the CCF party, to which Bethune had been invited as a special guest. During the course of the evening, he "scathingly denounced the CCF for harboring Trotskyites in their organization and for their refusal to cooperate with the Communists during the recent provincial elections,"[16] both of which were true, and both of which did serious harm to the building of the popular front Bethune thought so necessary to the antifascist struggle not only in Spain but at home.

After speaking in Vancouver for a second time, to a crowd of some one thousand who had been turned away the week before at the Orpheum, Bethune headed into the interior of British Columbia.[17] He traveled to Kamloops, Kelowna, Vernon, and Salmon Arm over the space of four days.[18] In Kelowna he spoke at the First United Church, explicitly raising the issue of China. "We must have a defense against our common enemy – fascism," Bethune announced. "The three great fascist countries are Japan, Germany, and Italy. We will be forced to fight these mad dogs for they will plunge us into a new age of barbarism unless we do something about it."[19] The listing of the fascist powers is here notable, reflecting a new re-ordering of importance in Bethune's thought: Japan first.[11]

In Salmon Arm, a small lakeside community, six hundred people occupied the Gymnasium Hall. The night was very hot. The hall was crammed, two deep standing all around, in the doorway, down the steps, and along the road in both directions. Loudspeakers had been placed under the roof of the hall, both inside and out. It was the largest meeting that had ever been held in the town on any occasion. The meeting had been organized by Elvira Stirling, a member of both the Women's League Against War and Fascism, and the Friends of the Mackenzie–Papineau Battalion. Stirling had written to Bethune that she had wanted to join him in Spain; she had some years of nursing experience, had traveled, and knew several languages. After the public meeting, a small gathering convened at Stirling's home; since the Party was well-developed in the region, there would certainly have been a number of Communists among them, as well as the inevitable secret police spy. Bethune told them he was not returning to Madrid, he was going to China; victory in Spain was by no means certain given Franco's powerful allies and the treachery of the non-intervention pact. It was in China that the antifascist struggle would now be fought out.[20] The police agent notified headquarters: "It is stated that Dr. Bethune is not returning to Spain but is considering a project to establish a blood transfusion service in China."[21] An important question arises: When Bethune made his decision, in California, to go to China did he inform the Party and seek its consent? If not, did he do so in Vancouver? And if it still remained a purely personal project, why would he announce it at a semi-public gathering in Salmon Arm in front of people some of whom, he must certainly have known, were Party members? To do so would have been an excessively serious breach of discipline, far more important than revealing his Party status from an auditorium platform, since it would have exposed what surely should not have been revealed on a tour ostensibly intended to raise funds for the blood transfusion unit in Spain. To state that he had no intention of returning to Spain would have vitiated the whole purpose of the tour. Much has been made of Bethune's intransigent independence; but equally he was a dedicated Party militant. It is entirely likely, then, that Bethune had notified the Party of his plans, and that they had accepted them in principle. Indeed, a document exists indicating that Bethune suggested to Tim Buck, sometime in August, that a medical unit be sent to China;[22] in all probability this would have been sent from either California, or more likely, Vancouver, prior to his arrival in Salmon Arm. After all, a return to Spain was not possible for Bethune; that much was understood. What's more, the Japanese invasion of China was quickly turning into a ferocious bloodbath. Mao needed doctors. The Communist International had put out the call to come to Mao's aid. That Bethune actively wanted to go to China would satisfy them all.

23

People Let Me Tell You, Now is the Time to Wake Up

From Salmon Arm, Bethune continued to travel east, often returning to towns and cities he had previously visited, and equally as often to communities that had not been scheduled on the westward leg: Canmore, in the shadow of the Rocky Mountains, Drumheller, Calgary, Edmonton; another two hundred, five hundred, a thousand people; workers, the unemployed, the few men, here and there, inspired by his words to get the necessary papers and tickets from the Communist Party, and join their comrades in the Mackenzie–Papineau Battalion.[1]

"Spain will be peaceful after my Canadian publicity tour," he said in Calgary, knowing he would never return.[2]

In Edmonton, Bethune spoke again at the Empire Theatre; bad weather reduced the numbers who came through the door, but the local radio station carried his words to a potential audience of thousands. He denounced the government's restrictions making it illegal for antifascist volunteers to go to Spain. A protest resolution opposing the government's actions was passed unanimously by a standing vote. Afterwards, at a social gathering held in the Albion Hall, Bethune once again proudly declared himself a Communist.[3]

Across the great Canadian prairies, Bethune traveled, through town after town, night after night, always speaking of the class struggle, of the worldwide conflict of fascism and democracy, of the blood transfusion unit in Madrid, of the refugees and the orphaned children, of the Japanese aggression, showing *Heart of Spain*, in Medicine Hat, Swift Current, Moose Jaw, Regina, Saskatoon, North Battleford, Prince Albert, Yorkton, Melville, sleeping in trains, in hotels, in the homes of strangers. Fifteen hundred came to hear him in Regina;[4] in Saskatoon the hall was jammed to the doors as hundreds jostled for chairs, stood in the aisles, even sat on the stage; everywhere the collection box was passed from hand to hand, to give a dollar, a quarter, a nickel, "to the Doctor."[5]

On 28 and 29 August, he spoke three times in Winnipeg; twice at the Starland Theatre to afternoon and evening gatherings, the latter drawing, according to a police report, an audience of almost ten thousand. At the Walker Theatre, the next night, he delivered one of his most important and revolutionary speeches. He began by warning the audience that much of what they read about Spain in the capitalist-controlled press should not be believed; that their correspondents and reporters seldom told the truth, and were purposely hired to distort the facts and tell misleading lies. Still, he said, "the Spanish people will eventually come out victorious no matter what the reporters try to make the people believe." But he said little about Spain that night, focusing instead on class-consciousness:

"I am a doctor," he said, "and a doctor after all is a worker just as any working man, and so are all the intelligentsia and professionals who work and depend on wages for their living. Even the small businessman is a worker as he is only working for the big concerns. I am a doctor, a mechanic or a carpenter of the human body."

And then, with a poetry born of his own immersion in the class struggle, Bethune said:

Man's eyes open twice only in his life; first when he is born, and secondly when he learns and becomes conscious of his position in society. . . . I am forty-seven years of age and my eyes opened just two years ago when I went with three other doctors from Montreal to the Medical-Physiological Congress in Moscow. There my eyes really opened after what I had seen. One seeing is worth more than hundreds and thousands of tellings. I visited many clinics and discussed the conditions of workers under the new social system, under socialism, where they have the security of economic democracy. . . . People let me tell you, now is the time to wake up and get together and elect *your* representatives to *your* government, who would really stand for your *interests*. Do it now. A little later might be too late. . . . The people could have stopped the last war, and could stop this war in Spain by only refusing to work at anything that helps war. . . . but the profits are far more important than human lives under this capitalist order.

Bethune spoke of the vastly increased shipments of nickel and of armaments from Canada to Spanish Morocco; shipments for Franco's fascists and blood money for Canadian capitalists. "It is a disgrace," Bethune continued,

in this present age and in a country like Canada to have unemployment and misery. There could be plenty for everybody if the toiling masses got their due share of the products of their labor. . . . The fascism menace is

People Let Me Tell You

creeping in and striving to enslave the people. It will come here and is coming. All these Orders-in-Council passed and put into effect are nothing else than fascist measures. An Order-in-Council was passed forbidding volunteers from Canada to Spain. . . . Even my name was mentioned during the last Parliament when I went over to Spain; that I was subject to cancellation of my citizenship and other penalties. I wrote to Minister LaPointe that if it is a crime to save some five hundred lives and punishable it is all right with me; he may exact the penalty.

He concluded with a ringing call for working-class unity. He traced the history of the rise of fascism in Germany and Italy; how the refusal of social democrats to cooperate with the Communists gave the ruling class the opportunity to install fascism. "They are trying to force it upon the Spanish people," he said, "and it will come here if you people do not unite into a People's Front and elect *your* government by you and for you."[6]

Bethune spent the last two days of August in Chicago, where he spoke at a gathering of the Medical Committee to Aid Spain.[7] The meeting was chaired by Walter B. Cannon, a politically progressive physiologist, Chair of the National Medical Bureau to Aid Spanish Democracy, and a personal friend not only of Ivan Pavlov, but Juan Negrín; he was soon also to be associated with the Medical Bureau for Medical Aid to China.[8]

At the beginning of September, Bethune returned to Ontario, speaking in Windsor, London, St. Catherines, and Niagara Falls. In London, according to a press report, "Dr. Bethune could see a connection between 'the man on the picket line in the Oshawa strike and the soldier fighting for his freedom in Shanghai; between the girl blinded by tear gas in a Montreal labor struggle, and the girl who was in the front line of Madrid's defense.' Similar politics united demagogues such as Mitchell Hepburn and Hitler, he added."[9] Giving credence to his claim that Hepburn was indeed a fascist, the Ontario government ordered the Board of Censors to delete certain sections of *Heart of Spain*: the image of a dead horse on a street, medical operations, and, notably, any unflattering references to Hitler and Mussolini, including the phrase "the war-mad fascist dictators of Germany and Italy."[10]

The lecture tour was coming to an end; sitting in his hotel room, he relished the few days off granted to him before the next speech; examining his itinerary it was happily obvious that the remaining lectures were spaced further and further apart. There was a little time now to answer the correspondence that had been accumulating: letters from the CASD, or from those who had heard him and been touched, from friends and, sadly, from Frances. What could he say to her? What did he *need* to tell her? It was well and truly over between them. But she was a wound that would not heal. "My path," he wrote, "is set on a strange road, but as long as I feel it is a good road I will go down it. And you must go down yours."[11]

For some time, and certainly after he joined the Communist Party, Bethune had felt that Frances was wasting her life. Coleman offered her nothing but a useless existence of consumption and political apathy. In the middle of a terrible economic crisis, surrounded by poverty and misery, she did nothing but display her aristocratic manners; ultimately, she had changed little since the early days in England. She distained the struggle that mattered most to Bethune, and the powerful attraction he had felt for her for so long was dying, if not yet entirely dead. The future which he was forging for himself included no role for Frances. He would write her one last time, but by then he had already left for China.

From Niagara Falls, Bethune returned to Toronto staying, again, with Paraskeva Clark and her husband. It was about this time that he encountered Edgar Snow's *Red Star Over China*, a groundbreaking book on Mao and the early years of the Communist Party of China. Bethune was much inspired by Snow's work, reading and re-reading it, and recommending it to everyone he knew. From time to time he would go to Party headquarters. Kate Bader, Tim Buck's secretary, recalled that "Dr. Bethune used to come to talk with Mr. Buck and I would have a few words with him; I think I typed some letters for him. . . . I remember him as a quiet man with a quiet voice and a complete absence of affectation or anything that would draw attention to himself." Now that he had settled on a course of action, he had found a certain inner resolve, a certitude without doubts or contradictions. A friend, Dr. Pauline Beregoff-Gillen, thought of him at this time as "extraordinary in every way and above all as a man. He would drop in, sit on the sofa, put his feet on the table, and talk of the revolution, of the wars, of China."[12]

During these weeks in September, Bethune was scheduled to speak in Detroit. He arrived on Saturday the 11th, to lecture at the Art Institute, under the sponsorship of the American Medical Bureau to Aid Spanish Democracy, but was unable to show *Heart of Spain* intact. Precisely as Hepburn had censored the film in Ontario, Detroit Police Commissioner Heinrich Pickert, had objected to any uncomplimentary references to Hitler or Mussolini.[13] After the meeting, Bethune had dinner with his old friend John Barnwell, and they had a vigorous conversation about communism. Dr. Robert Shaw, who was with them, recalled that "there was no doubt as to Dr. Bethune's political philosophy, and he more than held his own defending it."[14] On 15 September, he returned to Toronto. Speaking at Massey Hall, he addressed an audience of twenty-five hundred, along

People Let Me Tell You **221**

with Larry Ryan who had recently returned from fighting with the Mackenzie–Papineau Battalion.[15] The next day, in Ottawa, he spoke at the 53rd Annual Trades and Labor Convention in the afternoon,[16] and at the Chateau Laurier in the evening under the auspices of the CASD.[17]

The Communist Party announced that they were planning a series of meetings and demonstrations across Canada to protest the Japanese invasion of China.[18] In Moscow, the Executive Committee of the Communist International (ECCI) was preparing an appeal, uniting the conflict in Spain with that in China, and which read, in part:

> The struggle of the Spanish and Chinese peoples for liberation, independence, and peace is the vital concern of the international proletariat, of all peoples. Not a single worker, not a single toiler, not a single Socialist, not a single democrat can fail to assist in bringing about the victory of the Spanish and Chinese peoples. . . . There is no more urgent task facing all sincere supporters of democracy and peace than in every way to contribute to the defeat of German and Italian fascism in Spain, and of the Japanese fascist militarists in China. . . . Remember, working people, that it depends on the outcome of the struggle in Spain and China whether the fascist cutthroats succeed in driving mankind into a new world imperialist slaughter. . . . By defending Spain and China today, you defend the cause of world peace, you defend other peoples against fascist onslaught, you defend yourselves, your homes, your children against fascist brigandage. . . . Let the mighty voice of the peoples resound throughout the world with the words: Out with the fascist interventionists from Spain! Out with the Japanese usurpers from China![19]

The preparatory documents leading up to the ECCI appeal were being debated at the Central Committee meetings of every Party, including the Communist Party of Canada.

Bethune took the opportunity to make a formal request, in person, to Tim Buck that he be sent to China. Buck considered the matter. Neither the CASD nor the Party was in any position to fund a medical mission to China; the Party itself was stretched to its financial limits in funding the Mackenzie–Papineau Battalion in Spain. Buck promised to telephone Earl Browder, the leader of the Communist Party of the United States (CPUSA) to see what could be done. Browder was amenable to the proposal.[20] Bethune went immediately to New York City to consult with him. Years later, after Bethune's death, Browder said in his closing speech to the CPUSA convention of June 1940:

222   IN DEFENSE OF THE REPUBLIC

We sent our ambassador to China, one we need to mention very often, as
a symbol of what America should do for China – Dr. Norman Bethune. Dr.
Bethune was one of the greatest surgeons of the world. He went to Spain
also. He was not known as a Communist because in the kind of world we
live in today, the finest surgeons, the finest minds of all kinds are denied
the right to exercise their genius and their skills if they are known communists. But when Dr. Bethune, at my proposal, immediately and
unhesitatingly agreed to go to China to serve the Eighth Route Army with
the miserable equipment of five thousand dollars worth of drugs and tools,
he knew that the chances of his coming back were very small, and he said:
"I accept on one condition, that if I don't come back, you will let the world
know that Norman Bethune died a Communist Party member."[21]

Less than two months after meeting Browder, Bethune gave his forwarding
address to a friend in New York as: "c/o 8th Route Army, Medical Service,
Yenan (Fu Shih), North Shensi, China."[22]

There remained only a handful of meetings to complete Bethune's
speaking tour: a series of venues in the Maritime Provinces followed by a
final appearance in Philadelphia. On 26 September he spoke in Halifax, at
the Dalhousie University gymnasium to a large audience.[23] In Sydney, the
owner of the local radio station refused to announce Bethune's meeting,
claiming it was too "controversial"; local labor leaders were able to prevail
upon him, but only after agreeing to pay more than the usual fee for the
announcement.[24] From Sydney, Bethune traveled to Glace Bay, New
Waterford, and Moncton, before returning to Halifax.[25] Here again there
was radio censorship. The station, owned by the Conservative Party Senator,
W. H. Dennis, had interviewed Bethune but then informed him that they
would not broadcast one of the answers he had given to their questions.
Bethune responded by refusing to allow any of his scheduled address to be
heard. Explaining himself to the press, he held that he would not be
governed by "such intolerable dictatorship." There exists in Canada, he said,
"certain institutions beyond the pale of criticism, in short a privileged class.
This is in direct and violent conflict with the principles of free speech, and
I maintain it is one of the first evidences of dictatorship in Canada, and as
such must be opposed by every lover of democracy."[26] That evening he was
invited to dinner at a private golf club by a group of doctors to describe the
techniques employed at the blood transfusion service in Spain. When
Bethune returned to the home of Professor Mercer, where he was staying,
one of the doctors, in a true excess of cowardice, telephoned to say, "Please
let it not be known that we were entertaining him."[27]

On his way south to Pennsylvania, Bethune stayed overnight with

People Let Me Tell You

George and Jean Holt, artists whom he had known in Montreal, but who were living then in Boston. He spoke with them about communism and the Party, and confided to them precisely what he had written to Frances from South Porcupine: that he had not enjoyed the lecture tour; that he had disliked being confined to so much speaking when it was action that was needed and called to him.[28] Bethune had spoken in all the major cities in Canada, and virtually all the major cities in the United States that were close to the Canadian border; but there was no public speech in Boston. The decision not to speak there may well have been related to the very heavy influence of the Catholic hierarchy in the city and its open and enthusiastic support for Franco. In Philadelphia, Bethune stayed with Dr. Richard Meade with whom he had become close friends through the American Association of Thoracic Surgeons. He tried to convert Meade to communism, and left him a list of books he thought he should read. While in Philadelphia he addressed an audience at Witherspoon Hall, along with Victor Hirschfield, an ambulance driver with the Abraham Lincoln Battalion.[29] The tour was over.

Bethune's long months on the road were declared, accurately, a "great success" by the *Daily Clarion*.[30] He had asked the people to open their eyes, and they had opened them. He had told the people that it was time to wake up, and they had awoken. Well over thirty thousand people heard him speak; hundreds of thousands more read detailed reports of his speeches in the press. Not a few were inspired to volunteer for the Mackenzie–Papineau Battalion, and popular support for the combatants had steadily increased. In the deep heart of the Depression, thousands of dollars were raised for the antifascist struggle. The prestige of the Party was intensified; the inherent value of the concept of the Popular Front was everywhere evident. The CASD grew in strength and influence. And perhaps most gratifying to Bethune personally, the Committee had committed itself to feeding and sheltering the lonely and displaced Spanish orphans.[31] When asked how he felt about the tour, Bethune commented: "I have become for thousands of workers, a symbol – to contemplate this responsibility is terrifying! I feel a tremendous urge to get back into the mass and hide myself from this bright glare. . . . For me it has been a revelation of working class solidarity which will long live in my memory."[32]

24

Will You Come?

Over the first weekend of October, the Communist Party of Canada held its Eighth National Convention. Party membership was near its peak, and the Convention was well attended. The policy of the Popular Front assured there were many non-Party guests and observers. What's more, it was the twentieth anniversary of the Soviet Revolution.[1] The situation in Spain was the common concern of the whole Party membership, as was China. In its half-dozen Resolutions, the Convention called upon the government of Canada to "remove the ban on the export of arms and materials to the legal democratic Spanish government," to "give full support to China in its just resistance against Japanese invasion," and to "stop the shipment of war materials to Japan." The government, in all three cases, did precisely the opposite.[2]

Earl Browder arrived from New York to address the Convention as the leader of the Party's most significant fraternal ally, speaking passionately for a common front of every nation against the fascist warmongers. Although there is no record, it would seem improbable that Bethune would not have been present, and spoken with Buck and Browder. Browder had proposed to Bethune not only that he serve with the Eighth Route Army, but that he head a full surgical and medical mission; a replication of the blood transfusion service he had instituted in Spain would be inadequate to China's requirements.[3]

Accordingly, Bethune went to Michigan, to re-train with John Barnwell and recover the general surgical skills he had once learned in England and Europe, but which he had not practiced since he had begun to specialize in thoracic work.[4] In New York City, a few weeks later, Dr. Milton Feltenstein helped prepare him in general medicine,[5] while Dr. Louis Davidson reviewed anatomy.[6] The enormity of his self-imposed task was becoming evident to Bethune: compared to Spain, China was immense; doctors from around the world had hastened to Spain's aid, in China doctors were worse than scarce. If Bethune had to go alone, he would face that possibility with equanimity; he had made his decision and he was not afraid; the onslaught of global fascism had to be arrested, sacrifices would have to be made and were, in fact, being made daily. So many had already died in Spain; too many of the heroic volunteers of the Mackenzie–Papineau battalion would never come home. What was needed in China was a large team of professionals – a battalion of doctors – and if it were necessary he would recruit them himself.

Throughout the fall and early winter of 1937, Bethune moved frequently between Montreal, Toronto, and New York. Wherever he went, wherever he encountered an old friend, or a doctor he could talk to, he asked the same question: *will you come?* In Toronto, it was Dr. Ernest Struthers; he had been to China, and Bethune wanted his opinion on what medical equipment he should take with him. Would he come? No. In Montreal, it was Dr. Sclater Lewis, whom he had known at the Royal Victoria Hospital. Would he come? No.[7] In New York, Bethune consulted with Browder, who had not been idle. The situation in China was deteriorating; just as the major capitalist powers had betrayed Spain, they were now materially supporting Japan. Under these circumstances it was necessary to act quickly. Browder was eager to launch Bethune's China mission, but there was little money; the anti-Japanese campaign – mass meetings, demonstrations, political work – was expensive, and there remained the dominant financial commitment to Spain and the Abraham Lincoln Battalion. Browder turned to Philip Jaffe, a businessman with a strong political interest not only in the CPUSA, but in China. Jaffe had recently returned from Beijing, and was establishing a funding organization, the China Aid Council. Together with the League for Freedom and Democracy, and the New York section of the Committee to Aid Spanish Democracy, the China Aid Council guaranteed some degree of financial support for Bethune, but further independent fundraising would be required.[8] Meanwhile, in Toronto, Sam Carr, a member of the Central Executive of the Party, successfully recruited Jean Ewen, a seasoned nurse who had recently returned from China, to join Bethune's team.[9]

Toward the end of October, Bethune returned to Montreal, visiting the friends he had known before he went to Spain: Wendell MacLeod; George Mooney, Libbie Park, and many others. Bethune had sent Libbie Park a letter from Spain describing the nightmare of Malaga, but he had not seen her since his return to Canada. He telephoned her and asked if he could come over for tea. They talked together of friends and mutual interests as if they had never been apart. Afterwards they drove to the nearby city reservoir on the edge of Pine Avenue and stood looking down over the city lights spread below them to the shore of the St. Lawrence River, each one pointing to familiar landmarks. As Park wrote later, Bethune said, "he felt as if he were in limbo in an unreal world. He told me he was taking a medical team to China, including a nurse, Jean Ewen, and the team was to leave in a couple of months. Would I come too? I could join them in Vancouver. It was hard to say no, but I had to. We said goodbye. He took me home and as he drove off we waved to each other. I never saw him again."[10] In the morning he called George Deshaies at Sacré Couer and told him he was leaving for New York to raise funds.[11]

On 24 October, Dr. Edward Barsky, who had established the first American hospitals in Spain and was the chief medical officer for the American battalions of the International Brigades, was given a farewell dinner. He had come back to the United States for much the same reasons Bethune had, and was now returning to Spain. Among the speakers on the platform was Bethune himself;[12] it must have been, for him, an especially poignant and bittersweet moment – so many memories of Spain, of so much won and so much lost, the possibility of return forever foreclosed. Spain: the center of the earth, the tomb of fascism. No matter what he had said to Frances about how much he hated the cross-country tour, talking endlessly in town after town, he understood perfectly the necessity of arousing the people for the antifascist fight. He had done what he could do, what needed to be done, in defense of the Republic. For Barsky the road led back to Spain; for Bethune a new road led to China.

Not much later, Bethune met Hazen Sise. Both Sise and Sorensen had been planning to leave Spain as early as August. It had taken them some time to complete their affairs. Sorensen had gone to Denmark, soon to return to Canada. Sise had only recently arrived, and was back and forth between Toronto and New York. Of all the little band that had worked together in Madrid, only Allen May remained.[13] They met together, Sise and Bethune, two or three times, having a drink, talking about Spain, and then about China. Finally, Bethune put the question to him: *"Will you come?"* Would he go with him to shoot a film on the guerilla fighting near Yanan? No. Years later, Sise was to say: "I've always regretted that I didn't."[14]

Bethune appears to have spent most of November and December entirely in New York, staying with whoever could provide him with a bed and a meal. For a short while he lived with Elsie Siff with whom he had a pleasant but brief affair.[15] While he was boarding with Dr. Davidson, the doctor's wife went to tidy Bethune's room. His suitcase was open on the bed: there were almost no clothes; it was filled with Communist literature.[16] But perhaps most interestingly, he lived for a time with the legendary "Mother Bloor." Ella Bloor had a long radical history; she began in the women's suffrage movement, later she helped Upton Sinclair in exposing the filth and exploitation in the Chicago meatpacking industry. She organized solidarity with the United Mine Workers strike against Rockefeller in Colorado, and organized miners and other workers across the country into

Will you Come?

the Communist Party, of which she herself was a Central Committee member. In 1934 she led the American delegation to the Women's International Congress Against Fascism and War in Paris.[17]

During these final months of 1937, fundraising began in earnest, and medical supplies were purchased and warehoused.[18] In a quiet moment Bethune reflected on the new horizon he had set for himself. He knew that others thought him lonely; but that was of no true importance to him. He had many friends, but none of them were with him. And he had the Party. Spain was never a matter of his medical commitment; that was never an issue. Spain was a test of his *political* commitment; it forced upon him the difference between sympathy and generosity on the one hand, and solidarity on the other. It was a difficult lesson to learn, and he knew he was still learning it. Only a single question now occupied him: would he be good enough? He knew what he had accomplished in Spain, and he knew that he had, in some ways, let his Party and his comrades down. It must not happen again. He would not let it happen again. And it was not solely a matter of his impatience and his anger. He was haunted by the Norwegian boy who had died in his arms. And by the simple trust of the little lad in the middle of British Columbia who had heard him speak and had given him the dime that he was going to spend on a milkshake.[19] And by the small boy, not more than three feet tall, who had given five pennies "for the Doctor."[20] Would he be good enough for *them*? For all the wounded and the helpless and the kind-hearted and the poor; for those who would come to him in need of his skill; would he be *good* enough? And there were those other ghosts: Frances, and Marian, and Elizabeth, and Margaret, and Kajsa; all loved, all gone, all lost.

The preparations were almost complete. Near the end of December another volunteer for the mission was found: Dr. Charles H. Parsons. An American surgeon, he had practiced in the fishing village of Twillingate, on an islet off the northeastern coast of Newfoundland. He was, unfortunately, so often drunk that Bethune considered him a serious risk to the project; but since the group was already far smaller than he had hoped, Bethune decided to offer no objection.[21] On New Year's Eve there was a farewell party for Bethune in Manhattan. The next day, Bethune left for Toronto; he was to connect with Parsons in Vancouver. Jean Ewen would meet them there.[22]

Why Bethune went to Toronto is not clear; perhaps a last meeting with Tim Buck, or to clear up some personal affairs. In any event he stayed once more, for a day or two, with Paraskeva Clark. She wanted him to continue painting in China. "Take at least my little water colors," she implored, "maybe you'll do something; you have so much in your painting." Bethune was touched. "You know," he said, "praise from you means much to me." He bought the Clarks dinner at a restaurant the evening before he was to board the train to Vancouver. After dinner, they left in a rush. Paraskeva took him in a taxi to the train station, and as they passed the University of Toronto, he said, reminiscing, "Oh someday I studied in here." And then with sudden alarm, "My God, I forgot my surgical instruments!" He gave her some money to send the instruments by air in time to catch the ship. And then they were at the station and he was gone.[23]

On 8 January 1938 the *Empress of Asia* prepared to set sail from Vancouver harbor. Bethune was ebullient. A new world was about to begin. He stood leaning over the railing with Parsons, breathing in the brisk salt air. Ewen came up the gangplank while a fellow Scotsman, Jimmy Mitchell, in full Highland dress, played the bagpipes.[24]

Soon the Canadian shoreline disappeared in cloud and fog and they were heading out into open water.

*   *   *

For almost two years Bethune served with Mao's Eighth Route Army. One evening, hurrying to operate on the last of the wounded soldiers before the Japanese renewed their attack, his scalpel slipped and slashed his finger. He died of blood poisoning in Yellow Stone Village on 12 November 1939, surrounded by the love of his comrades. At the official funeral, ten thousand came to weep over his body.[25]

PART FIVE

Aubade

25
A Dream of Himself

Aubade: a curious word possessing a somewhat hybrid meaning: a hymn to daybreak, to the new dawn; but also the time when lovers must part . . .

Do we know Bethune better, now that we have told something of the story of his life? Yes; perhaps. We know what he *did*, to the extent that the historical record – the remaining documents and letters, testimonies and memoirs – allow us that privilege. And we know something of who he *was*, the interior of the man, as much as that can be revealed with our admittedly partial and imperfect analytic tools. But do we know him now, fully, and finally, and completely? An impossible task in any event, made more difficult since Bethune was the least introspective of subjects: he left no fragment of autobiography, his focus almost always turned outward toward the world. How can we know him, when, as his friend Paraskeva Clark put it with an air of strange profundity: "I don't know if he knew himself, anything about himself . . . he was a dream of himself . . . And it's sort of most wonderful, he wasn't a person, he was just a chapel, a university, I don't know what, a temple."[1]

Did he know himself? Perhaps no better than the rest of us know ourselves. But perhaps in those few months in Spain, purified in the struggle against fascism, and that interior struggle that was always with him, he became, as Mao said, *selfless*, and the meaning of his life became for him self-clarified.

Bethune died in 1939 as the world erupted into the very war that he predicted and tried to prevent. It could be said that he lived and died in his times, and that the times have changed: that he has nothing left to say to us; that he was a man of his century, and that century has passed.

But is this true? Has history nothing to tell us? Do men and women simply come and go like brief spray on pointless waves, their lives without value, receding into a meaningless and darkening mist? The ideology of capitalism is clear on this point: the present is all that matters; the human past and the human future have no meaning. And looking back on the whole of Bethune's century, what do we find? Brutality and death, endless war and vicious repression, gas chambers, torture cells and prison camps, police states, and everywhere the bloody advance of imperialism. But it was also the first century when the working class of the whole world began to stand up, to fight in earnest for a new society, a new dawn for humanity: a struggle which stumbled and fell, and was prematurely declared dead, but which may yet regain its feet: a struggle that, perhaps, has just begun.

Nearly twenty years after Bethune's death, Vittorio Vidali, "Comrade Contreras" of the Spanish war, was speaking with Jacques Duclos of the Communist Party of France at the International Conference of Communist and Worker's Parties in Moscow, in 1957. Mao recognized Vidali and came up to him, offering his hand. Vidali relates:

> His handshake was friendly, strong and warm. He is a great personage. Before the reception was over he came to us with an interpreter. Taking me by the hand, he asked: 'You were wounded at Madrid, weren't you?' 'Yes, I was,' I replied. He looked at me in a friendly way, held my hand in his own for a little while, as if to express his affection, and then explained that he had wanted to greet me a second time because he knew that I had once been engaged in helping those persecuted by Chiang Kai-shek and in assisting the red zones in China. I told him that I had known friends of China such as Dr. Bethune . . . I parted from him deeply moved.[2]

If we remember Bethune now, and repeat the story of his life for a new generation, it is not to lay him to rest, but to let him rise again. He was a man who was torn and damaged, tormented and wounded; and if he could heal himself, and change, and become whole, and through joining himself with the world's oppressed become selfless, then so can we all.

There are no spirits beyond the grave, but there are spirits who live in history. If we let Bethune beckon to us, and follow him into the fight, then we can say, with him:

> Whether we will ever live to see that peaceful and prosperous Republic of workers doesn't matter. The important thing is that we are making that new Republic possible, are assisting in its birth. But whether it will be born or not, depends on our actions today and tomorrow. It is not inevitable; it is not self-generating. It must be created by the blood and work of all of us who believe in the future; only in this way is it inevitable. In devotion to our great cause, let the living and the dying seal our comradeship. In struggle and sacrifice we shall have one purpose, one thought. Then we will be invincible. Then we will know that even if we do not live to see it, some day those who come after us will gather to celebrate a great and democratic republic for the liberated people.[3]

Notes

Preface

1 Sigmund Freud and Arnold Zweig, *The Letters of Sigmund Freud and Arnold Zweig* (New York: Harcourt, Brace & World, 1970), p. 127.

PART ONE   Wounded

I   A Rotten Childhood

1 Osler Library of the History of Medicine, Montreal [OLHM], 637 1/65. Dr. Richard Brown, 1963. [Unless otherwise noted, all material referenced as OLHM is to the Roderick Stewart Fonds.]

2 OLHM, 637 2-4. See also Roderick Stewart and Sharon Stewart, *Phoenix: The Life of Norman Bethune* (Montreal: McGill–Queen's University Press, 2011), p. 112. [SS]

3 OLHM 637 1/65. Archibald to Nadeau, 4 April 1941.

4 SS, p. 7.

5 Ibid.

6 OLHM, 637 1/106. Elizabeth Wallace to Ted Allan, [TA] no date.

7 SS, pp. 53, 55.

8 Roderick Stewart, *Bethune* (Toronto: New Press, 1973), p. 30. [SB]

9 Ted Allan and Sydney Gordon, *The Scalpel, the Sword: The Story of Dr. Norman Bethune* (Boston: Little, Brown, 1952), p. 36. [AG]

10 SB, p. 28.

11 Ibid., p. 29.

12 The murals are displayed in Eugene P. Link, *The T.B.'s Progress: Norman Bethune as Artist* (Plattsburgh: Center for the Study of Canada, State University of New York, 1991).

13 Ibid., p. 11.

14 AG, p. 10.

15 Ibid.

16 Hilary Russell, "'I Come of a Race of Men . . . '," in David A. E. Shephard and Andrée Levesque, eds., *Norman Bethune: His Times and his Legacy* (Ottawa: Canadian Public Health Association, 1982), p. 16. [SL]

17 AG, p. 10.

18 OLHM, Julie Allan Fonds. [JAf] TA's notes from a 1942 interview with Frances Penney. [FP]

19 AG, p. 13.

20 Ibid.
21 J. Wilbur Chapman, *The Life and Work of Dwight Lyman Moody* (London: James Nisbet, 1900), p. 235.
22 AG, p.10.
23 SS, p. 4.
24 LAC, MG30, D388, 30/19. Letter of Malcolm Bethune to his father. Unless otherwise noted, all material referenced as LAC, MG30, D388 is to the Ted Allan Fonds.]
25 AG, p. 10.
26 Ibid.
27 SB, p. 2.
28 SS, p. 5
29 LAC MG30 D388, 2/4. Janet Stiles notes.
30 Canadian Broadcasting Corporation [CBC] Radio Archives. Georges Deshaies. [GD]
31 LAC MG30 D388, 29/12.
32 OLHM, JAf. TA's notes from a 1942 interview with FP.
33 Ibid.
34 OLHM, 637 1/106
35 Ibid.
36 OLHM, JAf, TA's notes from a 1942 interview with FP.
37 CBC, GD.
38 OLHM, 637 1/65.
39 Russell, p. 13.
40 Ibid., p. 15.
41 Ibid.
42 LAC MG30 D388, 29/12.
43 Larry Hannant, *The Politics of Passion: Norman Bethune's Writing and Art* (Toronto: University of Toronto Press, 1998), p. 73.
44 Ibid.
45 Ibid., p. 78.
46 SS, p. 7.
47 SB, p. 2.
48 OLHM 637 1/65.
49 LAC MG30 D388, 29/12; also 30 / 5.
50 OLHM 637 1/65. Letter from Harriet Elliston Hammond to Roderick Stewart [RS], 28 June 1971.
51 Ibid.
52 OLHM, 637 1/65. Richard Brown.
53 Hannant, p. 38.
54 SB, p. 3.
55 LAC MG30 D388, 2/34. Janet Stiles.
56 Ibid.
57 AG, p. 10.

Notes to pp. 15–21

58 Ibid., p. 11.
59 LAC MG30 D388, 16/18. Letter of FP to TA 29 December 1942.
60 AG, p. 58.
61 SS, p. 11.
62 Russell, p. 19.
63 LAC MG30 D388, 29/12. Notes by Malcolm Bethune.
64 OLHM 637 1/48. Darley Gordon.
65 SS, p. 20.
66 SB, p. 2.
67 LAC MG30 D388, 29/12.
68 SS, p.19.
69 OLHM 637 1/48. Janet Cornell.
70 SS, p. 23.
71 Ibid., p. 20.
72 Ibid.
73 Ibid., p. 22.
74 Richard Allen, "The Religious Setting of Norman Bethune's Early Years," in SL, p. 22.
75 LAC MG30 D388, 29/12.
76 LAC MG30 D388, 2/34; 2/33.
77 LAC MG30 D 388, 30/5.
78 LAC MG30 D 388, 2/34; 2/33.
79 SB, p. 4.
80 Ibid.

2   Nothing He Would Not Do

1 AG, p. 14; LAC MG30 D388, 2/34.
2 AG, p. 15.
3 SS, p. 30.
4 SB, p. 9.
5 AG, p. 16.
6 Ibid.
7 Mary Larratt Smith, *Prologue to Norman: The Canadian Bethunes* (Oakville and Ottawa: Mosaic Press/Valley Editions, 1976), p. 80.
8 LAC MG30 D388, 29/12.
9 SB, p. 11.
10 OLHM, JAf. Folder 5. TA interview with FP.
11 SB, p. 11; OLHM, JAf. Folder 6. Letter of FP to TA 29 December 1942.
12 OLHM, JAf. TA interview with FP.
13 Ibid.
14 Ibid.
15 OLHM, JAf, letter of Marian Scott to TA.
16 LAC MG30 D388 29/12.
17 SB, p. 14.

18 Ibid., p. 15.
19 OLHM, 637 1/31, letter from Ralph C. Rueger, MD to RS. Paul Kavieff, *The Purple Gang: Organized Crime in Detroit 1910–1945* (Fort Lee: Barricade Books, 2000).
20 OLHM, 637 1/57. Letter of Coleman to John Kemeny [JK] 7 July 1963.
21 LAC MG30 D388 29/12.
22 Ibid.
23 AG, p. 25.
24 SB, p. 18.
25 Ibid.
26 Ibid., p. 17.
27 LAC MG30 D388 29/12.
28 SS, p. 53.
29 SB, p. 174.
30 Ibid., pp. 30–31.
31.Ibid., p. 32.
32 Ibid., p. 40.
33 OLHM, 637 1/28. Amy Russell to RS December 1971.
34 See for example, SB, p. 65; SS, p. 85.
35. OLHM, JAf, TA interview with FP.
36 Hannant, p. 40.
37 Ibid., p. 41.
38 OLHM, JAf, TA interview with FP.
39. LAC MG30 D388 3/28.
40 Ibid., 30/13.
41 Hannant, pp. 42–43.
42 SB, p. 62.
43 OLHM, JAf, TA interview with FP.
44 Ibid.
45 Ibid.
46 Ibid.
47 OLHM, 637 1/28. Amy Russell to RS December 1971.
48 OLHM, P89, File 1-48.
49 NFB research files, Hjalmar Larsson to JK, 29 June 1963.
50 LAC MG30 D388, 2/37; OLHM 637 1/106, Elizabeth Wallace to TA.
51 Wendell MacLeod, "Dr. Norman Bethune," in Wendell MacLeod, Libbie Clark, and Stanley Ryerson, *Bethune: The Montreal Years* (Toronto: Lames Lorimer, 1978), p. 40.
52 NFB research files, Ethan Flagg Butler to JK, 28 May 1963.
53 SB, p. 58.
54 Pierre Delva, "Norman Bethune: L'influence de L'hopital du Sacré Coeur," in SL p. 85.
55 Jean-Pierre Tetrault, "History of Canadian Anaesthesia: Georges Cousineau (1906–1987)," *Canadian Journal of Anaesthesia*, Vol. 40, 2, p. 188.

Notes to pp. 27–33

56 NFB research files, interview with Georges Deshaies 12 November 1963. [NFB/GD]
57 Delva, p. 89.
58 NFB/GD.
59 LAC MG30 D388, 1/7. Dr. M. McQuitty to TA, May 1942.
60 Delva, p. 89.
61 NFB research files, interview with Aubrey Geddes.
62 SB, p. 57.
63 Letter from H. J. Scott to Alexander Walt, 16 February 1963, courtesy Dr. Larry Stephenson.
64 Charles Hill, Louis Muhlstock, Marian Scott, Leo Kennedy, " 'They Could Split Rock . . . ': Painting in Montreal in the 1930s, and the Children's Creative Art Centre – A Conversation Piece," in SL, p. 114.
65 David Lethbridge interview with Delva, 14 December 2007; also, Delva unpublished manuscript.
66 Libbie Park, "Norman Bethune As I Knew Him," in MacLeod, Park, and Ryerson, p. 95.
67 Charles Hill et al., p. 118.
68 Ibid.
69 MacLeod, p. 59.
70 Ibid., p. 62; OLHM, 637 1/66. Hyman Shister's membership in the Communist Party is noted in an interview with Gordon McCutcheon.
71 AG, pp. 78–79; Stanley Ryerson, "Comrade Beth," in MacLeod, Park, and Ryerson, p. 147.
72 Park, pp. 92–93.
73 NFB, *Bethune*, post-production script, p. 11.
74 AG, p. 82; MacLeod, p. 64; Park, p.80; NFB research files, interview with Wendell MacLeod.
75 AG, p.83.
76 Norman Bethune, "Reflections on Return from 'Through the Looking Glass,'" *Bulletin of the Montreal Medico-Chirurgical Society,* March–April 1936.
77 Dr. Larry Stephenson interview with Irene Kon, 2000; Park, pp. 77–78.
78 Ryerson, p. 145.
79 Park, pp. 105–106.
80 Norman Bethune, "Take Private Profit Out of Medicine," *Canadian Doctor*, 3, no. 1, January 1937.
81 Park, pp. 126–127; Hannant, pp. 104–105.
82 Park, p. 114.
83 Park, p. 119; NFB research files, interview with Paraskeva Clark. [NFB/PC]
84 Letter of Wendell MacLeod to Vivian Schwartz, quoted in Louis Horlick, *J. Wendell MacLeod: Saskatchewan's Red Dean* (Montreal: McGill–Queen's University Press, 2007), p. 118.
85 SB, p. 68.
86 Park, p. 115; NFB, *Bethune*, post-production script, p. 10.

238 NOTES TO PP. 33–43

87 Hannant, pp. 76–77. The following letter appears on pp. 85–89.

88 Park, pp. 98–99

89 According to H.J. Scott, Marian Scott's nephew, in a 16 February 1983 letter to Alexander Walt, "[Bethune] had a cruel streak in his nature, but that he was very aware of this himself and was his own worse critic in this regard." Letter courtesy Larry Stephenson.

90 Patricia Whitney, "First-Person Feminine: Margaret Day Surrey," *Canadian Poetry*, Vol. 31, 1992. The succeeding paragraphs are based on Whitney's interview, and SS, p. 142.

91 MacLeod, p. 65.

92 Ibid.

3 Last Night Rose Low and Wild and Red

1 Tim Buck, *Thirty Years: 1922–1952* (Toronto: Progress Books, 1952), pp. 116–117.

2 George Dimitrov, *Two Years of Heroic Struggle of the Spanish People* (New York: Workers Library, 1938), p. 5.

3 Daily Clarion, 20–29 July 1936. [DC]

4 Ibid., 27 July 1936.

5 Ibid., 4 August 1936.

6 Ibid., 5, 6 August 1936.

7 Ibid., 8 August 1936.

8 Ibid., 13 August 1936.

9 Arthur H. Landis, *Spain: The Unfinished Revolution* (New York: International Publishers, 1972), pp. 215–218.

10 NFB research files. Fernand Dallaire interview.

11 NFB, *Bethune*, post-production script, p. 14.

12 NFB/PC.

13 LAC MG30 D297. Graham Spry papers. Vol. 1. File 1-25.

14 Rose Potvin, *Passion and Conviction: The Letters of Graham Spry* (Regina: Canadian Plains Research Center, 1992), p. 104.

15 DC, 3 September 1936.

16 Oscar Ryan, *Tim Buck: A Conscience for Canada* (Toronto: Progress Books, 1975), pp. 188–189.

17 SB, p. 89.

18 Tim Buck, "Soldiers of Democracy," *Marxist Quarterly*, Vol. 18, 1966, p.15. See also Buck, *Thirty Years*, p. 120; Oscar Ryan, p. 189.

19 *Toronto Star*, 15 September 1936; DC 16 September 1936.

20 *Toronto Star*, 16 September 1936.

21 DC, 22 September 1936.

22 DC, 24 September 1936.

23 *New Commonwealth*, 26 September 1936.

24 Henning Sorensen, "Henning Sorensen to Graham Spry: A Letter," in SL, p. 156.

Notes to pp. 43–57   **239**

25 SB, p. 89.
26 Potvin, p. 104.
27 DC, 29 September 1936; *New Commonwealth*, 3 October 1936.
28 NFB/GD.
29 DC, 7 October 1936.
30 OLHM, 637 2/6, tape 44.
31 Hannant, pp. 114–115.
32 DC, 22 October 1936.
33 Hannant, p. 116.
34 Pierre Berton, *The Great Depression* (Toronto: McClelland and Stewart, 1990), pp. 362–364. DC, 24 October 1936.
35 *New York Times*, 27 October 1936.
36 Berton, p. 365.

PART TWO   Capitalism Breeds Fascism the Way a Fly Breeds Maggots

4   The Double Pyramid

1 Quoted in Lawrence James, *The Rise and Fall of the British Empire* (New York: St. Martin's Press, 1996), p. 206. The literature on British imperialism is, of course, extensive. I have relied on James, and on James Morris, *Pax Britannica*, in three volumes (London: The Folio Society, 1992), in the following pages.
2 Morris, I, p. 158.
3 James, p. 198.
4 Ibid., p. 185.
5 Morris, I, p. 376.
6 James, p. 174.
7 Ibid., p. 262.
8 Ibid., p. 294.
9 Ibid. p. 193.
10 Morris, III, pp. 102–110.
11 James, p. 219.
12 Ibid.
13 Morris, I, pp. 376–393.
14 Ibid., p. 384.
15 Ibid., p. 392.
16 Karl Marx, "The Future Results of the British Rule in India," in Karl Marx and Frederick Engels, *The First Indian War of Independence 1857–1859* (Moscow: Progress, 1978), p.33.
17 Frederick Engels, *The Condition of the Working Class in England* (Moscow: Progress, 1977), passim. See especially pp. 59–103, 120–153. The term "social murder" is Engels'.
18 Morris, II, p. 19. Morris notes "most of the British possessions were acquired either for *Lebensraum* or for strategy."

5 Men of Iron, Men of Gold

1 Plato, *The Republic*, 414–415. (The citation employs the standard Stephanus numbering system here, and in the succeeding note.)
2 Plato, *The Laws*, 663–664, 903c and 739c; *Crito*, 50e.

6 The Frankenstein Project

1 Stefan Kuhl, *The Nazi Connection: Eugenics, American Racism, and German National Socialism* (New York: Oxford University Press, 1994).
2 Edwin Black, *The War Against the Weak: Eugenics and America's Campaign to Create a Master Race* (New York: Four Walls Eight Windows, 2003).
3 Catherine Clay and Michael Leapman, *Master Race: The Lebensborn Experiment in Nazi Germany* (London: Hodder and Stoughton, 1995).
4 Paul Preston, "The Answer Lies in the Sewers: Captain Aguilera and the Mentality of the Francoist Officer Corps." *Science & Society*, Vol. 68, #3, Fall 2004, pp. 277–312.

7 Imperialism Prefers Fascism

1 Berton, p. 97.
2 Ibid., pp. 140–147.
3 Ibid., pp. 120–127.
4 Lita-Rose Betcherman, *The Swastika and the Maple Leaf: Fascist Movements in Canada in the Thirties* (Toronto: Fitzhenry & Whiteside, 1975), pp. 10, 11, 42.
5 Dr. Terman, "Fascism in Canada: The Early Years," *Anti-Fascist Forum*, #3, 1998, p. 14.
6 Berton, pp. 464–465.
7 Ibid., p. 465.
8 Ibid., pp. 414–416.
9 Ibid.
10 Irving Abella and Harold Troper, *None Is Too Many: Canada and the Jews of Europe, 1933–1948* (Toronto: Lester and Orpen Dennys, 1982).
11 Berton, p. 468.
12 Winston Churchill, *The Hinge of Fate* (Boston: Houghton Mifflin, 1950), p. 475.
13 Margaret George, *The Hollow Men* (London: Leslie Frewin Publishers, 1967), p. 48. See also Clement Leibovitz, *The Chamberlain-Hitler Deal* (Edmonton: Les Editions Duval, 1993), Chapter IV.
14 Robert Rhodes James, *Churchill: A Study in Failure* (New York: World Publishing Company, 1970), pp. 330–331, 236.
15 Mark Curtis, *The Great Deception* (London: Pluto, 1988), p. 135.
16 Martin Gilbert, *Churchill and the Jews* (New York: Henry Holt, 2007), p. 182
17 G. Ward Price, *Extra-Special Correspondence* (London: George G. Harrap, 1957), p. 242.
18 Frances Stevenson, *Lloyd George: A Diary* (New York: Harper and Row, 1971), p. 259.

Notes to pp. 68–79   **241**

19 Joachim von Ribbentrop, 2 July 1945, Top Secret Interrogation Summaries, Vault 14, USNA. Quoted in Mark Aarons and John Loftus, *Ratlines* (London: William Heineman, 1991), p. 211, note 9.
20 Anthony Cave Brown, *C: The Secret Life of Sir Stewart Menzies* (New York: Macmillan, 1987), pp. 178–185.
21 Charles Higham, *Trading with the Enemy* (New York: Dell, 1984), pp. 201–211.
22 Leibovitz, p. 99.
23 Higham, p. 188.
24 *Nation's Business*, March 1935; May 1935.
25 *New York Herald*, 22 May 1932.
26 Higham, passim, but see especially pp. 55, 60, 95, 97, 113, 182–186.
27 Ibid., p. 183.
28 Ibid., p. 177.
29 Ibid., pp. 175–176.
30 Max Wallace, *The American Axis: Henry Ford, Charles Lindbergh, and the Rise of the Third Reich* (New York: St. Martin's Press, 2003), pp. 145–16.

8 The Butchers' Revolt

1 The literature on the Spanish war is extensive. I have largely relied on Landis in this chapter and the next.
2 Ibid., p. 17.
3 Dimitrov, *Two Years*, p. 6.
4 Ibid., pp. 4–5.
5 Landis, p. 64.
6 Ibid., pp. 69–70.
7 Oleg Rzheshevsky, *Europe 1939: Was War Inevitable?* (Moscow: Progress, 1989), p. 53.
8 Landis, p. 94, 104.
9 Ibid., p. 96.
10 Ibid., p. 117.
11 Franco's letters to Hitler are cited in John Somerville, *The Philosophy of Peace* (New York: Gaer Associates, 1949), pp. 35–36.
12 Jorge M. Reverte, "La Lista de Franco para el Holocausto," *El País*, 20 June 2010.
13 Mussolini cited in Allan Chase, *Falange: The Axis Secret Army in the Americas* (New York: G.P. Putnam's Sons, 1943), p. vi.

9 Imperialist Betrayal

1 Landis, p. 198.
2 Ibid., pp. 182–183.
3 Fyodor Volkov, *Secrets from Whitehall and Downing Street* (Moscow: Progress, 1980), p. 248.

242 NOTES TO PP. 80–90

4 Landis, p. 239.
5 Ibid., p. 183; 204–209.
6 Ibid., p. 203.
7 Ibid.
8 Ibid., p. 356.
9 Ibid., pp. 242–244; International Editorial Board, *International Solidarity with the Spanish Republic; 1936–1939* (Moscow: Progress, 1974), pp. 328–330. [IEB]
10 Quoted in Santiago Carrillo, *Eurocommunism and the State* (London: Lawrence and Wishart, 1977), pp. 124–125.
11 Victor Howard, *The Mackenzie–Papineau Battalion* (Ottawa: Carleton University Press, 1986), p. 16.
12 William Beeching, *Canadian Volunteers: Spain 1936–1939* (Regina: University of Regina, 1989), p. xxxv.
13 IEB, pp. 64 and 338; Michael Petrou, *Renegades: Canadians in the Spanish Civil War* (Vancouver: UBC Press, 2008).
14 William L. Shirer, quoted in Landis, p. 390.

10 They Killed My Soul

1 Sarah Wildman, "Spectres of Fascist Past Back to Haunt Spain." *The Guardian*, 7 November 2007.
2 Giles Tremlett, "Spain Poised to Seek the Graves of Franco's Disappeared." *The Guardian*, 23 August 2002. See also Landis, pp. 5, 405, 408–409; and Paul Preston, *The Spanish Civil War: Reaction, Revolution, and Revenge* (New York: W.W. Norton, 2007), p. 302. For a comprehensive treatment of the savagery of Franco's forces see Paul Preston, *The Spanish Holocaust: Inquisition and Extermination in Twentieth Century Spain* (New York: W. W. Norton, 2012). [PSH]
3 Ted Allan, "Battle for Spain, the Struggle Still Goes On," *Colliers*, 3 February 1945, pp. 11, 49.
4 Enrique Lister, "Guerrilla Warfare in Spain, 1939–1951," in William J. Pomeroy, ed., *Guerrilla Warfare and Marxism* (New York: International Publishers, 1968), pp. 139–145.
5 Giles Tremlett, "Children Stolen by Franco Finally Learn the Truth." *The Guardian*, 29 October 2002.
6 Somerville, p. 35. See also, United Nations Security Council Resolutions 4, 7, and 10; 29 April, 26 June, 4 November 1946.

PART THREE   Life's Blood

11 The Plan

1 SS, p. 157
2 PSH, p. xiii.
3 Ibid., p. 313.

Notes to pp. 90–99   **243**

4 Ibid., p. 293.
5 SB, p. 91.
6 SS, p. 158.
7 Paul Preston, *We Saw Spain Die* (London: Constable, 2008), p. 39. [WSSD]
8 LAC MG30 D388, 30/33, handwritten notes by Sorensen; Hannant, pp. 129–131.
9 Howard, p. 50.
10 SB, p. 93.
11 Patricia Albers, *Shadows, Fire, Snow: The Life of Tina Modotti* (Berkeley: University of California Press, 2002), p. 289.
12 SB, p. 93.
13 Hannant, p. 131.
14 SB, p. 93.
15 IEB, pp.157–175; Howard, p. 50.
16 Landis, pp. 244–272.
17 Howard, p. 50.
18 NFB research files. Hazen Sise interview. [NFB/HS]
19 SS, p. 162.
20 LAC MG30 D388, 30/33.
21 SS, p. 163.
22 SB, p. 93.
23 LAC, Henning Sorensen, File: Medical and Personnel 068900. RCMP File, secret document, 23 December 1942.
24 OLHM. 637 1/39, tape 2.
25 SS, p. 412.
26 SS, pp. 164–165.
27 AG, p. 125.
28 SB, p. 94.
29 NFB/HS.
30 SB, p. 95.
31 Ibid.
32 LAC, Activities of Sorensen in Spain, File: 631-B. Telegram from Vincent Massey to the Secretary of State for External Affairs, 28 November 1936.
33 Ibid. Telegrams of 17, 20, 26, and 27 October 1936.
34 Ibid. Memo from "L. C. C." 28 November 1936.
35 SB, pp. 95–96.
36 Ibid., p. 96.
37 Charles Hill, et al, p. 114.
38 From this point to the end of the chapter – with the exception of notes 39 and 40 – the narrative is based on NFB/HS; LAC MG30 D388, Vol. 30, File 30-26, HS Diary, 1936; HS Diary note, 7 February 1938.
39 SS, p. 414.
40 LAC MG30 D 187, HS Fonds, Vol. 43, File 22.

12 Based on Blood: A New Type of Human Relationship

1 Sise Diary.
2 Ibid.
3 PSH, 341.
4 Sise Diary; Howard, p.54; OLHM, 637, 2/2, tape 17; Anonymous report by a member of the Spanish authorities dated 3 April 1937, in LAC, Mackenzie–Papineau Collection (Moscow Archives), Fonds 545, file list 6, file 542, 1937–1940, in Hannant, pp. 361–364. [Anonymous report 1937]
5 NFB/HS.
6 Hannant, pp. 131–135.
7 SS, 420–421. There is some controversy concerning when the four doctors joined Bethune's unit. It may be that the "two medical students" referred to in Bethune's letter (see Ibid) were Sanz and de la Loma, and that the two senior physicians – Culebras and Goyannes – joined shortly thereafter. According to SS, p. 421, Sanz recalled joining the unit in December, and de la Loma in the winter of 1936.
8 Sise Diary.
9 Hannant, p. 144.
10 NFB/HS.
11 Albers, especially Chapter 13; Pino Cacucci, *Tina Modotti: A Life* (New York: St. Martin's Press, 1999), p. 148.
12 NFB/HS.
13 Ibid.
14 SS, p. 169.
15 Film, *Heart of Spain*, produced 1937, Bethune, Herbert Kline, and Geza Karpathi, released by Frontier Films.
16 CASD publication 1937, *This is Station EAQ, Madrid Spain*. [EAQ]
17 SS, p. 170.
18 EAQ, "Canada Greets Spain," Bethune, 24 December 1936.
19 Ibid. "Madrid: Peaceful Amid War," Bethune, 2 January 1937.
20 Hannant, pp. 147–148.
21 SS, p, 171.
22. EAQ, "Text Books in the Trenches," Sise, 30 December 1936.
23 NFB/HS.
24 Imperial War Museum (London), sound archives, Vera Elkan interview #16900 Reel 3.
25 Ibid.
26 SS, p. 172.
27 Imperial War Museum, Vera Elkan Collection, Photo Archive HU71499 – HU71698.
28 Hannant, pp. 131–135. Bethune's letter to Spence is dated 17 December, but this is clearly an error. The more likely date is 27 December, especially given the reference to the Guadarrama Mountains which he had visited on the 25th.
29 SS, p. 173.

Notes to pp. 111–119 **245**

30 Ibid., pp. 173–174.

31 Hannant, pp. 144–147.

32 Ibid., p. 146.

33 NFB/HS.

34 J. B. S. Haldane, "Madrid Against Fascism," DC, 20 January 1937.

35 Virginia Cowles, *Looking for Trouble* (New York: Harper, 1941), p. 36; "Kajsa kampade for Spaniens barn," in *Varmlands Folkblad*, 27 November 2004; Lucy Viedma, "Everything you have done for us Spanish children," *The World in the Basement* (Stockholm: Arbetarrrorelsens Arkiv och Bibliotek, 2003), p. 37.

36 Diaries of Priscilla Scott-Ellis, University of Cardiff Library Archive, Manuscript No. 3/233, 3 April 1939.

37 C. E. Lucas Phillips, *The Spanish Pimpernel* (London: Heinemann, 1960), pp. 85–88. For Rothman's detention see Hannant, pp. 361–364.

38 Kate Mangan, and Jan Kurzke, "The Good Comrade," unpublished memoir, Jan Kurzke papers, Archives of the International Institute for Social History, Amsterdam. Names in the memoir have been changed to protect their identity; Celia Greenspan is referred to as "Sarah." [MK] Also, Hannant, p. 126.

39 Anonymous report 1937. Handwritten notes by Henning Sorensen in his "Chronology" (LAC MG30 D1987, Vol. 43, File 18) refer to Lindbaek and Haldane; Elkan may be seen repeatedly with Jordan et al in photographs at the Imperial War Museum; Hartung's identification as press censor with the foreign propaganda services is evident in the postscripts of Bethune's letters to Spence of 17 December 1936 and 11 January 1937, which latter notes that Cockburn was staying at the Institute. There is some controversy about the fate of Hartung. According to Hans Landauer, *Lexicon der osterreichischen Spanienkampfer 1936–1939* (Vienna: Theodor Kramer Gesellschaft, 2008), p. 127, he survived the war.

40 OLHM, RS interview with Sorensen, tape 38.

41 EAQ, "Children's Day Celebrated," Sise, 12 January 1937.

42 Bethune's letter to Ben Spence of 11 January notes that Haldane had already returned to London.

43 Hannant, pp, 144–147, 135.

13   I Would Not Be Anywhere Else

1 NFB/HS.

2 Hannant, pp. 144–147.

3 Sise, CBC interview.

4 Griffin, "Canadians Lend a Hand," *Toronto Star Weekly*, 20 February 1937, in David Lethbridge, *Bethune: The Secret Police File* (Salmon Arm: Undercurrent, 2003), document 13. While the interview was published in February, it is clear from internal references that the interview was conducted in late December or very early January.

5 Howard, pp. 54–55.

6 NFB/HS.

7 Howard, p. 58.
8 SB, pp. 103, 107.
9 Letter of RS to Hannant, 14 January 1996.
10 Howard, p. 58.
11 SS, p. 177.
12 SS, p. 178.
13 Sise, CBC interview; NFB/HS; R. W. B. Ellis, "Blood Transfusion at the Front," *Proceedings of the Royal Society of Medicine*, 1938, 31 (6), 684–686.
14 Hannant, pp. 148–149.
15 Ibid.
16 Letters of RS to Hannant, 27 January 1996; 5 January 1996.
17 SS, p. 173.
18 OLHM, 637 1/39, tape 38.
19 Howard, p. 57.
20 LAC MG30 D187, vol. 43, file 18, Sise, "Outline," no date.
21 NFB/HS.
22 Ted Allan, "With Norman Bethune in Spain," in SL, p. 158.
23 A. Franco, J. Cortes, J. Alvarez, J.C. Diz, "The Development of Blood Transfusion: The Contributions of Norman Bethune in the Spanish Civil War (1936–1939)," *Canadian Journal of Anaesthesia*, 1996, Vol. 43, #10, p. 1077. Also letter from J.C. Diz to David Lethbridge, 7 July 2008.
24 LAC MG30 D187, vol. 43, file 18, "Outline," no date. Paulion's duties are recorded in Bethune, "Internal Organization of the Institute," no date.
25 Sorensen "Chronology," and Sise "Time Table" in Ibid. Also NFB/HS.
26 John Sutherland, *Stephen Spender: A Literary Life* (London: Oxford University Press, 2005), pp. 205–220.
27 Ibid.
28 Sise, "The Vivid Air Signed with his Honour: In Memory of Norman Bethune," in SL, p. 165.
29 SS, p. 180.
30 Paul Weil, "Norman Bethune and the Development of Blood Transfusion Services," in SL, p. 177, editors note.
31 SS, p. 180.
32 SS, p. 417.
33 Angela Jackson, *"For us it was Heaven": The Passion, Grief and Fortitude of Patience Darton* (Brighton, Portland, Toronto: Sussex Academic Press, 2012), p. 30; Preston, WSSD, p. 112.
34 MK.
35 Hannant, p. 150.
36 SS, p. 182.
37 Ibid., p. 181.
38 Hannant, p. 150.
39 SS, p. 183.

Notes to pp. 128–140   **247**

14 Slaughter of the Innocents

1 SS, p. 185.
2 SH, pp. 176–177; Claud Cockburn, *Daily Worker*, 8 February 1937.
3 Sorensen, "Chronology;" Sise, "Time Table;" "Outline."
4 Albers, p. 297.
5 Sise, Diary note, 7 February 1938, in LAC MG30 D187, Vol. 9 File 15; Cockburn, *Daily Worker*, 8 February 1937.
6 SS, p. 185.
7 Sise, "Outline;" Bethune to Spence, 9 March 1937, in Ontario Archives, A. A. MacLeod Papers F126, MU7390, File 12. [AMf]
8 SS, pp. 186–187.
9 MK.
10 NFB/HS.
11 SS, p. 186.
12 SS, p. 188.
13 Archives and Research Centre, University of Western Ontario, Victor Howard interview with Hazen Sise, 1966. [ARC]
14 Albers, pp. 297–298; Vittorio Vidali, *Retrato de Mujer* (Puebla: Universidad Autonoma de Puebla, 1984), p. 40.
15 Howard, p. 60.
16 Bethune, *The Crime on the Road: Malaga–Almeria* (Madrid: Publicaciones Iberia, 1937), reproduced in Hannant, pp. 151–154.
17 MK.
18 OLHM, 637 2/1, tape 6. Anne Taft interview with RS.
19 SS, p. 193.
20 Sorensen, "Chronology" and Sise "Time Table."

15 Every Minute is Beautiful

1 LAC MG 30 D388, 16/2.
2 Landis, pp. 281–289.
3 Hannant, p. 363; LAC MG 30 D187, HSf, Vol. 43, File 17.
4 Sutherland, p. 219.
5 Ibid.
6 Ione Rhodes, "Con la Espana Republicana en el Corazon," *Migraciones y Exilos*, Numero 5, 2004.
7 SS, p. 193.
8 AMf, F126, MU7590, File 12.
9 NFB/HS.
10 Ibid.
11 LAC MG 30 D388, 16/2.
12 No Author, *From Prairie Trails to the Yellowhead* (Winnipeg: Intercollegiate Press, 1984), p. 507. HS wrote to TA on 20 January 1945 that May had killed

himself, despondent that life was passing him by. LAC MG30 D187 HS Correspondence, Vol. 7 File 2.

13 LAC Activities of Sorensen in Spain, vol. 1801, file 631-B.

14 Ibid.

15 AMf, F126, MU7590, File 12.

16 SS, p. 182.

17 Ibid., p. 180.

18 AMf, F126, MU7590, File 12.

19 "Canadians in Spain," DC, 7 March 1937.

20 ARC, p. 63.

21 "Canadians in Spain."

22 NFB/HS.

23 *From Prairie Trails to the Yellowhead,* p. 507.

24 Sorensen, "Chronology" and Sise "Time Table."

25 Sorensen, "Chronology;" OLHM, 637 1/39, tape 38; SS, p. 203.

26 Anonymous report 1937.

27 SS, p. 195.

28 Dolores Ibarruri, *They Shall Not Pass: The Autobiography of La Pasionaria* (New York: International Publishers, 1966), 272–281.

29 SS, p. 195.

30 DC, 3 March 1937.

31 Hannant, pp. 123, 125.

32 LAC MG30 D187 HSf, Vol. 6, File 8.

33 Letter from RS to Hannant, 14 January 1996.

34 Sorensen, "Chronology."

35 SB, p. 104.

16   The Blood of the Dead

1 AMf, F126, MU7590, File 12, Bethune to Ben Spence, 9 March 1937.

2 Paul Preston, "Two Doctors and One Cause: Len Crome and Reginald Saxton in the International Brigades," *International Journal of Iberian Studies*, Vol. 19, 1, 2006, pp. 15–19.

3 Ibid.

4 Peter H. Pinkerton, "Norman Bethune, Eccentric, Man of Principle, Man of Action, Surgeon, and His Contribution to Blood Transfusion in War," *Transfusion Medicine Reviews*, 2007, 21, #3, p. 261.

5 OLHM, P89, Box 1, File 1-2.

6 R. S. Saxton, "The Madrid Blood Transfusion Institute," *The Lancet*, 4 September 1937, pp. 606–607.

7 Preston, "Two Doctors," p. 22. An obituary of Saxton, published in *The Independent* on 6 April 2004 by Patrick Reade, similarly states quite incorrectly that: "Saxton had also considered cadaveric transfusion . . . but ethical, practical and infection issues prevented it."

8 Frederic Duran-Jorda, *The Service of Blood Transfusion at the Front*, (No publisher;

Notes to pp. 149–154   **249**

no date. The pamphlet was published in English.) Marx Memorial Library, London; Box A-4, U/7-8.

9 Alexander Bogdanov, *The Struggle for Viability: Collectivism through Blood Exchange* (Philadelphia: Xlibris, 2001), Edited and translated by Douglas W. Heustis.

10 Charles, L. Drew, "The Role of Soviet Investigators in the Development of the Blood Bank," *American Review of Soviet Medicine*, 1, 1943, pp. 360–369.

11 Louis K. Diamond, "A History of Blood Transfusion," in Maxwell M. Wintrobe, ed., *Blood, Pure and Eloquent* (New York: McGraw-Hill, 1980), p. 679.

12 Heustis, in Bogdanov, p. 17.

13 Heustis, in Bogdanov, p. 274.

14 S. S. Yudin, "Transfusion of Cadaver Blood," *Journal of the American Medical Association*, 106, 12, 1936, pp. 997–999.

15 Ibid., pp. 998, 999.

16 S. S. Yudin, "Transfusion of Stored Cadaver Blood," *The Lancet*, 230, 5946, pp. 362–366.

17 SB, p. 72.

18 Ibid.

19 LAC MG30 D388, 25/1.

20 Elof Axel Carlson, *Genes, Radiation and Society: The Life and Work of H. J. Muller* (Ithaca: Cornell University Press, 1981), pp. 229–243.

21 H. J. Muller, Notes on Blood Transfusion. Notes for 30 March 1937, and undated notes. Muller Mss., Series: Research and Education; Box 3, 1937 March–April; Blood Transfusion File; Lilly Library, Indiana University, Bloomington, Indiana.

22 Muller, Notes for 29 March 1937.

23 Muller, Notes for 14 April 1937.

24 Muller, Notes for 20 April 1937.

25 Muller, Notes for 29 March to 4 April.

26 Ibid.

27 Muller, Notes for 14 April.

28 Muller, Notes for 16 April.

29 Carlson, p. 238–242.

30 NFB research files, Muller to Sise 22 November 1963; Muller to JK undated.

31 LAC MG30 D187 Vol 6. Sise. "Internal Organization of the Institute," (undated); "Preamble Confidential," (undated); "New Headquarters for the Institute," (undated); "Untitled: The Canadian comrades of the Institute . . . " (undated). All Sise documents circa April 1937.

32 Howard, p. 55.

33 James Neugass, *War is Beautiful: An American Ambulance Driver in the Spanish Civil War* (New York: New Press, 2008), pp. 128–129.

17 I Killed My Own Son

1 Preston, "Two Doctors;" Ian MacDougall, *Voices from the Spanish Civil War: Personal Recollections of Scottish Volunteers in Republican Spain 1936–1939* (Edinburgh: Polygon, 1986), pp. 8–10.

2 UCLA Special Collections. Kenneth MacGowan Papers, Collection 887, Box 30, Folder 1, Greg Moller to Hedda Hopper, 28 January 1943.

3 Anonymous report 1937.

4 SS, p. 193.

5 OLHM, 637/2/6, tape 37.

6 LAC MG30 D187 Vol 7 File 19, Sise, 21 November 1968; LAC MG30 D187 Vol 35 File 1, Sise, 13 March 1943.

7 Jean Watts, "Making a Movie of Dr. Bethune," DC, 5 May 1937.

8 Landis, pp. 290–298.

9 Ibid.

10 Ibid., pp. 295, 298.

11 Bethune, "With the Canadian Blood Transfusion Unit at Guadalajara," DC, 17 July 1937; Jean Watts, "Bethune Escapes Death," DC, 12 March 1937.

12 Watts, "Bethune Escapes Death;" SS, pp. 197–198.

13 SB, p. 103.

14 CBC Archives, interview with Haze Sise.

15 OLHM, 637/2/6, tape 38.

16 Mark Zuehlke, *The Gallant Cause: Canadians in the Spanish Civil War 1936–1939* (Vancouver: Whitecap, 1996), p. 112.

17 OLHM, 637/2/6, tape 38.

18 OLHM, 637 1/108, Jean Ewen Kovich to RS.

19 OLHM, 637/2/6, tape 41.

20 AMf, F126, MU7590, File 12.

21 ARC.

22 SS, p. 203.

23 Ibid., pp. 203–204.

24 ARC.

25 CBC Television Archives. "Henning Sorensen: One Man's Life," 30 November 1980; SS. p. 201.

26 Moller.

27 Jean Watts, "Bethune Gave Blood to 1500," DC, 12 March 1937.

28 Preston, WSSD, pp. 115–118.

29 "Kajsa kampade for Spaniens barn;" "Hon var sin tids mest kanda Karlstadsbo;" both in *Varmlands Folkblad*, 27 November 2004.

18 The Conspiracy

1 LAC MG30 D388, Vol.68, File 68-10. Interview with TA, 1992.

2 "Introduction," Julie Allan, Norman Allan, and Susan Ostrovsky, in Ted Allan and Sydney Gordon, *The Scalpel, the Sword* (Toronto: Dundurn Press, 2009).

Notes to pp. 167–173

3   D. P. Stephens, *Memoir of the Spanish Civil War: An American-Canadian in the Lincoln Battalion* (St. John's: Canadian Committee on Labour History, 2000), p. 26.

4   Ted Allan, "With Norman Bethune in Spain," in SL, p. 158. [WNB]

5   DC, 6 July 1937.

6   Allan, WNB p. 158.

7   LAC MG30 D388 Vol. 20 File 2 Correspondence 1949, Garner to TA.

8   "Introduction," Julie Allan, Norman Allan, and Susan Ostrovsky.

9   Ibid.; LAC MG30 D388, Vol.68, File 68-10. Interview with TA, 1992.

10 Dorothy Livesay Collection, Archives of British Columbia, Tape 1627:1, Interview with Jean Watts.

11 LAC MG30 D388, Vol. 30, File 30-26. Hazen Sise Diary.

12 LAC, MG30 D187, vol. 43, file 18; Sise, "Time Table;" Sorensen, "Chronology."

13 Dorothy Livesay Collection.

14 LAC MG30 D388, Vol. 68 File 68-10.

15 LAC MG30 D388, Vol. 67, File 67-28.

16 Ted Allan, "Blood for Spanish Democracy," *New Frontier*, Vol. 1, #10, pp. 12–13.

17 Moller.

18 Imperial War Museum, London, England, Box D-4, Cr 3. David Crook Diary, 14 March 1937.

19 Ibid., 3 April 1937.

20 Ibid.

21 Allan, WNB p. 158.

22 Ibid., p. 159. According to Hannant, "Sorensen scoffed at the idea that Allan was the unit's political commissar, going so far as to call Allan a liar to his face in the midst of a Toronto cocktail party;" and "In 1982 Communist Party of Canada leader William Kashtan would also dismiss Allan's assertion that he was the unit's political commissar." Draft notes for a proposal for a *Saturday Night* article.

23 SS, p. 203.

24 Allan, WNB p.158.

25 Ted Allan, *Canadian Magazine*, 6 July 1975.

26 SS, p. 201.

27 NFB Research files, Muller to JK, 17 October 1963; Muller to JK undated.

28 OLHM, 637/2/1, tape 6.

29 SS, p. 416.

30 A. Franco, J. Cortes, J. Alvarez, J.C. Diz.

31 OLHM, 637/2/6, tape 41.

32 OLHM, 637/2/ 6, tape 38.

33 Allan, WNB p. 158; Ted Allan, *Canadian Magazine*, 6 July 1975.

34 LAC, MG30 D187, vol. 43, file 18; Sorensen, "Chronology."

35 Ibid., Sise, "Time Table."

36 Anonymous report 1937.
37 LAC (Moscow) MG10 K2, 545/6/542. Norman Bethune's Personnel File, Undated report, circa July 1937.
38 Anonymous report 1937.
39 LAC (Moscow) Undated report.
40 Sorensen, "Chronology."
41 SS, p.203.
42 Vidali, *Retrato*, p. 40.
43 Ibid., p. 40. Cacucci, p. 170.
44 AG, p. 155.
45 Vidali, *Retrato*, p. 40.
46 SS, p. 200.
47 CBC Archives, interview with Sise.
48 NFB/HS.
49 Sorensen, "Chronology."
50 SS, p. 205.
51 Sorensen, "Chronology."
52 Vidali, *Retrato*, p. 40.
53 Sorensen, "Chronology."
54 Hannant, p. 158
55 Ibid., pp. 159–160.

19 They Are In Me, They Have Changed Me

1 George Steer, "The Tragedy of Guernica," *The Times*, 28 April 1937.
2 Preston, WSSD, p.59; 158; 166–168; 280–282; 312–313; 360–361.
3 Ibid. p. 59.
4 Sorensen, "Chronology." Sise, "Time Table."
5 ARC.
6 Cowles, pp. 31–32.
7 OLHM, 637/2/6, tape 38.
8 ARC.
9 OLHM, 637/2/6, tape 38.
10 ARC.
11 Amanda Vaill to David Lethbridge, 3 May 2012.
12 Martha Gellhorn, "Madrid to Morata," *The New Yorker*, 24 July 1937.
13 OLHM, P89, File 1/42. Cables 16 April; 7 May.
14 No Author, *Canada's Party of Socialism: History of the Communist Party of Canada, 1921–1976* (Toronto: Progress Books, 1982), p. 176.
15 OLHM, P89, File 1/42. Cable 12 April.
16 Ibid., Cables 6 April; 12 April; 18 April; 29 April; 5 May.
17 Ibid; Cable 5 May.
18 OLHM, 637/2/2, tape 17.
19 Landis, pp. 339–348.
20 OLHM, 637/2/2, tape 17.

Notes to pp. 182–199 **253**

21 Ibid.
22 OLHM, P89, File 1/42. Cable 7 May.
23 Ibid., Cable 8 May; 13 May.
24 Ibid.; Sorensen, "Chronology."
25 OLHM, P89, File 1/42. Cable 13 May.
26 Sorensen, "Chronology."
27 CBC Archives, Interview with Sorensen.
28 ARC.
29 LAC MG30 D187 Vol. 6. File 33. Undated notes.
30 OLHM, P89, File 1/42. Cable 27 May.
31 LAC RG 25, Vol. 1810, File 1937-11-BS, Canadian Minister in France to Secretary of State for External Affairs, 27 May 1937.
32 OLHM, P89, File 1/42. Cable 27 May.
33 LAC MG30 D388, Vol. 30, File 30-26, Sise Diary.
34 Ibid.
35 DC, 25 May 1937.
36 Lethbridge, Document 67.
37 OLHM, P89, File 1/42. Cable 2 June.
38 Ibid.
39 Norman Bethune, "An Apology for Not Writing Letters," *New Frontier*, May 1937.

PART FOUR   In Defense of the Republic

20   A Tumultuous Welcome

1 Lethbridge, Document 14.
2 Hannant, pp. 170–174.
3 NFB research files, interview with Irene Kon. See also, Larry W. Stephenson, "Two Stormy Petrels: Edward J. O'Brien and Norman Bethune," Journal of Cardiac Surgery, Vol. 18, #1, Jan/Feb 2003, p. 73.
4 AMf, F126, MU7390, File 12, Letter of Ben Spence to "Dear Comrades," 12 August 1937. Also, LAC MG30 D187 Vol. 6. Sise to Spence, 14 October 1937.
5 Spence to "Dear Comrades."
6 Jean Evens Shiels and Ben Swankey, *Work and Wages: A Semi-Documentary Account of the Life and Times of Arthur H. (Slim) Evans* (Vancouver: Trade Union Research Bureau, 1977), pp. 255–261.
7 Lethbridge, Document 15.
8 SS, p. 213.
9 Lethbridge, Documents 15, 16, 17. See also DC, 15 July 1937.
10 Hannant, pp. 175–179.
11 Ibid., pp. 179–181.
12 Jean Hamelin and Nicole Gagnon, *Histoire du Catholicisme Quebecois* (Montreal: Boreal, 1984), p. 383.
13 Lethbridge, Documents 18–21. See also, AG, pp. 157–158; DC 18 July 1937.

14 Dovid Kunigis, letter to David Lethbridge, 20 March 2008.
15 OLHM, 637 2/ 1-10. Interview with Robert and Thelma Ayres.
16 SS, p. 216.
17 NFB research files, interview with Marian Scott.
18 NFB/GD.
19 SB, p. 112.
20 Pierre Delva, letter to David Lethbridge, 26 May 2009.
21 Zuehlke, p. 129. See also, SS, pp. 217–218.
22 NFB/PC.
23 Horlick, p. 117.
24 NFB/PC.
25 SS, 216–217.
26 LAC MG30 D398 Vol. 4. File 4-16. Paraskeva Clark Fonds.
27 Hannant, pp. 181–182; Bethune to FP, 7 July 1937.

21 Sharply Raising the Question of Class Struggle

1 Horlick, p. 102.
2 Lethbridge, Document 22.
3 *Northern Daily News*, July 9 1937.
4 *North Bay Nugget*, July 14 1937.
5 Hannant, pp. 181–182.
6 *Sault Daily Star*, 15 July 1937.
7 LAC, MG30 D187, Vol. 6. HSf.
8 LAC, Norman Bethune Comintern File, MG 10-K2 545/6/542.
9 *Sault Daily Star*, 14 July 1937.
10 OLHM, Louis and Irene Kon Fonds, P162, Folder 2.11.
11 Fort William *Times Journal*, 16 July 1937.
12 Port Arthur *News Chronicle*, 16 July 1937.
13 Fort Frances *Times*, 18 July 1937. Fort Frances *Bulletin*, 18 July 1937.
14 Lethbridge, Documents 23, 24, 25.
15 Ibid., Documents 26, 28.
16 Ibid., Document 30.
17 Ibid.
18 Hannant, pp. 183–185.
19 Lethbridge, Documents 31, 32.
20 Ibid., Documents 33, 34. See also, Hannant, pp. 186–188.

22 You See Now Why I Must Go

1 DC, 7 July 1937.
2 DC, 14, 15 July 1937.
3 Winnipeg *Free Press*, 20 July 1937.
4 San Francisco *Chronicle*, 29 July 1937.
5 SS, pp. 242–243.

Notes to pp. 211–220

6 Hannant, p. 200.
7 San Francisco *Chronicle*, 29 July 1937.
8 NFB research files, letters from Leo Eloesser to JK, 1 May; 22 May 1963.
9 DC, 31 August 1937.
10 Los Angeles *Times*, 28 July 1937.
11 Lethbridge, Documents 35, 36, 37, 41.
12 Ibid., Documents 37, 38.
13 Ibid., Document 41; Victoria *Times*, 2 August, 3 August 1937.
14 DC, 31 August 1937. Nanaimo *Free Press*, 5 August 1937.
15 SB, p. 112.
16 Lethbridge, Document 39.
17 Ibid.
18 DC, 31 August 1937
19 Kelowna *Courier* 11 August 1937.
20 OLHM, 637 1/55, Letter of Elvira Stirling.
21 Lethbridge, Document 40.
22 SS, p. 228.

23   People Let Me Tell You, Now is the Time to Wake Up

1 DC, 31 August 1937.
2 Ibid.
3 Lethbridge, Document 42.
4 Regina *Leader-Post*, 22 August 1937.
5 Saskatoon *Star-Phoenix*, 23 August 1937.
6 Lethbridge, Documents 46, 45.
7 OLHM, 637 1/26, Rachel Levine to RS.
8 Walter B. Cannon. *The Way of an Investigator* (New York: W. W. Norton, 1945), pp. 165–174.
9 London *Free Press*, 3 September 1937.
10 DC, 3 September 1937.
11 Hannant, pp. 182–183.
12 OLHM, P89 Box 1 File 1-2.
13 Detroit *News*, 12 September 1937. *Daily Clarion*, 14 September 1937.
14 OLHM, P89, Dr. Robert Shaw, 12 December 1971.
15 Lethbridge, Document 48.
16 DC, 16 September 1937.
17 Lethbridge, Document 47.
18 DC, 30 September 1937.
19 *Communist International*, Vol. XIV, No. 12, 1937, pp. 1168–1169.
20 SB, p. 114.
21 *Daily Worker*, 6 June 1940.
22 LAC Microfilm K-169, letter from Bethune to Elsie Siff.
23 Halifax *Chronicle*, 27 September 1937.
24 DC, 2 October 1937.

25 Moncton *Daily Times*, 30 September 1937.
26 DC, 8 October 1937.
27 SB, pp. 112–113.
28 OLHM, 637/ 2/ 1-10. Interview with George and Jean Holt.
29 NFB Research Files, Richard H. Meade to JK, 9 May 1963.
30 DC, 7 September 1937.
31 AMf, F 126 MU 7591 File 10, File 16.
32 DC, 7 September 1937.

24 Will You Come?

1 Tim Buck, *Thirty Years*. pp. 155–156.
2 DC, 9 and 11 October 1937.
3 James G. Ryan, *Earl Browder: The Failure of American Communism* (Tuscaloosa: University of Alabama Press, 1997), pp. 128–129.
4 OLHM, 637 1/41.
5 OLHM, P89, Box 1, File 1-13.
6 OLHM, 637 1/57.
7 OLHM, 637 2/ 1-10. Interviews with Struthers, Lewis.
8 SB, pp. 114, 117.
9 Jean Ewen, *China Nurse: 1932–1939* (Toronto: McClelland and Stewart, 1981), pp. 43–46.
10 Park, pp. 131–133.
11 NFB/GD.
12 DC, 24 October 1937.
13 LAC MG30 D187, HSf, Vol. 6.
14 LAC MG30 D187, HSf, Vol. 35 File 1. Letter of 8 June 1943, Sise to MacGowan.
15 SS, pp. 245–246.
16 OLHM, 637 1/108.
17 OLHM, 637 1/26.
18 SS, pp. 243–244.
19 SB, p. 111.
20 Lethbridge, Document 28.
21 SS, pp. 247–248.
22 SB, pp. 118–119.
23 NFB/PC.
24 Ewen, p. 46.
25 SS, pp. 364–369.

Notes to pp. 229–230

PART FIVE Aubade

25 A Dream of Himself

1 NFB/PC.

2 Vittorio Vidali, *Diary of the Twentieth Congress of the Communist Party of the Soviet Union* (Westport: Lawrence Hill and Company, 1984), p. 136.

3 Hannant, p. 291.

Index

Abraham Lincoln Battalion, 83, 145, 168, 203, 223, 225
Afghanistan, 52
Aguilera, Gonzalo, 63, 64
Albacete, 93, 94, 96, 111, 136, 169, 170, 184, 208
Alexander, John, 3
Alfonso XIII, 72
Algoma, 18, 20
Alicante, 130
Allan, Ted, 151, 157, 168–173, 174, 175, 178, 180, 182, 183, 184, 185, 207
Almeria, 76, 130–137, 139
Almuzarza, Marcelino Gavilan, 63
Alvarez del Vayo, Julio, 84, 103
American Association for Thoracic Surgery, 26, 213, 223
Anarchists, 41, 76, 114, 183
Andalucia, 76
Araquistain, Gertrude, 139, 158
Araquistain, Luis, 91
Arcand, Adrien, 65–66
Archibald, Edward, 3
Arthur, George, 54
Ary, Sylvia, 32–33
Asensio, José, 143–144
Asturias, 73, 76
Atkins, Thomas, 53
Australia, 6, 52, 53, 54, 68
Ayres, Robert, 202
Ayres, Thelma, 202
Azaña, Manuel, 41, 42, 73, 74

Badajoz, 39
Bader, Kate, 220
Barcelona, 63, 64, 76, 84, 101, 114, 121, 122, 125, 126, 127, 129, 132, 134, 138, 139, 141, 143, 145, 169, 174, 182, 183
Barnwell, John, 220, 224
Barsky, Edward, 145, 146, 159, 172, 226
Bayonnes, 75
Beijing, 212, 225
Bennett, R. B., 65–66
Beregoff-Gillen, Pauline, 220
Berlin, 73, 77, 83
Bethune, Elizabeth, *see* Goodwin, Elizabeth
Bethune, Frances, Penney, Frances
Bethune, Janet, 6, 7, 8, 19, 205
Bethune, Malcolm, 6, 7, 9, 10, 12–15, 17, 19
Bethune, Malcolm, Jr., 7, 8, 19
Bethune, Norman (grandfather), 3, 10, 14–17
Bethune, Norman
  and atrocity on the Malaga road, 129–137, 139, 144, 169, 180, 192, 195, 201, 225
  and *Heart of Spain*, 158–159, 166, 172, 176, 180, 182, 183, 184, 186, 196, 203, 208, 214
  and Margaret Day, *see* Day, Margaret
  and Frances Penney, *see* Penney, Frances
  and Kasja Rothman, *see* Rothman, Kajsa
  and Marian Scott, *see* Scott, Marian
  and Elizabeth Wallace, *see* Wallace, Elizabeth
  anger, 8, 9, 13, 14, 16, 18, 23, 27, 34, 36, 46, 120, 133, 137, 144, 145, 165, 166, 167, 172, 215, 227
  attitude to children, 25, 27, 32–33, 35, 132, 133, 136, 139–140, 162, 163, 166, 180, 181–182, 184, 185, 192, 200, 201, 207, 210, 217, 223

Index **259**

attitude to patients, 22, 23, 26, 27, 30, 161, 162–163

cadaver blood transfusion research, 151–157, 166

childhood, 3–19, 122, 136

conspiracy to remove him from Spain, 168, 171–178

decision to go to China, 212–214, 215–216

decision to go to Spain, 39–40, 41–42, 43, 44

develops blood transfusion service in Spain, 95–96, 97, 100, 102–106, 111–113

drinking, 23, 36, 111, 164–174 *passim* , 204, 205

influence of grandfather, 3, 10, 14–16, 17

interest in art, 20, 28–29, 32, 120, 144, 166, 186–190, 227

joins Communist Party of Canada, 31

journey to Soviet Union, 30–31, 209, 218

medical and surgical innovations, 26, 27, 36, 96, 105, 119, 127–128

murals at Trudeau Sanatorium, 4–5

performs abortions, 24–25, 35

relations with father, 9–10, 12–14, 15

relations with mother, 3, 4, 5, 7–9, 10, 11, 13–19, 123, 163, 192

relations with sister, 19

reveals Communist Party affiliation, 209, 214, 217

writings:

An Apology for not Writing Letters, 187–190

Crime on the Road: Malaga-Almeria, 133–136

I Come from Cuatro Caminos, 109

Madrid: Peaceful Amid War, 107–109

Take the Private Profit out of Medicine, 31

Bieler, Jacques, 43

Biggar, J. L., 41

Bilbao, 64, 179, 180, 182, 184, 185, 186

Bloor, Ella (Mother Bloor), 226

Bogdanov, Alexander, 149–150, 151

Bogolomets, Alexander, 150

Bolin, Luis, 75

Boston, 3, 23, 223

Brandon, 209, 210

Brandtner, Fritz, 28, 32, 44, 202

British Battalion, 83

British imperialism, 51–57, 58–60, 61, 62, 199

Browder, Earl, 221–222, 224, 225

Brown, Richard, 3, 10, 13

Brussels, 41

Buck, Tim, 41, 98, 140, 200, 208, 216, 220, 221, 224, 227

Byrnne, Albert, 146

Caballero, Largo, 72, 74, 82, 143

Cadiz, 75, 79, 125

Calgary, 211, 217

California, 22, 62, 211, 212, 213, 216

Canary Islands, 75

Canmore, 217

Cannon, Walter B., 219

Carr, Sam, 200, 225

Catalonia, 84, 101

Cerrada, Colonel, 121–122, 126, 127, 128, 137, 143, 144, 164–165, 177

Chamberlain, Joseph, 52

Chaumont, Conrad, 200

Chicago, 23, 150, 219, 226

Children's Creative Art Center, 32–33, 44–45

Chilton. Henry, 79

China, 3, 52, 83, 95, 212–216 *passim*, 219, 220, 221–222, 224–225, 226, 227, 232

China Aid Council, 225

Churchill, Winston, 67

Clark, Ken, 198

Clark, Paraskeva, 32, 40, 204, 220, 227, 228, 230

Clark, Philip, 204, 220

Cockburn, Claud, 100, 102, 103, 116, 130, 185

Coleman, Albert Robert Ernest (A. R. E.), 22, 24, 25, 33, 35, 205, 220

Coleman, Frances, *see* Penney, Frances

Comfort, Charles, 46

Committee to Aid Spanish Democracy (CASD), 43–47 *passim*, 91, 95–99 *passim*, 104, 105, 111, 115, 120, 121, 122, 126, 127, 137, 141, 142, 143, 145, 158, 164, 174, 177, 178, 181–186 *passim*, 196, 197, 198, 200, 203, 205, 206, 207, 219, 221, 223, 225

Communist Party of Canada, 7, 29, 30, 31, 39–45 *passim*, 65, 95, 96, 98, 120, 140, 145, 151, 168, 174, 175, 181, 195, 203, 208, 212, 214, 215, 217, 220, 221, 224

Communist Party of France, 83, 232

Communist Party of Great Britain, 100, 125, 147

Communist Party of Spain, 73–74, 76, 78, 82, 86, 87, 96, 124, 127, 143, 174, 175, 208

Contreras, Carlos, *see* Vidali, Vittorio

Cooperative Commonwealth Federation (CCF), 38, 39, 40, 41, 42, 46, 199, 215

Cordoba, 75, 122

Cousineau, Georges, 27, 28

Cowles, Virginia, 166, 180

Crome, Leonard, 157, 166, 167, 172

Crook, David, 171

Culebras, Antonio, 103, 121, 123, 124, 126, 141, 144, 148, 160, 162, 164, 165, 166, 172, 176, 180

Cumberland, 215

Czechoslovakia, 84

Dale, Clunie, 98, 99

Dallaire, Fernand, 39

Darwin, Charles, 5, 18, 54, 56

Davidson, Louis, 224

Day, Margaret, 34–37, 227

Denmark, 158, 226

Dennis, W. H., 222

Deshaies, Georges, 27, 44, 163, 164, 202, 226

Detroit, 21–23, 92, 136, 162, 220

Diaz, José, 41, 42

Dilke, Charles, 52

Dimitrov, George, 38

Dodd, William E., 69

Domingo, Marcelino, 45

Drew, Charles, 150

Drumheller, 217

Duclos, Jacques, 232

Duplessis, Maurice, 31, 39, 40, 44, 46

DuPont, Irénée, 70

Duran-Jorda, Frederic, 121, 122, 125–127, 129, 144, 145, 149, 151

Eden, Anthony, 79, 210

Edinburgh, 20, 21, 24, 153

Edmonton, 210, 217

Edward VIII, 68–69

Egypt, 52

Elkan, Vera, 110, 111, 115, 116

Eloesser, Leo, 213–214

Espanola, 208

Ethiopia, 68, 81, 195

Eugenics, 61–64

Evans, Arthur, 197

Ewen, Jean, 225, 227, 228

Executive Committee of the Communist International, 221

Eyre, Edward, 52

Falange, 73, 74, 75, 77, 78, 87

Farah, Ted, 120

Feltenstein, Milton, 224

Fifth Regiment, 38, 94, 104, 118, 159, 175, 176

Ford, Henry, 69, 70

Forrest, Willie, 166

Fort Frances, 208

Fort William, 208

France, 20, 75, 79, 84, 87, 97, 99, 100, 101, 142, 166, 168, 179

Franco, Francisco, 20, 33, 39, 44, 46, 47, 60, 63, 68, 73–91 *passim*, 94, 95, 98, 100, 102, 103, 110, 111, 114, 115, 118, 124, 125, 129, 138, 147, 148, 159, 160, 176, 179, 180, 183, 195, 200, 203, 212, 216, 218, 223

Friends of the Mackenzie–Papineau Battalion, 216

Friends of the Soviet Union, 31, 208

Freud, Sigmund, xvi

Galicia, 76

Galton, Frances, 56, 61, 62

Gariépy, Roger, 203

Index

Garner, Hugh, 168
Gellhorn, Martha, 181
Germany, 38, 41, 57, 61–73 *passim*, 77–86
    passim, 91, 102, 111, 118, 126, 129,
    133, 135, 142, 159, 179, 180, 195,
    207, 215, 219, 221
Gibraltar, 79, 125, 129
Gil Robles, José, 72–73
Glace Bay, 222
Goodwin, Elizabeth, 3, 4, 5–10, 11–19
    passim, 22, 26, 34, 36, 115, 123, 163,
    192
Goodwin, Henry, 5, 7
Gorbunov, N. F., 152
Goyanes, Vicente, 103, 121, 123, 124,
    126, 141, 144, 147, 165, 166, 176
Granada, 75, 76
Grande Covian, Francisco, 152, 153, 154
Gravenhurst, 3, 10, 25, 200
Greenspan, Celia, 103, 105, 122, 126, 127
Griffin, Frederick, 118, 119, 120, 151
Guadalajara, 76, 159–162, 164, 166, 170,
    174, 176, 190
Guadarrama mountains, 109, 110, 112,
    161
Guernica, 80, 83, 179, 180, 181, 186,
    191, 195
Guerrilla war, 87–88

Haldane, J. B. S., 103, 106, 110, 113, 115,
    116, 117, 120, 151, 152, 181
Halifax, 222
Hammond, Harriett, 3
Hartung, Herrmann, 115, 116
Hawaii, 5, 6
Hemingway, Ernest, 180, 181
Hepburn, Mitchell, 206, 208, 219, 220
Herbst, Josephine, 166
Hill, Charles, 28
Himmler, Heinrich, 77
Hirschfield, Victor, 223
Hirohito, 70
Hitler, Adolf, 33, 41, 47, 60–70 *passim*,
    77, 83, 84, 85, 94, 141, 207, 210,
    212, 219, 220
Holt, George, 223
Holt, Jean, 223
Howard, Victor, 154

Huelva, 76
Huot, Louis, 120
Huxley, Julian, 152
Hyndman, Tony, 126, 138

Ibarruri, Dolores, 76
India, 52, 53
International Brigades, 41, 83, 84, 93–95,
    99, 102, 107, 111, 113, 118,
    125–127, 130, 136, 138, 140, 145,
    147, 154, 157–163, 168, 169, 171,
    181, 184, 197, 208–212, 226
International Medical Center, 83
Italy, 41, 67, 68, 69, 73, 77, 78, 80, 81,
    84, 104, 198, 215, 219

Jacobsen, Fernanda, 114, 157
Jaen, 76, 122, 142, 143, 176
Jaffe, Philip, 225
Jamaica, 52–53
Japan, 212, 213, 215, 216, 217, 221, 224,
    225, 228
Jarama river, 138, 147, 157, 159, 160,
    164, 166, 174, 181
Jewish Anti-Fascist Conference, 41, 42
Jolly, Douglas, 111, 161, 174
Jordan, Phillip, 116, 166

Kamloops, 215
Karpathi, Geza, 157–160, 162, 167, 182,
    186, 196
Kashtan, William, 181, 184, 185
Kelowna, 215
Kerrigan, Peter, 169
Kirkland Lake, 206
Kleber, Emilio, 93, 94, 140
Kline, Herbert, 157–159, 171, 182, 186
Kon, Irene, 31, 196
Kon, Louis, 31, 208
Kulcsar, Ilsa, 92
Kunigis, Dovid, 202
Kurzke, Jan, 126–127, 130, 136

Landa, Mathilde, 130, 133
League Against War and Fascism, 41, 198,
    216
League for Freedom and Democracy, 225
League of Nations, 45, 84, 160, 185, 210

Lee, Norman, 96, 142
Lenin, V. I., 149, 150
Leningrad, 30, 150, 151, 152
Lenthier, John, 168
Leon, 76
Lerroux, Alexandre, 72–73
Lewis, Sclater, 225
Lindbaek, Lise, 115
Lindbergh, Charles, 69
Linden, Maurice, 157
Lloyd George, David, 68, 80
Loma, Valentin de la, 103, 121, 123, 126, 154
London, 5, 6, 11, 20, 21, 28, 35, 81, 83, 97–100, 110, 117, 120, 125–127, 136, 139, 179, 209
Longo, Luigi, 169
Lopokova, Lydia, 20
Lord Chatfield, 79
Lord Curzon, 53
Lord Halifax, 84
Lord Palmerston, 52
Los Angeles, 214
Lyman, John, 28, 33, 98

MacDonald, Ramsay, 68
MacFarquhar, Roderick, 157
Mackenzie King, 66–67, 83, 141, 206, 210
Mackenzie–Papineau Battalion, 83, 175, 181, 184, 201, 208, 210, 215–217, 220, 223, 225
MacLeod, A. A., 41, 42, 44, 45, 46, 142, 144, 181, 184–186, 196, 197, 207
Madrid, 20, 39, 42, 43, 45, 46, 63, 64, 73, 75, 76, 81, 83, 85, 91–130 passim, 133, 137–185 passim, 195, 201–210 passim, 216, 217, 219, 226, 232
Malaga, 76, 80, 81, 104, 128, 129–137, 139, 143, 144, 145, 158, 169, 176, 180, 184, 192, 200, 201, 225
Malraux, André, 91, 132, 185, 186
Manchuria, 195
Mancini, Roatta, 159, 161
Mangan, Kate, 126–127, 130
Mao Zedong, 212, 213, 215, 220, 228, 230, 232
Marion, George, 103, 116

Marseilles, 122, 125
Marx, Karl, 54
Massey, Vincent, 97
Matthews, Herbert, 116, 166
May, Allen, 93, 141, 142, 143, 153, 158, 160, 171, 173, 180, 182, 185, 207, 226
Meade, Richard, 223
Medical Bureau for Aid to China, 219
Medical Bureau to Aid Spanish Democracy, 213, 219, 220
Medicine Hat, 217
Melville, 217
Mexico, 81, 104, 166
Mitchell, Jimmy, 228
Modotti, Tina, 104, 130, 133, 176
Mola, Emilio, 91, 118
Moller, Greg, 157, 158, 160, 165, 166, 167, 170, 172
Molotov, Vyacheslav, 82
Moncton, 222
Montreal, 3, 21, 22, 23, 24, 28, 30, 31, 35, 36, 39, 40, 42, 43, 44, 46, 91, 92, 98, 109, 116, 136, 142, 162, 168, 169, 186, 195, 196, 200–208 passim, 218, 219, 223, 225
Montreal Group for the Security of the People's Health, 31, 36. 40
Montreal Medico-Chirurgical Society, 31
Moody, Dwight Lyman, 5, 6, 7
Mooney, George, 30, 40, 225
Moose Jaw, 217
Morgan, Nigel, 215
Morocco, 39, 75, 76, 77, 79, 218
Morris, James, 52
Morris, Leslie, 168
Moscow, 38, 83, 97, 104, 150, 151, 152, 153, 154, 209, 218, 220, 232
Motril, 130, 134
Muhlstock, Louis, 28
Muller, Hermann, 151–155, 157, 160, 166, 167, 172, 180
Munich, 83, 84
Murcia, 126, 127, 130, 131, 136
Mussolini, Benito, 33, 41, 47, 60, 65, 67, 68, 70, 72, 77, 78, 81, 83, 85, 78, 200, 212, 219, 220

Index

Nanaimo, 215
Navarre, 76
Negrín, Juan, 74, 84, 212, 219
Neugass, James, 154–155
New York, 23, 168, 169, 186, 194, 195, 196, 205, 213, 221, 222, 224–226
New Waterford, 222
New Zealand, 52, 111
Newman, Percy, 41
Niagara Falls, 219, 220
Non-Intervention Committee, 79, 80, 81, 84, 106, 111, 160, 176, 180, 195, 198, 199, 201, 209, 216
North Battleford, 217
North Bay, 207
Nova Scotia, 22
Nurenberg, 73

Owen Sound, 18

Palencia, Isabella de, 45
Palermo, Louis, 198
Paris, 21, 83, 91, 97–101, 114, 120, 122, 125, 128, 129, 137–143, 147, 153, 158, 168, 169, 173, 174, 181–185, 197, 207, 227
Park, Libbie, 31, 34, 44, 225
Parsons, Charles, H., 227, 228
Pavlov, Ivan, 30, 151, 219
Pearson, Lester, 98
Peisy, Charles, 39
Penney, Frances, 9, 11, 13, 16, 17, 20–26, 33–36, 44, 123, 165, 202, 205, 207, 219, 220, 223, 226, 227
  abortion, 24–25
  divorces Bethune, 23, 24
  marries Bethune, 21, 23
  relations with A. R. E. Coleman, 22, 24, 25
Perron, Jean, 39
Philadelphia, 222, 223
Pickert, Heinrich, 220
Picone, Jean, 154
Piero, Tomas, 186
Planelles, Juan, 175
Plato, 58–59
Pollard, Hugh, 75
Pollitt, Harry, 100, 125

Popular Front (in Spain), 38, 39, 41, 73, 74, 76, 78, 80, 82, 86, 87, 106, 121, 128
Port Arthur, 208
Portugal, 20, 52, 79, 81
Preston, Paul, 149, 154
Prince Albert, 217
Purple Gang, 21, 92

Quebec City, 46
Queipo de Llano, Gonzalo, 76, 129

Regina, 208, 210, 217
Rhodes, Ione, 139, 158
Rhodes, Peter, 139, 158
Rivera, Diego, 104
Roatta, Mario, 129
Robinson, George, 54
Rolland, Gerard, 27
Rome, 67, 77, 78, 150
Rosales, Ignacio, 63
Rose, Fred, 168
Rothman, Kajsa, 114, 115, 116, 121–125, 138, 140, 141, 143, 145, 147, 157, 158, 165, 166, 167, 172, 173, 174, 177, 180, 183, 227
  affair with Bethune, 115, 122, 123, 158, 165, 166, 173
  suspicion of spying, 116, 143, 158, 165, 173, 174, 177, 183
Rouquès, Pierre, 93, 95
Rouyn, 207
Royal Victoria Hospital, 3, 23, 26, 27, 35, 213, 225
Russell, Amy, 25
Ryan, Larry, 221

Sacré Coeur Hospital, 27, 29, 32, 39, 44, 96, 136, 163, 202, 203, 213
Salazar, Antonio de Olivera, 78
Salmon Arm, 215–216, 217
Salsberg, Joseph, 41, 203–204, 205
San Esteban de Pravia, 87
San Francisco, 212, 213, 214
Sanjurjo, José, 38, 73, 75
Santander, 81
Sanz, Andrés, 103, 121
Sarasola, Luis, 45, 46

Saskatoon, 210, 217
Sault Ste. Marie, 208
Saxton, Reginald, 147–149, 151, 154,
155, 157, 160, 166, 167, 172
Scotland, 23, 25
Scott, Frank, 33, 43, 46
Scott, Marian, 11, 28, 32–37 passim, 44,
98, 123, 202, 213
Scottish Ambulance Service, 114, 157, 169
Seville, 39, 75, 86, 129
Shaw, Robert, 220
Shister, Hyman, 29, 31
Siff, Elsie, 226
Sise, Hazen, 28, 98–106 passim, 109–144
passim, 153, 154, 162–185 passim,
207, 208, 226
at Almeria, 131–133
declines to accompany Bethune to
China, 226
meets Bethune, 99–100
plans for expanded research center,
153–154
relations with Rothman, 124–125, 140,
141
Smedley, Agnes, 212
Smith, A. E., 208
Smith, Stewart, 198
Snow, Edgar, 220
Socialist Party of Spain, 72, 73, 74, 75, 76,
78
Socorro Rojo Internacional (SRI), 97, 101,
102, 104, 115, 116, 117, 121, 130,
131, 133, 135
Sorensen, Henning, 43, 92–104 passim,
109–127 passim, 138, 141, 142, 143,
144, 145, 146, 157–185 passim, 207,
226
communist party affiliation, 96, 120
letter to Spry, 43
meets Bethune in Madrid, 92–93
role in conspiracy to eject Bethune from
Spain, 173–178, 179, 183
suspicious of Rothman and of spies,
115–116, 143, 158, 165, 166, 173,
177, 183
South Porcupine, 205, 207, 223
Soviet Union, 27, 30, 35, 70, 80, 81, 82,
150, 153

Spence, Benjamin, 98, 111, 115, 117, 118,
122, 142, 164, 184, 185, 186, 195,
196, 197, 198, 199, 207, 208
Spencer, Herbert, 56
Spender, Stephen, 125–126, 138, 139
Spry, Graham, 40, 41, 42, 43, 44
Stalin, Joseph, 82, 152
St. Catherines, 219
Steer, George, 179
Stephens, Pat, 168
Stevens, Dolly, 215
Stirling, Elvira, 216
Stolen children, 87
Struthers, Ernest, 225
Sudan, 52
Sudbury, 207, 208
Swift Current, 217
Sydney, 222

Taft, Anne, 136, 172
Tasmania, 53–54
Teruel, 87, 154
Thaelmann Battalion, 94, 138, 161
Thorez, Maurice, 83
Thorning, Joseph, 179
Tibet, 53
Timmins, 42, 206, 212
Toronto, 3, 6, 10, 13, 18, 20, 23, 32,
40–45 passim, 97, 122, 140, 141,
142, 186, 196, 197, 198, 200, 201,
203, 205, 206, 207, 213, 220, 225,
226, 227, 228
Trudeau Sanatorium, 3, 4, 23, 24
Tuberculosis, 3, 7, 23, 25, 26, 27, 30, 31,
35, 55, 136, 206, 213

UK economic and military aid to fascism,
79–80, 81
University of Toronto, 18, 19, 20, 228
US economic and military aid to fascism,
69–70, 80

Valencia, 94, 95, 96, 101, 103, 121,
122, 126, 127, 129, 130, 137,
138, 139, 140, 143, 147, 159,
164, 169, 175, 176, 179, 182,
183, 184, 185, 207
Valladares, Portela, 73

Index

Vancouver, 213, 214, 215, 216, 225, 227, 228
Vatican, 46, 74, 85, 200
Vavilov, Nikolai, 151, 152, 153
Verdun, 30, 36
Vernon, 215
Victoria, 215
Vidali, Vittorio, 78, 104, 130, 133, 175, 176, 177, 180, 232
Vienna, 21
Villarejo, 147, 148, 157, 166
Villeneuve, Cardinal, 46
Voroshilov, Kliment, 82

Wallace, Elizabeth, 3, 25–26, 33, 115, 123
Watson, George, 198
Watts, Jean, 157, 168–171, 182, 185
Weaver, Dennis, 157
Welles, Sumner 69
Windels, Erich, 66
Windsor, 219

Winnipeg, 207, 208, 212, 217
Wintringham, Tom, 116
Women's General Hospital, 29
Women's International Congress Against Fascism and War, 227
Women's League Against War and Fascism, 216
World Peace Congress, 41
Worsley, Thomas, 125–126, 127, 129–133, 135, 136, 137, 138, 141, 143, 169

Yellow Stone Village, 228
Yorkton, 217
Ypres, 20
Yudin, S. S., 148, 149, 150, 151, 152, 154, 155

Zamora, Alcalá, 72
Zweig, Arnold, xvi

About the Author

David Lethbridge is a college professor of psychology with BA and MA degrees from Concordia University in Montreal, and a PhD from the University of Regina. He began researching Bethune's life in 1998, discovered an original 16mm copy of Bethune's 1937 documentary film *Heart of Spain*, and has lectured on Bethune's life across Canada. As well as his many scholarly and scientific publications, Prof. Lethbridge has authored *Bethune: The Secret Police File* and an article on Bethune's role in cadaver blood transfusion in the *Canadian Bulletin of Medical History*.